Current Clinical Practice

Series Editor
Tommy Koonce, Family Medicine
University of North Carolina at Chapel Hill
Chapel Hill, USA

Current Clinical Practice provides an array of practical resources for primary care clinicians. Designed for internists, family physicians, physician assistants, and nurse practitioners, the Current Clinical Practice series offers evidence-based, easy-to-read titles covering a broad range of disorders commonly presented in the primary care setting. Series editor Tommy Koonce, MD, is an Associate Professor of family medicine and Vice Chair of education at UNC School of Medicine in Chapel Hill, North Carolina.

More information about this series at https://link.springer.com/bookseries/7633

Robert Hudak • Jessica M. Gannon

Handbook of Psychiatric Disorders in Adults in the Primary Care Setting

Humana Press

Robert Hudak
Psychiatry
University of Pittsburgh
Pittsburgh, PA, USA

Jessica M. Gannon
Psychiatry
University of Pittsburgh
Pittsburgh, PA, USA

ISSN 2364-1150 ISSN 2364-1169 (electronic)
Current Clinical Practice
ISBN 978-3-030-98708-4 ISBN 978-3-030-98709-1 (eBook)
https://doi.org/10.1007/978-3-030-98709-1

This Humana imprint is published by the registered company Springer Nature Switzerland AG
The registered company address is: Gewerbestrasse 11, 6330 Cham, Switzerland

Introduction

This book is written for primary care physicians and advance practice providers specializing in primary care. It is dedicated to these PCP friends and colleagues who are the first to evaluate and treat mental illness and who implicitly understand that conventions separating medical from psychiatric treatment are as nonsensical as they are outdated. It is written to help empower PCPs with practical knowledge and advice on diagnosis and treatment of common mental illness as part of routine healthcare, as mental health is the cornerstone of good health.

This book is not a comprehensive review of all psychiatric treatment. The material presented here is only that which is essential to primary care management of mentally ill patients. Information that would only be of interest to mental health professionals was left out. For ease of use, algorithms encompassing assessment and treatment of patients in the primary care setting are included where appropriate, as are medication reference tables. Note that medication information provided is disorder specific and not exhaustive of all uses of the medication. It is focused on high yield information needed to prescribe for that particular disorder.

Furthermore, this book is designed to serve different purposes for the evaluation and treatment of different psychiatric disorders.

1. Some common disorders are typically recognized, diagnosed, and successfully treated in medical settings. In many cases, psychiatric treatment can often be withdrawn after symptom remission. This book will provide a guide to managing these relatively straightforward patients.
2. Other common disorders may be treated initially in the primary care setting but will often necessitate referral to specialty care. The appropriate recommendations for initial treatment are given, along with information on how and when to appropriately refer these more complex patients.
3. Some psychiatric disorders will initially present in the primary care setting, but almost always require psychiatric referral. Steps on how to recognize, accurately diagnose, and initially manage these patients are given.

4. Certain psychiatric illnesses (e.g., anorexia nervosa) should almost never be treated in the primary care setting. After appropriate guidance on recognition and diagnosis, a review of psychiatric guidelines is given so as to familiarize PCPs with the treatment that their patients will be receiving.

Management of Common Mental Illnesses

The authors of this book well recognize that, for better or worse, the proportion of patients with diagnosable mental illnesses who engage with specialty behavioral health care is small. Some of this is because the illnesses are often successfully managed by PCPs. In other cases, impediments to good mental health treatment exist. A common reason is that patients who would benefit from psychiatric care may decline due to lack of insight into their illness, denial about the severity of their condition, or stigma associated with seeking mental health treatment. While stigma around acknowledging mental health conditions and seeking treatment has become less pronounced in recent years, it still exists, and is more pronounced in some communities than others. Insurance and payment issues, lack of qualified mental health practitioners in a given region, and long wait lists to see a psychiatrist are common problems. Given these constraints, and because PCPs are first line in treating common psychiatric disorders, much of this book's focus is to provide PCPs with easily accessible information on diagnosing and treating common mental illnesses. We emphasize the importance of the following:

1. Making a correct, accurate, and exact diagnosis of your patients using established DSM criteria.
2. Communicating that diagnosis to your patient. For example, telling a patient they have "depression" is not the standard of care. Rather, engaging a patient in an informed discussion of their diagnosis of "major depressive disorder" better serves both you and the patient.
3. Providing your patient with the appropriate resources for education about their illness.
4. Initiating evidence-based treatment that conforms to established practice and/or guidelines.
5. Referrals for psychotherapy in appropriate disorders, as medications alone are not sufficient for most mental health care.

We hope that this information will provide PCPs with further confidence in initiating evidence-based treatment for conditions like major depressive disorder, generalized anxiety disorder, obsessive compulsive disorder, and others while also knowing when to refer to behavioral health.

Management of Serious Mental Illness

This book's authors also acknowledge the unfortunate fact that barriers to successful referral impact the care of even the most severely ill, including those with schizophrenia, bipolar disorder, post-traumatic stress disorder, and severe eating disorders. This has led PCPs to sometimes manage far more serious behavioral health conditions than for which they were trained. While this book does not aim to replace psychiatric residency nor suggest that PCPs should solely manage severe mental illness, we do hope to provide PCPs with knowledge critical for recognizing and diagnosing serious mental illness and acquaint them with some of the treatments for these conditions. While we do not recommend that PCPs initiate or even continue treatment for schizophrenia or bipolar disorder, for example, we recognize that when patient access to care is limited, the benefits of primary care management of these conditions may far outweigh the risks. As such, this book was written to provide information on commonly recommended treatments and side effect management. It also reviews how to work with psychiatrists and other behavioral health professionals to achieve best outcomes for mutual patients.

Preventative Healthcare and Medical Treatment in Patient with Mental Illness

Patients with mental illness who are connected with specialty behavioral care, even of the highest quality, still require excellent PCPs. Such PCPs champion preventative healthcare, provide ongoing care of comorbid medical illness, and partner with behavioral healthcare teams on engaging patients in their care. Patients with mental illness die most often of common medical illnesses, have a higher burden of medical illnesses, and die far sooner than the general population [3]. Estimated length of life lost is up to 25 years for individuals with serious mental illness [1]. While 30–40% excess deaths are attributable to suicide and accidental injuries, 60–70% are due to medical illnesses [2]. The reasons for this are complex but include disparities in medical care driven by a multitude of factors that can be divided into patient, healthcare professional, and systems levels [3]. For example, a patient may not obtain screening lab work as they feel too depressed to get up in the morning; a physician may skip smoking screening on a patient with a history of schizophrenia as they don't believe the patient will ever quit smoking; and lack of care integration may make it challenging to target services and track outcomes in mentally ill populations. Patients with mental illness also face social challenges associated with employment, resulting in low to no income and inadequate health insurance coverage. These factors compound to impact care access and provision in a multitude of ways. Given these challenges, it is particularly important for PCPs to have an understanding both of potential care barriers as well as of some specific health comorbidities individuals with mental illness may face. In this book, these topics are explored in more detail where particularly meaningful, for example, in the schizophrenia and bipolar chapters. Serious side effects of psychotropic medication, the sequalae of which are often managed by PCPs, and drug-drug interactions between psychotropics and other commonly prescribed medications are also explored throughout the text.

Book Structure

This book is divided into chapters based on patient diagnosis. Much of these chapters are self-contained and so serve as an accessible reference for diagnosis and treatment of that specific mental illness. While the structure of each chapter varies to some degree, they each start with a patient case as an anchor and proceed with:

- An introduction to each illness, including common presentations and symptoms, as well as information of course and risk factors, where appropriate
- Basic epidemiology
- Diagnosis
- Presentations in a medical setting, including of comorbid medical illness
- Treatment, including basic information on psychotherapy pertinent to referral, as well as on psychotropic prescribing, side effect screening/monitoring, and ongoing management

We hope that the information we provided will give you more confidence in treating psychiatric disorders and will empower you in treating patients who are in mental health care.

References

1. Colton CW, Manderscheid RW. Congruencies in increased mortality rates, years of potential life lost, and causes of death among public mental health clients in eight states. Prev Chronic Dis. 2006;3(2):A42. Epub 2006 Mar 15. PMID: 16539783; PMCID: PMC1563985.
2. Harris EC, Barraclough B. Excess mortality of mental disorder. Br J Psychiatry. 1998;173:11–53. https://doi.org/10.1192/bjp.173.1.11. PMID: 9850203.
3. Viron MJ, Stern TA. The impact of serious mental illness on health and healthcare. Psychosomatics. 2010;51(6):458–65. https://doi.org/10.1176/appi.psy.51.6.458. PMID: 21051676.

Contents

Chapter 1
Major Depressive Disorder

1.1 Introduction and Epidemiology

Case Example 1.1
Mr. W. was a 72-year-old male who was admitted to the general medical floor in an academic medical center for dizziness and falls. Initial labs showed that he had hyponatremia which was determined to be secondary to SIADH. He had been placed on citalopram 20 mg from his primary care physician 18 months ago, and the renal service wanted that medication discontinued, so psychiatry was consulted. The history they gathered indicated that he was placed on citalopram by his PCP for "depression and anxiety" after his wife died. Psychiatry asked him if he had received a specific psychiatric diagnosis such as major depressive disorder. He said that he had not. Mr. W. also did not remember if he had been placed on the medication immediately his wife's death while he was acutely grieving (making a diagnosis of MDD less likely) or if it was late enough that someone could normally be expected to be recovered from the grieving process (meaning a diagnosis of MDD at that time would be more likely). Psychiatry stated that if he had been started incorrectly on the medication due to grief rather than meeting criteria for MDD, he could safely be taken off. However, if he did indeed have MDD at that time, discontinuing the medication would be high risk for an exacerbation, and that may not outweigh the risk of the SSRI contributing to the SIADH which is typically greatest in the first weeks after initiation. Unfortunately, no further history was obtainable, and the SSRI was discontinued due to the lack of solid information regarding its target symptomology.

R. Hudak, J. M. Gannon, *Handbook of Psychiatric Disorders in Adults in the Primary Care Setting*, Current Clinical Practice,
https://doi.org/10.1007/978-3-030-98709-1_1

Major depressive disorder (MDD) is a serious health problem with significant morbidity and mortality accompanying it. According to the World Health Organization, it is the fourth leading cause of disability in the world [9] and is associated with a significant burden of disease, including the fact that about 1% of Americans die by suicide [23]. MDD has a 12-month prevalence of 6.6% and a lifetime prevalence of 16%, effecting twice as many women as men [14]. It has a significant burden on its own as a severe condition but also increases the morbidity when it is present with other chronic medical conditions including diabetes, asthma, angina, COPD, and arthritis [19]. Since MDD presents most commonly in primary care settings (most patients with MDD are seen initially by non-psychiatric physicians), it is crucial that MDD is properly recognized, diagnosed, treated, and referred by non-psychiatric physicians and that they are skilled in the fundamentals of this disease. In fact, many patients, especially older adults, prefer to discuss their mood or mental health issues—including suicidal thoughts—with their primary physician rather than being referred out to a psychiatrist [25] and half of suicide completers often visit their primary care physician 1 month prior to their suicide [23].

Patients with MDD often do not present with complaints of depression or depressed mood. If they do have a mental health-related chief complaint, the physician is as likely to hear complaints of "anxiety" as they do of "depression." Patients are likely to present with vague, somatic complaints or a worsening of their underlying medical conditions. Stressful life events may be present prior to the onset of the symptoms, but symptoms can appear spontaneously as well. External stressors can increase the risk for MDD, but MDD also increases the susceptibility to dysfunction secondary to stressful life events [24].

> Environmental stressors play a role in the development of MDD as do genetic and biological factors.

Response to stress can present as a decrease in mood, as can grief or other significant loss. If the dysfunction is clinically relevant, a diagnosis of an adjustment disorder may be appropriate. An adjustment disorder entails that the reaction to the stress is out of proportion to the stressor, and with grief, the person typically does not have suicidal thoughts and the symptoms tend to improve over time. With adjustment disorder, the symptoms should improve as the external stressor recedes. In both cases, the patients will not meet criteria for MDD. DSM 5 removed bereavement from its list of psychiatric conditions in order to ensure that MDD is not underdiagnosed after significant loss. If someone with a loss of a loved one or significant external stressor meets criteria for MDD, the diagnosis is considered appropriate, and treatment should be initiated. Suicidal thoughts, feelings of extreme guilt or worthlessness, psychomotor retardation, psychosis, and prolonged or marked functional impairment are NOT typical of bereavement or grief. If thoughts of death are present in grief, it is usually confined to thoughts of "joining" the deceased. Mood in grief is usually described as feeling of emptiness and loss, rather than persistent depressed mood and anhedonia. However, since modern antidepressants such as the SSRIs and other atypical antidepressants (e.g., bupropion) are safe with a low clinical risk of harm, prescribing medications where any uncertainty is present may be a prudent clinical decision. However, as the case of Mr. W. illustrates, doing the best job possible in making an accurate diagnosis and communicating that diagnosis to the patient is critical.

If the diagnosis of grief or adjustment is clear, and the person does not meet criteria for MDD, symptoms will typically clear on their own without pharmacological treatment. Short-term symptomatic treatment (e.g., for insomnia) may be indicated, however.

A first episode of MDD can occur at virtually any age although onset prior to puberty is rare; however, the average age of onset is in the late 20s with onset in the teen years very common [16]. The symptoms usually develop over a period of days to weeks and are often preceded by prodromal symptoms such as anxiety, phobias, or depressive symptoms that do not meet full MDD criteria [10]. Untreated episodes of major depression can last several months, sometimes years, and even with treatment full recovery can take up to a year, with about half of patients at risk for relapse [16].

1.2 Major Depressive Disorder in the Medical Setting

Major depressive disorder can present on its own in the primary care setting but is often seen comorbid with chronic medical illness as well (see Table 1.1).

The presence of co-occurring MDD with medical disorders has numerous implications for medical practice. A brief summary of some of these is as follows:

Table 1.1 Prevalence of MDD in patients with chronic medical conditions

General population	8%
Rheumatoid arthritis	13–20%
Stroke	22%
Coronary artery disease	15–20%
End stage renal disease	17%
Cancer	20–25%
COPD	20%
Parkinson's disease	25–45%
Huntington's disease	50%

Severance and Hope [24]

- *Hypertension*: Some antidepressants have been known to increase blood pressure, especially the SNRIs venlafaxine and duloxetine. Lowering the SNRI may decrease the blood pressure; however, if the patient is well-controlled, adding an antihypertensive may be preferred [10].
- Many antihypertensives can trigger depressive-like symptoms, and this has been classically most associated with beta blockers, especially propranolol. Physician awareness is vital if a patient on antihypertensives starts to develop MDD like symptoms; a change in antihypertensive may then be in order.
- *Insomnia* is a symptom of MDD, but the presence of MDD can complicate patients with chronic insomnia and vice versa. The symptoms of obstructive sleep apnea (OSA) and MDD can look similar, and either syndrome can exacerbate the other. Chronic insomnia is a risk factor for suicide, and patients with OSA have greater rates of mood disorders. Careful screening and evaluation of insomnia patients is essential.
- *Cardiac Disease*: The fact that MDD can worsen symptoms of cardiac disease has been well established [19, 21]. Patients who had a status of post-myocardial infarction with comorbid MDD have decreased survival rates, and patients with MDD and cardiac symptoms should be monitored for the development of new cardiac symptoms. The use of SSRIs or bupropion may be the safest options in this group.
- *Stroke*: Depression is observed in up to 50% of individuals in the weeks to months following a stroke [10] and is associated with a decrease in the quality of life and an increase in mortality. SSRIs have been studied in post-CVA patients to good effect; however, be aware that the effect of SSRIs on platelet function, and/or the fact that they are protein bound and therefore can interfere with anticoagulants may lead to an increase in bleeding risk [10].
- *Obesity* is a common medical comorbidity often seen in clinical practice, and many patients with MDD will also have comorbid obesity. Many antidepressants can lead to weight gain; therefore, medication choice can be important in this subgroup. Bupropion is arguably the most weight-neutral antidepressant and is an appropriate first choice in these patients. It should be noted that bupropion is an antidepressant that has minimal effects on anxiety disorders. The use of SSRIs in patients with comorbid mood and anxiety issues may be a better initial choice.
- *Chronic Pain* and MDD share biological pathways and neurotransmitters, and chronic pain is associated with higher rates of depression [1] with MDD being twice as common in primary care settings among individuals with pain [11]. Tricyclic antidepressants (TCAs) are most effective for the prevention of migraines and for treating pain associated with fibromyalgia as well as neuropathic pain. However, as SNRIs (e.g., venlafaxine, duloxetine) may be better tolerated at antidepressant doses than TCAs, they may be given first line in patients with comorbid pain and MDD with TCAs a secondary choice. It should be noted that the effective analgesic doses of TCAs are lower than the antidepressant dose in most circumstances, and TCAs may be a good first choice med in many pain patients in the absence of MDD.

- Other common medical conditions including Parkinson's disease, HIV, hepatitis C, seizure disorder, and diabetes appear to be associated with higher rates of MDD. Appropriate screening and treatment/referral are recommended.

Therefore, for both mental and physical health, proper recognition of major depressive disorders is vital in the primary care setting. Screening tools can assist in this, and research has validated the use of depression screening tools such as the PHQ-9 in primary care setting [7]. However, just asking a two-question screen ("In the last month, have you been bothered by little interest or pleasure in doing things" and "In the last month, have you been feeling down, depressed, or hopeless") is an effective and easy screening tool [15]. There are a number of risk factors for depression that should cause clinicians to screen their patients more closely (see Table 1.2).

The list of medications that have been implicated in triggering or causing depression is extensive. Physicians should always check for recently added medications when there is a new onset of a major depressive episode. Common medications that are known to be risk factors can include the following:

A. Cardiovascular drugs; ACE inhibitors, calcium channel blockers, clonidine, digitalis, hydralazine, methyldopa, procainamide, beta blockers (especially propranolol), reserpine, acetazolamide
B. Chemotherapeutics: asparaginase, azathioprine, bleomycin, cisplatin, cyclophosphamide, doxorubicin, vinblastine, vincristine
C. Antiparkinsonian drugs: amantadine, bromocriptine, levodopa
D. Stimulants: Caffeine, amphetamines, methylphenidate, and cocaine (either active use or from withdrawal)
E. Antibiotics and antivirals: various penicillins, chloramphenicol, dapsone, antituberculin drugs, metronidazole, nitrofurantoin, streptomycin, sulfonamides, tetracycline, antiretroviral drugs
F. Hormonal agents: adrenocorticotropin, anabolic steroids, glucocorticoids, oral contraceptives
G. Sedatives: barbiturates, benzodiazepines, ethanol

Table 1.2 Risk factors for depression

Clinical factors	Symptoms factors
History of depression	Unexplained physical symptoms
Family history of depression	Chronic pain
External stress or adversity	Fatigue
High utilizer of medical resources	Insomnia
Chronic medical disorders	Anxiety
Comorbid psychiatric disorders	Substance use disorders (SUDs)
Peripartum or postpartum period	

Adapted from [15]

H. Anticonvulsants: ethosuximide, phenobarbital, phenytoin, primidone, tiagabine, valproic acid, vigabatrin
I. Miscellaneous: cimetidine, phenylephrine, ranitidine, statins, tamoxifen

Adapted from [9].

1.3 Diagnosis and Presentation of Major Depressive Disorder

The diagnosis of major depressive disorder is a standard categorical diagnosis in which there are nine diagnostic criteria for MDD; for a patient to meet the criteria, they must have a minimum of five present. All five criteria must be present during the same 2-*week period*, and it must represent a *change from prior functioning*. In other words, MDD represents an acute illness that is a change from baseline. Of the five criteria, one of them must be either (1) depressed mood or (2) anhedonia (loss of interest or pleasure). Symptoms that are clearly attributable to another medical condition are not included (e.g., weight loss during chemotherapy where nausea is a main side effect).

It is possible for someone to meet the criteria for MDD and NOT have a depressed mood. Anhedonia must be present in those cases.

If the patient does not meet five of the MDD criteria but has a depressed mood with an identifiable stressor, consider a diagnosis of an adjustment disorder. The change in mood or functioning must occur within 3 months of the stressor and not persist for more than 6 months.

If the patient has five of the nine required criteria, but they have been present for less than a 2-week period, monitor the patient very closely. In patients with a history of recurrent MDD, immediate treatment is encouraged. In patients with no prior history of psychiatric issues, close monitoring may be warranted until they meet the 2-week threshold.

If the patient does not have at least five of the criteria but the depressed mood has persisted for 2 or more years, consider a diagnosis of persistent depressive disorder (dysthymia).

If the patient has recently experienced the loss of a loved one, bereavement or grief may be the diagnosis. However, suicidal ideation, feelings of extreme worthlessness or guilt, psychomotor retardation, psychosis, or prolonged functional impairment is not typically seen in bereavement. Consider MDD instead. **Note:** psychomotor retardation is an objective physical finding, and subjective complaints of feeling slowed down is not considered evidence of psychomotor retardation. The case example of Mr. W. illustrated the real-world consequence of not attempting to make the distinction between MDD and grief, as the current treatment team had to make clinical decisions without a clear understanding of what the patient had experienced 18 months earlier.

See Table 1.3 for the full diagnostic criteria for MDD.

When insomnia occurs in MDD, it is typically middle insomnia (i.e., awakening in the middle of the night with difficulty in falling back to sleep) or early morning awakening (i.e., terminal insomnia). Difficulty falling asleep (i.e., initial insomnia) can also occur, but terminal and middle insomnia are more common. Hypersomnia can also occur and can be a sign of atypical depression. Appetite loss and weight loss is more common in MDD, but appetite increase can also occur, and like hypersomnia, can be a sign of *atypical depression*.

Anxiety is a common feature in MDD with a majority of patients complaining of increases in anxiety. Often, the presenting chief complaint for patients suffering from MDD is, in fact, "anxiety."

> Patients with suspected MDD should have an appropriate physical exam and lab workup as indicated by the clinical picture. Routine metabolic and thyroid screening would be indicated in most patients and in particular those with no prior history.

MDD can have a *seasonal pattern* in which sufferers experience depression during a particular season, usually the winter. Informally, this is often called seasonal

Table 1.3 DSM criteria for major depressive disorder—must meet five of the nine following criteria

1. Depressed mood most of the day, nearly every day, as indicated by subjective report or objective report from others
2. Markedly diminished interest or pleasure in all, or almost all, activities, most of the day, nearly every day
3. Significant weight loss when not dieting, or weight gain (e.g., a change of more than 5% in body weight in a month) *or* decrease or increase in appetite nearly every day
4. Insomnia or hypersomnia nearly every day
5. Psychomotor agitation or retardation nearly every day (observable by others, **not** merely subjective feelings of restlessness or feeling slowed down)
6. Fatigue or loss of energy nearly every day
7. Feelings of worthlessness or excessive guilt nearly every day (not merely guilt about being sick)
8. Diminished ability to think or concentrate, or indecisiveness nearly every day (either subjective or objective and observable by others)
9. Recurrent thoughts of death, recurrent suicidal ideation, suicide attempt, or specific plan for suicide

Note: The disorder can be given a modifier of peripartum onset if the MDD occurs during the pregnancy or within 4 weeks of delivery

affective disorder although that phrasing is not recognized DSM 5 terminology. Symptoms of MDD with a seasonal pattern often have atypical depression features (e.g., hypersomnia and weight gain). To meet criteria, there have to be at least two seasonal depressive episodes (usually in the winter) that fully resolve when the season changes (usually in the spring). Light therapy with a 10,000 lux light source is often effective treatment for MDD with seasonal pattern.

Psychotic features can occur with MDD. The psychosis usually has mood congruent features. For example, the person may have auditory hallucinations of voices telling them that they are a bad, worthless individual, or delusions that they have cancer or rotting insides, or that their family does not love them. Psychosis in MDD should trigger an immediate referral to a psychiatric specialist in most cases. The addition of an antipsychotic to an antidepressant is the usual treatment in these cases.

While most patients with MDD should be alert and oriented x3 (although psychomotor slowing may cause a decrease in motivation to answer questions), about 50% of patients with MDD will report some sort of cognitive dysfunction or memory problem [17]. The most common complaints are of memory problems or forgetfulness. The problems can occasionally be quite severe with clinically significant symptoms; in such cases, it is termed pseudodementia. These symptoms typically resolve upon resolution of the mood disorder.

Patients who you suspect or diagnose with MDD should be screened for suicidality, which can be done either by clinical interview or by the use of a screening instrument such as the Patient Health Questionnaire (PHQ). Most primary care settings use the two-question PHQ-2 as a screening tool and if positive, follows-up with the PHQ-9 which assesses the rest of the depressive symptoms [23]. Patients with passive suicidal ideation (e.g., "Sometimes I think my family would be better off if I died of a heart attack in my sleep") should be seen and followed more frequently including a follow-up within a week [23]. Patients who have suicidal intent or who have specific plans require immediate referral to the appropriate crisis service in your area. Depending on your locale, this may be a mobile crisis service, a psychiatric emergency room, or a medical emergency room. Suicide by hanging and by gun are particularly lethal methods, and ideation that involves either of those should be considered a medical emergency.

Substance use disorders (SUDs) are commonly seen in MDD, and studies have shown that up to 36% of patients with MDD have a comorbid alcohol use disorder [12] with other illicit drug use, as well as cannabis use, being very common comorbidities. Screening for SUDs in MDD patients is therefore vital.

Persistent depressive disorder (formally called dysthymia) is another mood disorder that requires attention. Patients with PDD have a depressed mood for most of the day, for more days than not for a 2-year period. While depressed, they will have at least two of the six symptoms:

1. Poor appetite or overeating
2. Insomnia or hypersomnia
3. Low energy or fatigue
4. Low self-esteem

5. Poor concentration or difficulty making decisions
6. Feelings of hopelessness

PDD usually has an early and insidious course with a high rate of comorbid substance use disorders. It is less likely than MDD to resolve on its own. Recommendations for treatment, including pharmacotherapy and psychotherapy, are similar to that for MDD.

1.4 Treatment

Patients with MDD who are treated in the primary care setting will typically have a mild to moderate level of illness. Patients with a severe level of illness—especially with associated suicidal ideation—will need to be referred for specialty psychiatric care and often inpatient treatment. People with severe levels of depression and suicidality may be eligible for somatic treatments such as electroconvulsive therapy (ECT) that are beyond the scope of this book as they are not typically used in primary care settings. The choice of initial treatment in the primary care setting will depend on numerous factors, including severity of symptoms, comorbid conditions, seasonal pattern, patient preference, past history of treatment, and family history. Multiple modalities are often used, especially in the presence of comorbid conditions. Psychotherapy alone can be used in the treatment of mild to moderate illness, with cognitive behavioral therapy (CBT), behavioral activation, and interpersonal psychotherapy (IPT) commonly used [10, 16]. Psychotherapy alone may be preferred by patients who are breastfeeding, who are pregnant, or who wish to become pregnant. If significant psychosocial stressors are present, psychotherapy alone may also be appropriate as a first-line treatment. As the delivery of psychotherapy changed dramatically during the COVID pandemic, it should be noted that psychotherapy delivered remotely via video technologies appear to have the same positive outcomes as therapy delivered in person [16]. Patients with moderate to severe levels of depression should be offered medication management as psychotherapy alone is not preferred; however, many of these patients will choose both medication management as well as adjunct psychotherapy which may be preferred in most circumstances. Figure 1.1 presents an algorithm that can be followed by primary care physicians when presented with complaints of depression by their patients.

Mild cases of MDD may be treated either with meds or psychotherapy alone. While some moderate cases may be appropriate for psychotherapy alone, people with moderate to severe MDD will require medications either alone or with psychotherapy.

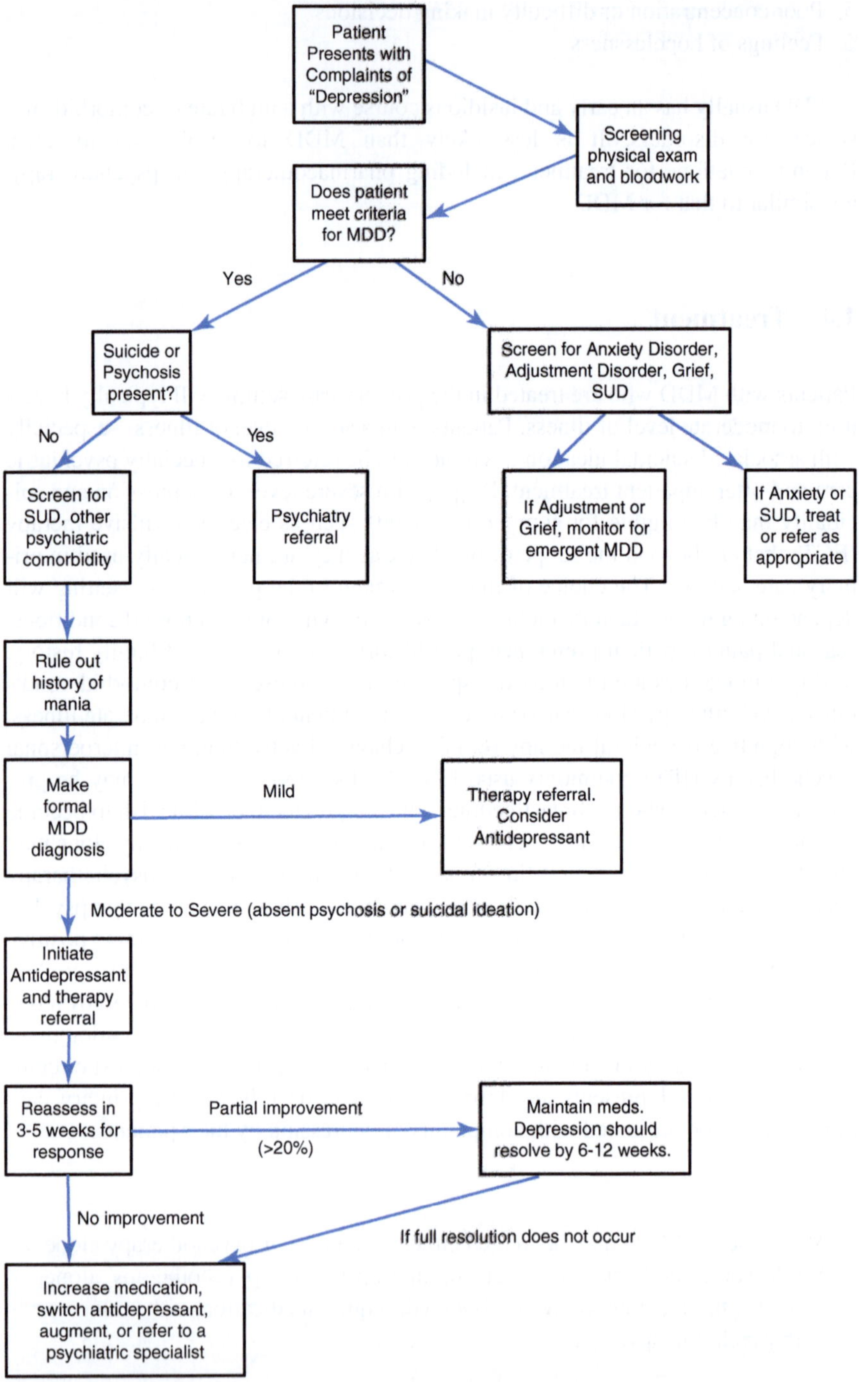

Fig. 1.1 Algorithm for approach to complaints of depression in the primary care setting

1.5 Treatment

1.5.1 Pharmacotherapy

Prior to the initiation of an antidepressant for MDD, the patient should be screened for mania to rule out bipolar disorder, to prevent antidepressant-induced mania. Asking about past instances of euphoria and instances of *decreased need* (not decreased amount) for sleep for >1 week are good screening questions.

The choice of medication for patients with MDD depends on numerous factors. Some of the factors that should be considered when choosing a medication are the following:

- Patient's past history of medication use and response
- Consideration of side effects from antidepressants
- Drug interactions
- Comorbid psychiatric or medical conditions (including pregnancy)
- Safety of the medication in overdose (especially in patients who have suicidal ideations or a history of overdose attempts)
- Family history of medication response
- Cost of medication and insurance formulary
- Patient and provider preference

Past history of response is vital. If a patient has a history of good response to a certain medication, that medication deserves strong consideration. Likewise, past failure of a medication indicates a different medication should be used and if possible, an antidepressant from a different class of medications should be considered. *Side effects* are often a top concern of patients. An atypical antidepressant such as bupropion makes an ideal first choice for MDD due to its low incidence of sexual side effects, sedation, and weight gain, all of which are problematic issues of antidepressant use. *Drug interactions* are a concern as some antidepressants are strong cytochrome p450 inhibitors and strong plasma protein binding can change the levels of meds such as coumadin. See Tables 1.4, 1.5, and 1.6 for a list of important antidepressant CYP inhibitors and substrates. At the end of the chapter, Table 1.13 contains a comprehensive list of CYP inhibitors and inducers in order to facilitate better recognitions of potential drug-drug interactions. The presence of *comorbid psychiatric conditions* should be considered. If the patient has a comorbid anxiety or obsessive-compulsive related disorder, they may benefit from an SSRI over other classes of medications. Patients with uncontrolled HTN may want to avoid SNRIs if possible. In pregnancy or breastfeeding, sertraline is the preferred medication by many clinicians [29]. *Safety* is a concern in a disorder in which suicidal ideations

Table 1.4 CYP450 inhibitory potential of SSRIs and SNRIs

CYP isoenzyme	Citalopram	Fluoxetine	Fluvoxamine	Paroxetine	Sertraline
CYP1A2	+/−	+	+++	+	+/−
CYP2C19	?	++	+++		+
CYP2D6	+	+++	+	+++	+
CYP3A4	?	++	++	+/−	+/−

CYP isoenzyme	Venlafaxine	Desvenlafaxine	Duloxetine
CYP1A2	+/−	+/−	?
CYP2C19	+/−	+/−	?
CYP2D6	+/−	+/−	++
CYP3A4	+/−	+/−	?

Key: +/− unlikely; ? unknown; + mild; ++ moderate; +++ substantial
Table adapted from [22]

Table 1.5 Important substrates of CYP isoenzymes

1A2	2C19	2D6	3A4
Caffeine, theophylline, clozapine, clomipramine, duloxetine	Proton pump inhibitors, diazepam,	Many tricyclic antidepressants (TCAs), beta blockers, antiarrhythmic agents, atomoxetine, duloxetine, risperidone, codeine, hydrocodone, oxycodone, vortioxetine, dextromethorphan	Calcium channel blockers, erythromycin, alprazolam, midazolam, triazolam, statins (HMG-CoA reductase inhibitors), HIV protease inhibitors, venlafaxine, mirtazapine, trazodone, levomilnacipran, vilazodone, ziprasidone

Table adapted from [13, 27]

Table 1.6 Other important CYP isoenzyme inhibitors

1A2	2D6	3A4
Ciprofloxacin, cimetidine	Cimetidine	Erythromycin, ketoconazole, ritonavir, amiodarone, grapefruit

Table adapted from [27]

play a major role. SSRIs are the safest drug class in terms of overdose. However, if possible, have a trusted family member take control of medications including locking them up, in patients who are at risk for self-harm. SNRIs and atypical antidepressants may not be as safe in overdose, and TCAs are potentially lethal with just a week's worth of a therapeutic dose. The provider should always check *family history*; if a first-degree relative has responded well to a particular medication, there is a greater chance that the patient will as well. Finally, cost as well as patient and provider preference are important—a patient is more likely to stick with a medication that they are agreeable with, that are able to afford, or that the doctor has confidence in.

There is a high comorbidity between MDD and substance use disorders. Substance-induced depressive episodes are also consideration in such patients. MDD patients should be screened for substance use disorders and substance withdrawal syndromes and referred appropriately, if present.

Once the antidepressant has been started, the medication should be increased to a therapeutic dose as soon as tolerability allows. Once a therapeutic level has been achieved, some therapeutic response should be observed within 3–5 weeks. Once they obtain that initial response, maintaining the medication at the initial dose and waiting is then typically sufficient to achieve remission. A > 20% improvement at the initial stage of 3–5 weeks correlates to response and remission within 6–12 weeks [13].

The initial response to antidepressant therapy is often objective and not subjective. In other words, family, friends, or the physician may see a brightening of the affect before the patient notices the improvement themself.

If a patient has not achieved a moderate level of improvement by 3–5 weeks, a change in treatment plan in indicated. Patient should be assessed for accuracy of the initial diagnosis, medication compliance, side effects, and any potential complicating comorbid conditions, either psychiatric or medical. At this point, an adjustment in the dose is indicated. If the patient again has minimal response after a 4–8 week trial, further action is indicated [10]:

Increase of the medication to the highest dose tolerated if not already done.

Switch the antidepressant. A switch to a medication in the same class (e.g., SSRI to SSRI) or switch from one class to another (SSRI to SNRI) is permissible.

Augmentation of the antidepressant. This typically involves the addition of another antidepressant from a different class of antidepressants (e.g., addition of bupropion to an existing SSRI) or the use of lithium, triiodothyronine (T3), or a second-generation antipsychotic. The second-generation antipsychotics with the best evidence include aripiprazole and quetiapine, with risperidone, olanzapine, and brexpiprazole showing some efficacy despite being less studied [4, 13]. Obviously, the use of lithium or antipsychotics warrants strict monitoring; T3 is only typically used for 2 months due to potential medical complications. See Chap. 4 for the instructions on the appropriate use and monitoring of antipsychotics.

Referral to a psychiatrist or mood disorders specialist. If possible, most non-psychiatric physicians should strongly consider referral if the patient fails an antidepressant trial—called treatment-resistant depression (TRD).

Antidepressants have been shown to potentially increase suicidal risk in adolescents and young adults; hence a black box warning in the United States for anyone under the age of 25. Close monitoring is advised when starting them in this age group. Antidepressants do, however, reduce the suicide risk in older adults.

1.6 Pharmacotherapy: Continuation, Maintenance, and Discontinuation

Once a patient has responded to antidepressant therapy, the next question is how long to continue medications. While noting that different published guidelines have different names for the phases of antidepressant therapy, after someone has responded in the acute phase, the antidepressant should be continued at the same dose for at least 6–9 months [13]. If the patient is not already in psychotherapy, the addition of CBT can improve outcomes during this time.

After a 6–9-month period of remission, the decision point than is whether maintained is required or if the medication can be discontinued. If the patient has had three or more episodes of MDD, or if they are being treated for persistent depressive disorder, ongoing maintenance therapy would be the preferred treatment. The dose that was used to achieve remission is the dose that should be continued. Regular monitoring to ensure that depressive symptoms have not reoccurred is recommended.

Patients with less than three major depressive episodes can be considered for medication discontinuation if the MDD has been in remission a minimum of 6–9 months. Geriatric patients (such as Mr. W.) may be at greater risk of relapse that younger patients, even with a single episode, and ongoing treatment in that group may be necessary [8]. There is always a risk of relapse, and this should be thoroughly discussed with the patient. It is recommended to taper the medication very slowly which not only helps minimize the risk of relapse but can help minimize discontinuation syndrome, which can occur with most antidepressants, especially the SSRIs (with the possible exception of fluoxetine) and the SNRIs. We recommend tapering by one titration dose per month, and once the low end dose is reached, using a half dose every other day for a month before stopping completely. For example, a patient who has been stabilized on 150 mg sertraline would take 100 mg daily for 1 month, then 50 mg daily for 1 month, then 25 mg daily for 1 month, and then finally 25 mg every other day for 1 month, and then discontinue.

Below are table of the various classes of antidepressants, covering the most common ones used in primary care settings. These tables are specific for the use in MDD—the treatment of other disorders may require different protocols—and these tables are not meant to be complete synopses of the medications but a summary (Tables 1.7, 1.8, 1.9, 1.10, and 1.11). Table 1.12 covers antipsychotic augmentation of antidepressants.

Table 1.7 Atypical antidepressants—often an excellent first-line choice for uncomplicated MDD

Medication	Starting dose (mg)	Usual dose (mg/day)	Notes
Bupropion	75 daily or bid: IR 150 daily: SR 150 daily: XL	150–450	Low incidence of sexual side effects, sedation, and weight gain. Contraindicated with seizures and eating disorders (anorexia and bulimia). SR is dosed bid above 200 mg daily
Mirtazapine	15 qhs	15–45 qhs	Sedation may lessen >15 mg. Lower incidence of sexual side effects, higher incidence of weight gain
Vortioxetine	5–10 daily	10–20 daily	Tolerability worsens at 20 mg. Do not use higher than 10 mg in patients who are on CYP 2D6 inhibitors
Trazodone	50 tid	150–600	Typically used as a sleep agent rather than an antidepressant
Nefazodone	50 bid	300–600 daily given bid	Black box warning of acute hepatic failure has limited usage
Vilazodone	10	20–40	Requires dose adjustments with drugs that inhibit or induce CYP 3A4

Key: *IR*, immediate release; *SR*, sustained release; *XL*, extended release

Table 1.8 Serotonin selective reuptake inhibitors—good when there is co-occurring anxiety. If patient fails one SSRI for MDD, a second may be tried prior to switching classes

Medication	Starting dose (mg/day)	Usual dose (mg/day)	Notes
Fluoxetine	10–20	20–80	Long half-life means it is less likely to cause discontinuation syndrome. Potent CYP 2D6 inhibitor
Sertraline	25–50	50–200	Should be taken after a meal. A preferred medication during pregnancy and/or breastfeeding
Paroxetine	10–20	20–60	Very potent CYP 2D6 inhibitor. Sedation and weight gain are more likely than other SSRIs. Concerns about malformations in pregnant woman. Significant discontinuation symptoms possible
Fluvoxamine	50	100–300	Dosed daily or bid. Potent CYP 3A4 inhibitor. Not approved in the US for MDD but effective
Citalopram	10–20	20–60	Black box warning regarding QTc prolongation. Use of greater than 40 mg in adults or 20 mg in elderly cautioned
Escitalopram	5–10	10–20	

MAO-I diet includes avoiding the following: aged cheeses, cured or processed meats, fermented foods, sauces (soy, miso, teriyaki, fish), soybeans, fava beans, yeast spreads, brewer's yeast (e.g., draft or bottle conditioned beers), and aged red wines.

Medications to avoid include the following: meperidine, tramadol, methadone, other antidepressants of any class, all sympathomimetics (including pseudoephedrine), stimulants, and St John's Wort.

Table 1.9 Serotonin norepinephrine reuptake inhibitors

Medication	Starting dose (mg/day)	Usual dose (mg/day)	Notes
Venlafaxine	37.5–75 XR daily 25 IR bid-tid	225–375 XR daily 375 IR (divided doses)	Low CYP interactions. Significant discontinuation symptoms
Duloxetine	20–30	30–60 (occasional use at 120)	Also approved for neuropathic pain at 60 mg daily
Desvenlafaxine	50	50–100	Patients with renal impairment should dose 50 mg every other day to 50 mg daily maximum. Patients with hepatic impairment should use no more than 50 mg daily
Levomilnacipran	20 × 2 days, then 40	40–120	40 mg daily for severe renal impairment. 80 mg daily for moderate renal impairment

Key: *XR*, extended release; *IR*, immediate release
Note: SNRIs may be less safe than SSRIs in overdose

Table 1.10 Commonly used tricyclic antidepressants

TCA	Starting dose (mg/day)	Usual dose (mg day)	Notes
Amitriptyline	25–75 qhs	150–300 qhs	Marked anticholinergic properties
Imipramine	25–75 qhs	150–300 qhs	Significant potential for orthostasis
Nortriptyline	25–50 qhs	50–150 qhs	Blood levels useful for therapeutic window. Lower potential for orthostasis
Desipramine	25–75 qhs	150–300 qhs	Lower potential for anticholinergic side effects
Clomipramine	25–75	150–250 qhs	Approved for OCD

Notes: Due to the fact that 1 weeks' worth of a therapeutic dose of a TCA is a potentially lethal dose in overdose, TCAs should generally be reserved for psychiatry use for MDD. Doses that are used for non-psychiatric conditions (e.g., pain, migraines) are given at doses much lower than therapeutic doses for MDD and are commonly and appropriately used by non-psychiatric specialists

Table 1.11 Commonly used MAO inhibitors. These medications should typically only be prescribed by psychiatric specialists due to dietary reactions (tyramine crisis) and significant drug interactions

MAO-I	Starting dose (mg/day)	Usual dose (mg/day)	Notes
Phenelzine	15 daily-tid	60–90	MAO diet and no sympathomimetics
Tranylcypromine	10 bid	30–60	MAO diet and no sympathomimetics

Table 1.12 Dosing of antipsychotics for MDD augmentation

Recommendation	Medication	Dose (mg/day)
First-line agents	Aripiprazole	2–5
	Quetiapine	150–300
Second-line agents	Risperidone	1–3
	Brexpiprazole	1–3
	Olanzapine	2.5–10

Prior to prescribing medication to a patient on an MAO-I, please check with the prescribing psychiatrist or obtain appropriate consultation with any questions or concerns.

1.7 Side Effects of Common Antidepressants

1.7.1 SSRI and SNRI Side Effects

Typical side effects of SSRIs/SNRIs include excessive yawning, headache, GI distress (nausea, dyspepsia, constipation, diarrhea), vivid dreams or nightmares, and tremors [2]. These side effects often are transient, and are usually managed conservatively, using over-the-counter analgesics for headache, stool softeners for constipation, and H2 blockers for dyspepsia. Starting at a lower dose and maintaining that dose for a few weeks prior to titration are often sufficient for symptom management.

- *Sexual side effects* are among the most troubling side effects that can occur with chronic, ongoing use of SSRI therapy and are reported in approximately a third of patients on SSRI therapy [6]. The most common reported problems are loss of libido, delayed orgasm or anorgasmia, erectile dysfunction (males), and lack of lubrication (females). Often, a careful history will determine that the complaints of erectile dysfunction or lack of lubrication are not primary issues per se but are the result of severe anorgasmia. There are numerous strategies that can be used in patients suffering from sexual side effects and a careful history regarding the nature of the actual side effects, their usual sexual habits, and their partner's (if there is one) knowledge of the situation. It should be noted that many patients state that the sexual side effects can remit over time, often taking many months or more; as a result, further intervention other than patience may not always be necessary. The addition of bupropion at a dose of 300 mg daily has been shown to reduce sexual side effects from SSRIs [2]. Buspirone can be used safely at doses between 20 and 60 mg daily and can help reverse sexual side effects. If the patient does not wish to take a medication chronically in order to reverse sexual side effects, the use of cyproheptadine 4 mg orally 1–2 hours prior to sexual activity can reduce sexual side effects [26]. We recommend this be used no more than 3 times per week. Another method that can be used is the drug holiday method. We recommend that the patient's medication be stopped the day before planned sexual activity. On the day that sexual activity occurs, the person can delay their dose until afterward. The medication can then be resumed on a normal basis the following day; this results in only one total missed dose. Patients should not do this more than one time per week in order to minimize missed dosages. The drug holiday method is not recommended with fluoxetine (due to its long half-life) and caution should be used with paroxetine and venlafaxine due to their potent discontinuation syndrome (see below).

- *Movement disorders such as myoclonus* are defined as sudden, abrupt, shock-like involuntary movements caused by muscle contractions. Nocturnal jaw clenching may also occur. Usually, lowering the dose or switching meds can help, but these side effects may spontaneously remit as well [28].
- A *frontal lobe amotivational syndrome* can occur, characterized by apathy, affective blunting, and memory issues. Complaints of sedation may accompany this. (Note: excessive yawning is also a side effect of SSRIs and is not associated with fatigue.) This side effect may be more common in OCD patients as it may occur at higher doses and may not improve with time as opposed to some other SSRI side effects [20]. The most common strategies to manage this include lowering the dose or switching agents. In our practice, we have had success using modafinil at usual therapeutic doses to counteract this side effect.
- Any of the SSRIs or SNRIs may lead to *weight gain* with long-term usage. This side effect may be associated with long-term use. Management of this side effect is usually conservative, with recommendations given around lifestyle changes such as appropriate diet and exercise.
- *Excessive sweating* is a common complaint. Conservative management works in most cases, which simply involves recommending the patient have a change of bed clothes available to change into in the middle of the night. While there is little data on pharmacological management of these side effects, benztropine at 0.5 mg nightly can be tried [2].
- *Hyponatremia* is a rare (0.5% per year incidence) problem that can occur with SSRIs or SNRIs; elderly, female, and patients using concomitant diuretics are in the highest risk category. This typically occurs within a few weeks of medication initiation or dose increase [18]. Symptoms typically include muscle cramps, fatigue, delirium, and seizures.
- *SSRI discontinuation syndrome* can occur with the abrupt discontinuation of many antidepressants, including the SSRIs (with the possible exception of fluoxetine due to its extended half-life) and the SNRIs, especially venlafaxine. While it does not demand medical intervention, the symptoms can be quite distressing and even disabling; dizziness, light-headedness, insomnia, fatigue, anxiety, headache, nausea, and sensory disturbances described as electric sensations in the head or limbs (colloquially known as "brain zaps") are reported most commonly [30]. While symptoms are acute, resolution can be achieved rapidly by reinstating the full dose of the medication. Very slow and extended tapers can

ameliorate this problem in most patients. In the case of someone on a maximum dose of an SSRI, the taper period may last 6 months or longer to reduce the risk of discontinuation syndrome. This also has the side benefit of decreasing the risk of relapse, as slower tapers of medications can reduce the possibility of Major Depression reoccurring after medications are stopped.

- *Serotonin syndrome* is a rare but serious medical condition that includes symptoms such as mental status changes, gastrointestinal symptoms, autonomic instability (tachycardia, hypertension, and hyperthermia), and neuromuscular abnormalities including myoclonus, hyperreflexia, hypertonicity, and rigidity; clinically, it presents very much like neuroleptic malignant syndrome [3, 5]. It has been most commonly associated with combinations of serotonergic agents but has been reported to occur with single agents. Treatment is usually supportive and includes discontinuation of the serotonergic agent; the addition of the 5-HT 2a antagonist cyproheptadine may also be of benefit [5].
- *Gastrointestinal bleeding* is a potential side effect of SSRI or SNRI use and may be exacerbated with the concomitant use of non-steroidal anti-inflammatory agents [18]. The use of medications to reduce the risk of GI bleeding may be warranted in high-risk patients (Andrade and Sharma 2016).

1.8 When to Refer

As usual, when to refer a patient to a psychiatric specialist is always dependent on the comfort and skill level of the treating physician. MDD is a common issue and the average provider in a primary care setting sees it as much as psychiatrists do and quite possibly even more often. In many rural settings, there is likely to be a dearth of psychiatric referrals, meaning that patients in the primary care setting may require more sophisticated psychiatric management prior to utilizing limited referrals sources than in other settings. Some general rules do apply, however.

Patients who have active suicidal ideation, or express suicidal intent, or discuss a specific plan should be immediately referred for emergency psychiatric evaluation and potential psychiatric hospitalization. If the patient is deemed a high risk of harm to self and transfer from the office setting to an emergency room cannot be done safely, crisis services appropriate to your local community may be activated, including 911. For example, a patient who says that they are not suicidal at this time but state that they have saved up medication to take in case they change their mind demands emergency evaluation by psychiatry.

The presence of psychotic symptoms also demands immediate psychiatric referral in most instances.

If there are other comorbid, serious psychiatric disorders present, that would also lower the threshold for psychiatric referral. Certainly, the presence of an eating disorder means the patient should see a psychiatric specialist as may other illnesses such as OCD. Again, much of that depends on the comfort level of the primary care physician.

Treatment-resistant depression is also a reason for referral. It would certainly be appropriate after the failure of one antidepressant to refer. Many physicians may feel comfortable trying a second medication from a different class, or even a third, but evaluation should strongly be considered after that many failures. Once a patient has had nonresponse to more than four antidepressants, many expert guidelines in psychiatry recommend considering TCAs or MOA-I for treatment, and that would typically be done by a psychiatrist.

If there are diagnostic concerns, such as being unable to rule out bipolar disorder, personality disorder, or other psychiatric disorders or comorbidity, the patients should be seen by a psychiatrist prior to starting medication therapy. Mr. W. is an example of a patient who was started on SSRI treatment where there was apparent diagnostic uncertainty (or a diagnosis was not properly communicated to the patient), and this created a significant medical conundrum down the road as a result.

If the patient is having side effects to the medication that may lead to non-compliance, referral is important in those cases, as early or abrupt discontinuation of medication can trigger a reoccurrence.

1.9 Addendum (Table 1.13)

Table 1.13 Inhibitors and inducers of CYP enzymes

CYP	Strong inhibitors	Moderate inhibitors	Inducers
1A2	Ciprofloxacin Fluvoxamine	Amiodarone Capmatinib Cimetidine Deferasirox Estrogens (hormone Replacement therapy and Oral contraceptives) Mexiletine Norfloxacin Ofloxacin Rucaparib Tacrine Thiabendazole Vemurafenib Zileuton	Carbamazepine[a] Rifampin[a] Smoking Tetrahydrocannabinol

Table 1.13 (continued)

CYP	Strong inhibitors	Moderate inhibitors	Inducers
2B6		Clopidogrel Crizotinib Mifepristone Ticlopidine	Artemisinin Carbamazepine[a] Efavirenz Isavuconazonium Nevirapine Phenobarbital Phenytoin derivatives Rifampin Ritonavir
2C8	Abiraterone Clopidogrel Gemfibrozil	Deferasirox Lapatinib Leflunomide Letermovir Mifepristone Sorafenib Teriflunomide Trimethoprim Trimethoprim/sulfamethoxazole	Dabrafenib Rifabutin Rifampin[a] Rifapentine[a]
2C9	Fluconazole Miconazole	Abiraterone Alcohol (intoxicating dose) Amiodarone Capecitabine Ceritinib Delavirdine Efavirenz Etravirine Fenofibrate Floxuridine Fluorouracil Fluvastatin Imatinib Metronidazole Mifepristone Rucaparib Sorafenib Sulfadiazine Sulfamethoxazole Sulfisoxazole Trimethoprim/sulfamethoxazole Valproate Voriconazole Zafirlukast	Aprepitant[a] Bosentan Carbamazepine[a] Dabrafenib Enzalutamide Letermovir Phenobarbital[a] Phenytoin derivatives[a] Primidone[a] Rifabutin Rifampin[a] Rifapentine[a]

(continued)

Table 1.13 (continued)

CYP	Strong inhibitors	Moderate inhibitors	Inducers
2C19	Delavirdine Fluconazole Fluvoxamine Ticlopidine	Abiraterone Armodafinil Bortezomib Cimetidine Efavirenz Eslicarbazepine Esomeprazole Etravirine Felbamate Fluoxetine Isoniazid Luliconazole Modafinil Omeprazole Oxcarbazepine Voriconazole	Carbamazepine Dabrafenib Enzalutamide Letermovir Phenytoin derivatives Rifampin[a] Saint John's wort Tipranavir/ritonavir
2D6	Bupropion Cinacalcet Fluoxetine Paroxetine Quinidine Quinine Terbinafine Tipranavir/ritonavir	Abiraterone Amiodarone Artemether/lumefantrine Celecoxib Chloroquine Chlorpheniramine Chlorpromazine Cimetidine Clobazam Clomipramine Cobicistat Darifenacin Darunavir Desvenlafaxine Diphenhydramine Dronedarone Duloxetine Eliglustat Haloperidol Imatinib Lorcaserin Mirabegron Promethazine Propafenone Ritonavir Rolapitant Rucaparib Sertraline	

Table 1.13 (continued)

CYP	Strong inhibitors	Moderate inhibitors	Inducers
2E1	Disulfiram		
3A4	Atazanavir Boceprevir Clarithromycin Cobicistat Conivaptan Idelalisib Imatinib Indinavir Isoniazid Itraconazole Ketoconazole Lopinavir/ritonavir Nefazodone Nelfinavir Posaconazole Ritonavir Telaprevir Telithromycin Tipranavir/ritonavir Voriconazole	Abiraterone Amiodarone Aprepitant Ceritinib Clotrimazole Crizotinib Cyclosporine Darunavir Delavirdine Diltiazem Dronedarone Erythromycin Fluconazole Fluvoxamine Fosamprenavir Fostamatinib Grapefruit juice Isavuconazonium Ivacaftor Letermovir Lomitapide Miconazole Netupitant Nilotinib Quinupristin/dalfopristin Saquinavir Verapamil Zafirlukast	Apalutamide[a] Armodafinil Artemether/lumefantrine Bexarotene Bosentan Carbamazepine[a] Dabrafenib Deferasirox Dexamethasone Efavirenz Elagolix Enzalutamide[a] Etravirine Mitotane[a] Modafinil Nafcillin Nevirapine Oxcarbazepine Phenobarbital[a] Phenytoin derivatives[a] Primidone[a] Rifabutin[a] Rifampin[a] Rifapentine[a] Rufinamide Saint John's wort[a]

[a]Strong inducer
Reprinted with special permission from [33]

1.10 Conclusion

Major depressive disorder is commonly encountered in the primary care setting. Proper screening, diagnosis, and treatment are within the purview of the primary care physician. Taking care to ensure a proper diagnosis, patient education, and appropriate referrals for psychotherapy can ensure good outcomes in your practice.

References

1. Bair MJ, Robinson RL, Katon W, Kroenke K. Depression and pain comorbidity: a literature review. Arch Intern Med. 2003;(20):2433–45. https://doi.org/10.1001/archinte.163.20.2433. PMID: 14609780.

2. Borue X, Sharma M, Hudak R. Biological treatments for obsessive-compulsive and related disorders. J Obsessive Compuls Relat Disorders. 2015;6:7–26.
3. Boyer EW, Shannon M. The serotonin syndrome. N Engl J Med. 2005;352(11):1112–20. https://doi.org/10.1056/NEJMra041867; Erratum in: N Engl J Med. 2007;356(23):2437; Erratum in: N Engl J Med 2009;361(17):1714. PMID: 15784664.
4. Cantù F, Ciappolino V, Enrico P, Moltrasio C, Delvecchio G, Brambilla P. Augmentation with atypical antipsychotics for treatment-resistant depression. J Affect Disord. 2021;280(Pt A):45–53. https://doi.org/10.1016/j.jad.2020.11.006. Epub 2020 Nov 5. PMID: 33202337.
5. Caroff SN, Watson CB, Rosenberg H. Drug-induced hyperthermic syndromes in psychiatry. Clin Psychopharmacol Neurosci. 2021;19(1):1–11. https://doi.org/10.9758/cpn.2021.19.1.1. PMID: 33508784; PMCID: PMC7851465.
6. Clayton AH, Pradko JF, Croft HA, Montano CB, Leadbetter RA, Bolden-Watson C, Bass KI, Donahue RM, Jamerson BD, Metz A. Prevalence of sexual dysfunction among newer antidepressants. J Clin Psychiatry. 2002;63(4):357–66. https://doi.org/10.4088/jcp.v63n0414. PMID: 12000211.
7. Costantini L, Pasquarella C, Odone A, Colucci ME, Costanza A, Serafini G, Aguglia A, Belvederi Murri M, Brakoulias V, Amore M, Ghaemi SN, Amerio A. Screening for depression in primary care with patient health Questionnaire-9 (PHQ-9): a systematic review. J Affect Disord. 2021;(279):473–83. https://doi.org/10.1016/j.jad.2020.09.131. Epub 2020 Oct 6. PMID: 33126078.
8. Frank C. Pharmacologic treatment of depression in the elderly. Can Fam Physician. 2014;60(2):121–6. PMID: 24522673; PMCID: PMC3922554.
9. Gautam S, Jain A, Gautam M, Vahia VN, Grover S. Clinical practice guidelines for the management of depression. Indian J Psychiatry. 2017;59(Suppl 1):S34–50. https://doi.org/10.4103/0019-5545.196973. PMID: 28216784; PMCID: PMC5310101.
10. Gelenberg AJ, Freeman MP, Markowitz JC, et al. Practice guidelines for the treatment of patients with major depressive disorder. 3rd ed. American Psychiatric Association; 2010.
11. Gureje O, Von Korff M, Simon GE, Gater R. Persistent pain and Well-being: a World Health Organization study in primary care. JAMA. 1998;280(2):147–51. https://doi.org/10.1001/jama.280.2.147. Erratum in: JAMA 1998;280(13):1142. PMID: 9669787.
12. Hunt GE, Malhi GS, Lai HMX, Cleary M. Prevalence of comorbid substance use in major depressive disorder in community and clinical settings, 1990-2019: systematic review and meta-analysis. J Affect Disord. 2020;1(266):288–304. https://doi.org/10.1016/j.jad.2020.01.141. Epub 2020 Jan 26. PMID: 32056890.
13. Kennedy SH, Lam RW, McIntyre RS, Tourjman SV, Bhat V, Blier P, Hasnain M, Jollant F, Levitt AJ, MacQueen GM, McInerney SJ, McIntosh D, Milev RV, Müller DJ, Parikh SV, Pearson NL, Ravindran AV, Uher R; CANMAT Depression Work Group. Canadian Network for Mood and Anxiety Treatments (CANMAT) 2016 Clinical Guidelines for the Management of Adults with Major Depressive Disorder: Section 3. Pharmacological treatments. Can J Psychiatry. 2016;61(9):540–60. https://doi.org/10.1177/0706743716659417. Epub 2016 Aug 2; Erratum in: Can J Psychiatry. 2017;62(5):356. PMID: 27486148; PMCID: PMC4994790.
14. Kupfer DJ, Frank E, Phillips ML. Major depressive disorder: new clinical, neurobiological, and treatment perspectives. Lancet. 2012;379(9820):1045–55. https://doi.org/10.1016/S0140-6736(11)60602-8. Epub 2011 Dec 19. PMID: 22189047; PMCID: PMC3397431.
15. Lam RW, McIntosh D, Wang J, Enns MW, Kolivakis T, Michalak EE, Sareen J, Song WY, Kennedy SH, MacQueen GM, Milev RV, Parikh SV, Ravindran AV; CANMAT Depression Work Group. Canadian Network for Mood and Anxiety Treatments (CANMAT) 2016 Clinical Guidelines for the Management of Adults with Major Depressive Disorder: Section 1. Disease burden and principles of care. Can J Psychiatry. 2016;61(9):510–23. https://doi.org/10.1177/0706743716659416. Epub 2016 Aug 2. PMID: 27486151; PMCID: PMC4994789.
16. Malhi GS, Bell E, Singh AB, Bassett D, Berk M, Boyce P, Bryant R, Gitlin M, Hamilton A, Hazell P, Hopwood M, Lyndon B, McIntyre RS, Morris G, Mulder R, Porter R, Yatham LN, Young A, Murray G. The 2020 Royal Australian and new Zealand College of Psychiatrists clinical practice guidelines for mood disorders: major depression summary. Bipolar Disord. 2020;22(8):788–804. https://doi.org/10.1111/bdi.13035. PMID: 33320412.

17. McIntyre RS, Xiao HX, Syeda K, Vinberg M, Carvalho AF, Mansur RB, Maruschak N, Cha DS. The prevalence, measurement, and treatment of the cognitive dimension/domain in major depressive disorder. CNS Drugs. 2015;29(7):577–89. https://doi.org/10.1007/s40263-015-0263-x. PMID: 26290264.
18. Moret C, Isaac M, Briley M. Problems associated with long-term treatment with selective serotonin reuptake inhibitors. J Psychopharmacol. 2009;23(8):967–74. https://doi.org/10.1177/0269881108093582. Epub 2008 Jul 17. PMID: 18635702.
19. Moussavi S, Chatterji S, Verdes E, Tandon A, Patel V, Ustun B. Depression, chronic diseases, and decrements in health: results from the world health surveys. Lancet. 2007;370(9590):851–8. https://doi.org/10.1016/S0140-6736(07)61415-9. PMID: 17826170.
20. Murphy TK, Segarra A, Storch EA, Goodman WK. SSRI adverse events: how to monitor and manage. Int Rev Psychiatry. 2008;20(2):203–8. https://doi.org/10.1080/09540260801889211. PMID: 18386213.
21. O'Connor CM, Jiang W, Kuchibhatla M, Silva SG, Cuffe MS, Callwood DD, Zakhary B, Stough WG, Arias RM, Rivelli SK, Krishnan R; SADHART-CHF Investigators. Safety and efficacy of sertraline for depression in patients with heart failure: results of the SADHART-CHF (Sertraline Against Depression and Heart Disease in Chronic Heart Failure) trial. J Am Coll Cardiol. 2010;56(9):692–9. https://doi.org/10.1016/j.jacc.2010.03.068. PMID: 20723799; PMCID: PMC3663330.
22. Page SA, Hudak R. Selective serotonin reuptake inhibitors in the treatment of obsessive-compulsive disorder. In: Hudak R, Dougherty DD, editors. Clinical obsessive compulsive disorders in adults and children. Cambridge University Press; 2011.
23. Raue PJ, Ghesquiere AR, Bruce ML. Suicide risk in primary care: identification and management in older adults. Curr Psychiatry Rep. 2014;16(9):466. https://doi.org/10.1007/s11920-014-0466-8. PMID: 25030971; PMCID: PMC4137406.
24. Severance AJ, Hope CR. Mood disorders and insomnia in the general medical setting. In Psychosomatic medicine. Ackerman KD, Dimartini AF, Oxford University Press 2015. 57–74.
25. Skultety KM, Rodriguez RL. Treating geriatric depression in primary care. Curr Psychiatry Rep. 2008;10(1):44–50. https://doi.org/10.1007/s11920-008-0009-2. PMID: 18269894.
26. Schweitzer I, Maguire K, Ng C. Sexual side-effects of contemporary antidepressants: review. Aust N Z J Psychiatry. 2009;43(9):795–808. https://doi.org/10.1080/00048670903107575. PMID: 19670052.
27. The medical letter on drugs and therapeutics. 2020;62(1607):e152–3.
28. Vandel P, Bonin B, Leveque E, Sechter D, Bizouard P. Tricyclic antidepressant-induced extrapyramidal side effects. Eur Neuropsychopharmacol. 1997;7(3):207–12. https://doi.org/10.1016/s0924-977x(97)00405-7. PMID: 9213080. Reprinted with Special Permission.
29. Womersley K, Ripullone K, Agius M. What are the risks associated with different selective serotonin re-uptake inhibitors (SSRIs) to treat depression and anxiety in pregnancy? An evaluation of current evidence. Psychiatr Danub. 2017;29(Suppl 3):629–44. PMID: 28953843.
30. Zajecka J, Tracy KA, Mitchell S. Discontinuation symptoms after treatment with serotonin reuptake inhibitors: a literature review. J Clin Psychiatry. 1997;58(7):291–7. https://doi.org/10.4088/jcp.v58n0702. PMID: 9269249.

Chapter 2
Excessive Anxiety

2.1 Introduction and Epidemiology

Case Example 2.1
Mrs. A. is a 59-year-old female who comes into her family doctor's office with a 1-week history of "severe depression" since she was laid off from her job. Her mood prior to 1 week ago was reported to be baseline. She is crying in the office and states that she is having trouble falling asleep at night and then sleeps until late in the morning as a result. She is pacing and restless most of the day and cannot stop thinking about work and possible financial difficulties if she does not find a new job. She had a panic attack while worrying about all of this but has had no resultant change in behavior. She denies suicidality. She is subsequently diagnosed as having situational anxiety and is placed on lorazepam 0.5 mg prn for sleep or for daytime restlessness. She is given 20 tablets and told that she should seek occupational counseling and unemployment insurance and to consider a psychotherapy referral if the symptoms last longer than a week or so.

Anxiety is unique among psychiatric symptoms in that it also occurs in people with no psychopathology. No other psychiatric symptom (e.g., delusions, hallucinations, obsessions, clinical depression, mania) is a typical part of the human experience, whereas anxiety is something that everyone experiences, not just those with anxiety disorders. Without normal, appropriate anxiety, people would feel no need to look

R. Hudak, J. M. Gannon, *Handbook of Psychiatric Disorders in Adults in the Primary Care Setting*, Current Clinical Practice,
https://doi.org/10.1007/978-3-030-98709-1_2

both ways before crossing the street or study for their gross anatomy final in medical school. Anxiety is not just normal but is a vital part of human evolution. Therefore, complaints from patients of anxiety are very common across all medical disciplines. When patients complain of anxiety, that is just the beginning of the medical differential. The person may have an anxiety disorder, anxiety secondary to environmental stressors, anxiety as a symptom of a different psychiatric condition, or anxiety as a sequela of a medical condition. Therefore, in this chapter, I will refer to any complaints of anxiety that are clinically notable as excessive anxiety regardless of the etiology. In other words, excessive anxiety is a symptom rather than a diagnosis in and of itself.

Anxiety can be considered to have two components: a mental (worry) aspect and a physical aspect. Generalized anxiety disorder can be considered to be the disorder of the worry aspect and panic disorder the dysfunction or disorder of the physical aspect of anxiety.

Despite the fact that it is such a common part of the human experience, anxiety can nonetheless be difficult for people to describe accurately or put into words. Therefore, patients' chief complaints are not straightforward in such a way that makes excessive anxiety easy to recognize. Anxiety can be defined as either a psychological or physiological state—or most commonly both—which is characterized by somatic, emotional, cognitive, and behavioral complaints. In other words, anxiety is experienced by both the mind and by the body and is expressed in a wide variety of ways in different individuals. Typically, anxiety is experienced by the mind as worry, fear, or a sense of doom or apprehension. Because these feelings of worry and doom can be dysphoric, people will often complain of "depression" or depressed mood. Anxiety is experienced somatically in numerous ways including arousal of the sympathetic nervous system: palpitations, shortness of breath, dry mouth, sweating, globus, dizziness, and gastrointestinal symptoms such as nausea and abdominal distress. Panic attacks can occur if anxiety is significant, and a panic attack in and of itself can be a normal phenomenon and not necessarily a sign of an underlying anxiety disorder.

One of the most common chief complaints of someone suffering from excessive anxiety is "depression," due to the fact that excessive anxiety can be very dysphoric. Therefore, when patient present with a chief complaint of "depression," careful screening to rule out excessive anxiety is imperative as the treatments can involve very different pharmacology.

Excessive anxiety can arise from different causes including the following:

1. Appropriate anxiety secondary to situational stressors (e.g., medical illness, marital or family stress, death of a loved one, test anxiety, etc.)
2. Anxiety stemming from an anxiety disorder, especially generalized anxiety disorder and panic disorder.
3. Anxiety as a result of symptoms of other psychiatric disorders (e.g., anxiety secondary to OCD, anxiety in someone with psychosis with delusions that they are going to be assassinated).
4. Anxiety as a primary symptom of an underlying medical condition (e.g., thyroid disorders, pheochromocytoma, etc.)

2.1.1 Panic Disorder

Panic disorder (PD) is characterized by recurrent and unexpected panic attacks, which are characterized by an abrupt surge in of intense fear that reaches a peak within minutes accompanied by physical symptoms such as palpitations or GI distress [10]. It affects 2.7% of individuals during any 12 month period and has a lifetime prevalence of 4.7% [11]. It is more common in women than men, and the typical age of onset is late adolescent or early adulthood [21] while a smaller number of people can have initial onset of panic disorder after the age of 45 [6]. The onset of panic disorder can therefore be considered to be bimodal with one peak of onset around age 20 and a smaller one at age 50. If left untreated, PD is often chronic with a waxing and waning course and only a minority of patients achieving complete remission [21]. The presence of comorbid agoraphobia, major depressive disorder, or personality disorders is a negative prognostic indicator [20]. With appropriate, evidence-based treatment, about one third of patients can achieve complete remission of symptoms while approximately 50% of patients will still have some subclinical level of symptoms [4]. Appropriate evidence-based care can potentially improve outcomes in these patients and reduce their overutilization of healthcare resources, a common issue in the medical setting.

Panic attacks are not by themselves indicative of a psychiatric disorder. As anxiety is a normal emotion, this extreme manifestation of anxiety may be either normal or pathological.

2.1.2 Generalized Anxiety Disorder

Generalized anxiety disorder (GAD) is a common disorder characterized by symptoms of chronic and persistent worry. It affects about 2% of the population, and its age of onset is 20–29, with a 2:1 ratio of females to males. People with GAD tend to report that they have always been anxious or will say that they are described as a "worrier" by family and friends. The symptoms tend to be chronic and will wax and wane over the course of their lives [6]. These patients tend to be high utilizers of the healthcare system and are much more likely to see primary care physicians or specialists than other patients [9].

2.1.3 Social Anxiety Disorder

Social anxiety disorder (SAD) is another common anxiety disorder that is characterized by a fear of being scrutinized or watched in public settings. It is much more severe than typical shyness and is a very common condition that affects as much as 10% of the population [18]. It affects more women than men and is the most common of the anxiety disorders [22]. The majority of patients have onset of symptoms in the pre-teen or early teen years, the course tends to be chronic, and it affects females more than males [22].

2.1.4 Specific Phobia

Phobias are a common condition and can affect up to 10% of the population. There is a bimodal peak for age of onset of specific phobias [23]. DSM 5 recognizes four different categories of specific phobias. Phobias involving *animals*, *natural environment*, or *blood-injection-injury* tend to have a childhood onset, whereas *situational* phobias are more likely to develop during early adulthood [23]. Phobias may result from specific occurrences such as being attacked by an animal; however, many people with phobias are unable to remember any traumatic antecedent.

> Blood-injection-injury phobia is the only instance in which anxiety can lead to fainting or loss of consciousness.

2.2 Anxiety in the Medical Setting

The vast majority of patients with excessive anxiety will initially be seen by a primary care physician or non-psychiatric specialist prior to seeing either a psychiatrist or psychotherapist. As people with excessive anxiety are noted to have increased healthcare usage across all medical settings [9], it is vital that all physicians are familiar with the myriad ways that anxiety presents. Due to the fact that symptoms of excessive anxiety can present with chief complaints matching virtually any other psychiatric or medical illness, we call anxiety the great imitator. As seen in Case Example 2.1, people suffering from excessive anxiety rarely present with anxiety as a chief complaint; depression is a common complaint due to the dysphoric effect that anxiety has on mood. Other psychiatric complaints are possible as well, including:

- "Racing thoughts"
- Insomnia or hypersomnia
- Increased energy or anergia
- "Paranoia"
- Panic attacks
- Hopelessness or helplessness
- Poor concentration
- "Mania" or "bipolar"
- Thoughts about death or dying

Symptoms of excessive anxiety can also present not as mental health-related complaints but as physical complaints as well. While anxiety can mimic virtually any physical complaint, some of the more common ones seen in the medical setting include:

- Chest pain.
- Shortness of breath.
- GI distress.
- Dizziness, vertigo, or light-headedness.
- Vague somatic complaints.
- Hair loss or skin, gum, or lip lesions (from increased body-focused repetitive behaviors, discussed in Chap. 6).

Numerous medical conditions will present with symptoms of excessive anxiety, or with physical symptoms that can be confused with excessive anxiety. Some of the more notable ones include the following:

- Endocrine disorders: for example, hyperthyroidism, pheochromocytoma, hypoglycemia.
- Cardiac: for example, angina, arrhythmia.
- Pulmonary: for example, COPD, asthma, weaning from respirators.
- Neurological: for example, migraines, vestibular dysfunction, balance disorders, stroke.
- Metabolic: for example, porphyria.
- Gastrointestinal: for example, irritable bowel syndrome, inflammatory bowel disease.
- Medication induced: for example.
  - Anesthetics and analgesics.
  - Anticholinergics.
  - Anticonvulsants.
  - Antidepressants (especially in the context of akathisia).
  - Antiemetics (especially in the context of akathisia): metoclopramide, promethazine, and prochlorperazine.

Table 2.1 Common causes of substance induced anxiety

Substances capable of producing anxiety with use or intoxication	Substances capable of producing anxiety upon withdrawal
Alcohol	Alcohol
Caffeine	
	Opioids
Cannabis, THC, CBD	
	Barbiturates
Benzodiazepines (paradoxical)	Benzodiazepines
Non-benzodiazepine hypnotics (e.g., zolpidem)	Non-benzodiazepine hypnotics (e.g., zolpidem)
LSD and other hallucinogens	
Stimulants/amphetamines/cocaine	Stimulants/amphetamines/cocaine
Inhalants	

- Other antipsychotics (especially in the context of akathisia).
- Antihypertensives, including beta blockers and ACE inhibitors.
- Antiparkinsonian medications (particularly compounds containing levodopa).
- Asthma medications, especially albuterol and theophylline.
- Benzodiazepines (seen as both a paradoxical reaction and as a symptoms of withdrawal).
- Corticosteroids.
- Lithium.
- Nasal decongestants, including phenylephrine and pseudoephedrine.
- Sympathomimetics and stimulants, including amphetamines and methylphenidate.
- Thyroid medication.

Substances of abuse can present with anxiety symptoms either due to normal use/intoxication or from withdrawal symptoms. See Table 2.1.

Anxiety is also known to worsen outcomes in numerous medical conditions including epilepsy, pain, fibromyalgia, non-cardiac chest pain, diabetes, irritable bowel syndrome, GERD, coronary heart disease, and asthma [13].

2.3 Diagnosis and Presentation of Anxiety Disorders and Excessive Anxiety from Environmental Factors

An accurate diagnosis is absolutely critical in the treatment of excessive anxiety. For example, the treatment of generalized anxiety disorder versus anxiety with panic attacks secondary to job loss or financial stressors is markedly different. A successful outcome is not likely if the proper diagnosis is not made.

The key to the recognition and proper diagnosis of anxiety disorders is to be mindful of the appropriate differential diagnosis. As noted above, anxiety should be a consideration with many of the common mental health complaints that a patient may present with. Anxiety can be the underlying cause of many physical chief complaints as well, and complaints of anxiety can also mask underlying medical conditions. Certainly, any patient who either complains of excessive anxiety or whom an anxiety disorder is suspected deserves an appropriate medical screening and workup. At a minimum, this would typically include:

- History and physical exam.
- Complete blood count with differential.
- Basic metabolic profile/complete metabolic profile as indicated.
- TSH or thyroid panel.
- EKG.
- Other tests if medically indicated.

People with an anxiety disorder may or may not report a precipitating event at the onset of illness. In contrast, patients with excessive anxiety secondary to a social stress (i.e., death of a loved one, financial difficulties) are usually able to give history of a clear antecedent, making the distinction between secondary anxiety and an anxiety disorder more readily apparent (especially if they report appropriate levels of anxiety prior to the event). The presence of acute anxiety secondary to situational stressors can also be formally diagnosed as adjustment disorder using DSM terminology.

2.3.1 Generalized Anxiety Disorder

The diagnosis of generalized anxiety disorder is dependent on a presentation of pervasive anxiety and worry (defined as apprehensive expectation—sometimes described as "doom" or "impending doom") about a number of events or activities. The worry is out of proportion to the actual likelihood of the anticipated event and the individual finds it difficult to control the worry. It must occur for more days than not for at least a 6-month period (DSM 5). Please see Table 2.2 for diagnostic criteria. The worry an individual with GAD has typically focuses on numerous activities, often on whatever is currently going on with them at that time. Often the worry takes the form of catastrophizing, in which the person imagines events in a worst-case scenario.

> Note that many of the associated physical symptoms of GAD are similar to physical symptoms seen in major depressive disorder. Ensuring a proper diagnosis is critical as the two disorders use different pharmacological treatment protocols.

Table 2.2 DSM 5 diagnostic criteria for generalized anxiety disorder

A. Excessive anxiety and worry (apprehensive expectation) occurring more days than not for at least 6 months about a number of events or activities such as work or school performance.
B. The individual finds it difficult to control the worry.
C. The anxiety and worry are associated with three or more physical symptoms, including: 1. Restlessness or feeling keyed up or on edge. 2. Being easily fatigued. 3. Difficulty concentrating or mind going blank. 4. Irritability. 5. Muscle tension. 6. Sleep disturbance (difficulty falling or staying asleep, or restless unsatisfying sleep).
D. The anxiety, worry, or physical symptoms cause clinically significant distress or impairment in social, occupational, or other important areas of functioning.
E. The disturbance is not attributable to the physiological effects of a substance (e.g., a substance of abuse or a medication) or another medical condition (e.g., hyperthyroidism).
F. The disturbance is not better explained by another mental disorder.

2.3.2 *Panic Disorder*

Panic disorder is defined as recurrent unexpected panic attacks which are characterized by an abrupt surge of intense fear or intense discomfort that reaches a peak within minutes. This is accompanied by physical symptoms such as palpitations, dizziness, or GI distress. Panic attacks can be normal and non-pathological; however, patients with panic disorder will have persistent worry about further attacks or maladaptive changes due to the attacks. Panic attacks can occur from a calm state, or from an anxious state. Panic attacks often will awaken someone from sleep in panic disorder. People with panic attacks, and especially those with panic disorder, will often present to emergency rooms to rule out myocardial infarction. Many cardiologists report that they see more panic attacks in the emergency setting than they do actual heart attacks. See Table 2.3 for the diagnostic criteria for panic disorder.

The symptoms of panic attacks can mimic those of many other medical disorders. However, there are some clues to look for that can make the diagnosis of a panic attack more likely. For example, symptoms that appear unrelated to the primary medical condition being ruled out (e.g., the presence of paresthesias in someone complaining of chest pain or palpitations). Other symptoms only occur in medical conditions and not in anxiety/panic. For example, suspect a cardiac arrhythmia in someone with tachycardia with abrupt offset.

> The symptom of feeling that one is suffocating or needing to consciously to remember to breathe as one is falling asleep is pathognomonic for anxiety.

Table 2.3 DSM 5 diagnostic criteria for panic disorder

A.	Recurrent and unexpected panic attacks. A panic attack is an abrupt surge of intense fear or intense discomfort that reaches a peak within minutes and during which four (or more) of the following symptoms occur: 1. Palpitations, pounding heart, or accelerated heart rate. 2. Sweating. 3. Trembling or shaking. 4. Sensations of shortness of breath or smothering. 5. Feelings of choking. 6. Chest pain or discomfort. 7. Nausea or abdominal distress. 8. Feeling dizzy, unsteady, light-headed, or faint. 9. Chills or heat sensation. 10. Paresthesias (numbness or tingling sensations). 11. Derealization (feelings of unreality) or depersonalization (being detached from oneself). 12. Fear of losing control or going crazy. 13. Fear of dying.
B.	At least one of the attacks has been followed by 1 month or more of one or both of the following: 1. Persistent worry about additional panic attacks or their consequences. 2. A significant maladaptive change in behavior related to the attacks (such as avoidance behaviors).
C.	The disturbance is not attributable to the physiological effects of a substance (e.g., a drug of abuse) or another medical condition (e.g., hyperthyroidism or cardiopulmonary disorders).
D.	The disturbance is not better explained by another mental disorder.

2.3.3 Social Anxiety Disorder

Social anxiety disorder (SAD) is characterized by excessive fear of embarrassment, humiliation, or rejection when exposed to possible negative evaluation by others when engaged in a public performance or social interactions [18]. The individual is concerned that they will be judged in some way when out in public or that they will act in some way that is socially unacceptable (e.g., stumbling over words, sweating, trembling, or appearing stupid or boring). The disorder can be confused with psychotic disorders on initial exposure due to the fact that patients will report that they are "paranoid" when out in public and fear that people are watching them. Patients often do not report symptoms as they simply believe that they are shy and do not realize that they have a treatable, medical condition [22]. DSM 5 criteria for social anxiety disorder contain a qualifier for "performance only" subtype for people whose fear is limited to public speaking. This subtype acts more like a specific phobia and carries less disability than the generalized disorder. As with other specific phobias, the fear or anxiety out of proportion to the real danger is posed by the specific object or situation [23].

Propranolol is often prescribed for people with fear of public speaking. As the drug has little anxiolytic effect and is primarily used to treat cosmetic manifestations of anxiety (e.g., tremulous voice), it is not recommended for this purpose. Cognitive Behavior Therapy is far more effective for fear of public speaking as well as other specific phobias.

2.3.4 Treatment

The treatment of anxiety and anxiety disorders typically involves psychotherapy with or without the use of medication. Many patients with anxiety disorders, particularly panic disorder, do not wish to take medications at all (often due to an outsized fear of side effects) and opt instead for psychotherapy [25]. The use of psychotherapy alone as first-line treatment for panic disorder is appropriate as it may be better than pharmacotherapy alone. In fact, therapy alone may be equal to combined treatment of medications plus therapy [7]. However, a combined approach (i.e., medications and psychotherapy) is commonly used for panic disorder and is clinically appropriate in many instances. A combined approach is preferable for generalized anxiety disorder and social anxiety disorder. For specific phobias, psychotherapy alone is indicated, although the judicious use of benzodiazepines may be warranted under certain circumstances (e.g., someone with a flying phobia who needs to board an airplane for a work-related trip may be given a few benzodiazepine pills).

Therapy for anxiety disorders typically involves cognitive behavioral therapy (CBT). CBT is a family of therapies that work on changing maladaptive patterns of behavior and cognition that contribute to the disorders. Talk-based therapies that try to determine "underlying causes" of the anxiety disorder have minimal efficacy and are generally not recommended. CBT usually involves specific cognitive and behavioral exercises performed in the office with the therapist and also given as homework in-between sessions. Therapy for anxiety disorders can be done in a protocolized format, and there are good workbooks available that therapists and patients can use in order to progress through treatment. Figure 2.1 presents an algorithm that can be used in the primary care setting when patients complain of excessive anxiety.

Referring a patient with excessive anxiety to therapy is a first-line treatment that can be done with or without pharmacotherapy. However, ensure that the therapist practices CBT and is familiar with treating anxiety.

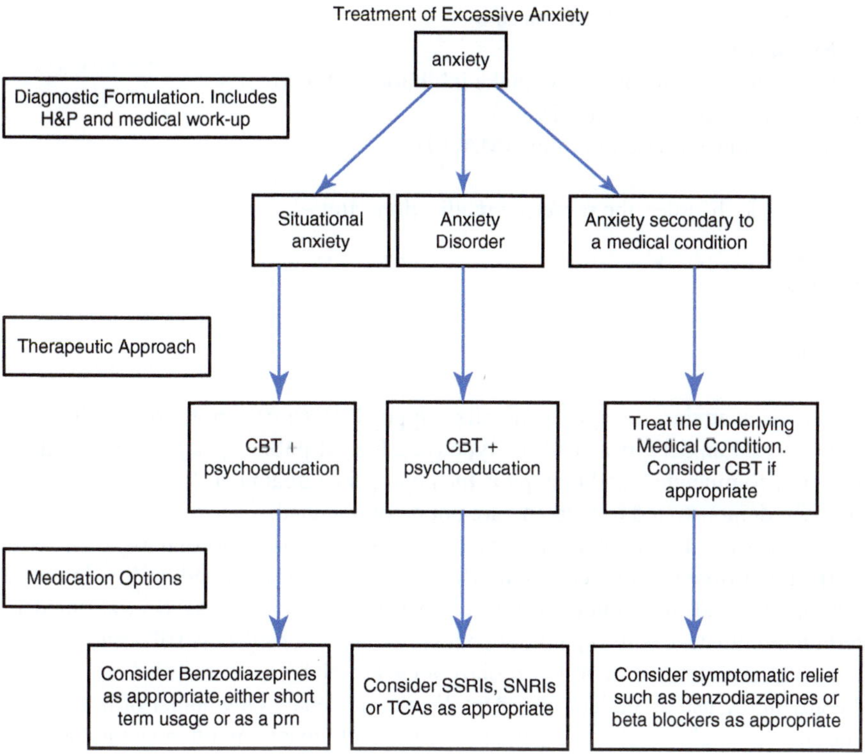

Fig. 2.1 Approach to complaints of anxiety in the primary care setting

2.4 Treatment

2.4.1 Pharmacotherapy

As a general rule of thumb, the first-line medication treatment for *anxiety disorders* are SSRIs. The first-line medication treatment for *situational anxiety* is benzodiazepines.

Proper medication treatment of excessive anxiety is reliant on the accuracy of the diagnosis, as the treatment for anxiety disorders is wholly distinct from medication use for anxiety secondary to psychosocial stressors. People with anxiety disorders should be offered antidepressant medications with SSRIs considered first line. Other classes of medications have been shown to work and can be considered when the patient is nonresponsive to or intolerant of SSRIs. Specifically, the recommended drug classes for generalized anxiety disorder include:

1. SSRIs (can be considered first line).
2. Buspirone.
3. Serotonin norepinephrine reuptake inhibitors (SNRIs).
4. Tricyclic antidepressants (TCAs).
5. Monoamine oxidase inhibitors (MAO-I).

For panic disorder, the preferred medications are:

1. SSRI.
2. SNRI.
3. TCA.
4. MAO-I.

For social anxiety disorder, generalized type, SSRIs are the preferred medication.

For social anxiety, performance type (i.e., fear of public speaking) medications are not recommended, and therapy is the appropriate treatment. Beta blockers have not been demonstrated to help and are not recommended.

By contrast, the pharmacotherapy for excessive anxiety secondary to stress is markedly different. Antidepressant (SSRI) therapy has limited utility in those patients. Instead, the judicious use of prn benzodiazepines may be warranted in certain circumstances for symptom control. While this subject is still controversial and without definitive data, benzodiazepines are NOT recommended as first-line therapy in the use of anxiety disorders. While the debate on whether or not benzodiazepines should be given to patients with anxiety disorders often centers around their potentially addictive qualities, that discussion is somewhat of a red herring. Since there is evidence that benzodiazepines have limited efficacy for anxiety disorders and potentially can interfere with treatment [12, 17, 27], they may worsen outcomes in patients. The authors themselves find that benzodiazepines are rarely needed in their anxiety disorders practice, especially in the presence of appropriate CBT. The treatment of excessive anxiety in patients with anxiety secondary to medical syndromes is generally symptomatic. Beta blockers may be useful in treating excessive anxiety in certain of these patients (e.g., pheochromocytoma).

In Case Example 2.1, the patient is suffering from situational anxiety secondary to a job loss. Her dysfunction is significant enough that a diagnosis of adjustment disorder would be appropriate. Adjustment disorder is defined as emotional or behavioral symptoms in response to an identifiable stressor that occurs within 3 months of the onset of the stressor. She was seen by a third year resident in the Family Medicine program, who initially considered an SSRI but quickly realized that a therapy referral was the treatment of choice. Short-term symptomatic treatment of her insomnia and restlessness/anxiety is indicated as well; a short-term prescription for benzodiazepines is appropriate in this instance. Simply relieving the insomnia may cause a marked short-term improvement. Of note, she has symptoms of major depressive disorder (MDD) but does not qualify for that diagnosis due to only a 1-week time course. Continued monitoring to ensure that patient does not develop MDD is warranted.

Case Example 2.2
Mr. B is a 48-year-old male referred to your office as his previous PCP has retired. He states that he has a marked fear of medical procedures, especially ones that involve injections. Going to the dentist is particularly difficult. He was in cognitive behavioral therapy for this many years ago which improved his fears to the point that he no longer skips routine medical care. He goes to the dentist routinely, gets blood draws when necessary, and accompanied his wife into the hospital when she had gall bladder surgery. However, he has taken 1 mg lorazepam prior to the situations which he is exposed to a needle or dental drill, either used on himself or his wife. You diagnose him with specific phobia, blood-injection-injury subtype. As his current level of symptoms is not causing dysfunction, you both agree to continue prescribing lorazepam prior to triggering situations. If, in the future, lorazepam stops working or he is avoiding triggering situations, he will be referred to a CBT therapist.

In Case Example 2.2, the patient has phobias that were significant enough to prevent him from seeking appropriate medical care. However, with the use of a benzodiazepine as pre-treatment, he is able to schedule medical visits appropriately. Continued use is appropriate; however, if patient desires therapy so as not to have to rely on medications, a referral is very appropriate. Usually, shorter to intermediate half-life benzodiazepines are appropriate in these patients. See Table 2.4 for a list of recommended medications and dosages:

2.4.1.1 SSRI Treatment for Anxiety Disorders

The treatment of anxiety disorders can be accomplished with a variety of groups of medications (see above); however, SSRIs are recommended as first-line treatment due to their proven efficacy. In addition, since there is a clinical relationship between GAD and OCD with some similar phenomenology, SSRIs should be used at the occasional dose for 12–16 weeks before being considered a treatment failure (same as OCD protocol). The choice of SSRI is up to the physician and patient and is usually based on side effect profile, drug interactions, family history (an SSRI that has worked for a family member is more likely to be efficacious), or simply personal preference. It is not unusual in treating anxiety disorders that SSRI dosing needs to be increased above

Table 2.4 Commonly used benzodiazepines for short-term situational anxiety and associated symptom management

Benzodiazepine	Half-life	Relative potency	Usual initial dose (mg)	Adult dosage range (mg/day)
Alprazolam	12–15	0.5	0.25	0.25–4
Diazepam	20–80	5	2–5	2–40
Lorazepam	10–20	1	0.5	0.5–4
Oxazepam	5–20	15–30	15	15–120
Clonazepam	18–50	0.25–0.5	0.5	0.5–8

Table 2.5 Medications for anxiety disorders

Anti-anxiety	Starting and titration dose (mg/day)[a]	Maximum dose (mg/day)	Occasional dose (mg/day)
SSRI[b]			
Fluoxetine	20	40	80
Sertraline	50	100–200	400
Paroxetine	20	20–40	80
Fluvoxamine	50	100–200	400
Citalopram	20††	20–40[d]	40[d]
Escitalopram	5–10	10–20	40
SNRI			
Venlafaxine	37.5	150	225
Duloxetine	20–30	60	20
Atypical			
Buspirone[c]	7.5 bid	30 bid	30 bid

[a] Medications may be started at this dose and titrated by the same amount until maximum dose is reached. In elderly or sensitive patients, considering using half this dose, but the maximum dose remains the same

[b] It is recommended that patients should be offered SSRIs as a first line, and the occasional dose be used for 12–16 weeks prior to considering a medication trial to be a failure

[c] For generalized anxiety disorder only. For panic disorder, social anxiety, please use SSRIs. For situational anxiety, consider therapy or short-term benzodiazepine

[d] Doses higher than 40 mg cannot be used due to issues with QTc prolongation

[††] Medication generally not recommended as effective dose may be above the dose that can be safely prescribed

what is used for major depressive disorder, and often OCD dosing (e.g., higher than normally used for Major Depression) is required (see Table 2.5 for list of medications and dosing). Patients are typically seen every 2–4 weeks while the dose is being titrated until the patient has achieved a therapeutic response. For patients with generalized anxiety disorder or panic disorder, the use of an SNRI may be appropriate if they have failed at least two SSRIs. For GAD, the use of buspirone is also appropriate and may be a preferred medication due to its relative lack of side effects.

Buspirone is approved for use in GAD and may be a preferred option due to its relative lack of side effects. Because it is approved for GAD, many textbooks compare it to benzodiazepines and call it an anxiolytic. However, buspirone is more properly thought of as an atypical antidepressant and should be used as such: prescribed with daily dosing and allowing 4–8 weeks or more to achieve a clinical effect. PRN dosing similar to benzodiazepines does not work and is cautioned against.

2.4.1.2 SSRI and SNRI Side Effects

Typical side effects of SSRIs/SNRIs include excessive yawning, headache, GI distress (nausea, dyspepsia, constipation, diarrhea), vivid dreams or nightmares, and tremors [1]. These side effects often are transient and are usually managed conservatively, using over-the-counter analgesics for headache, stool softeners for constipation, and H2 blockers for dyspepsia. Starting at a lower dose and maintaining that dose for a few weeks prior to titration are often sufficient for symptom management.

- *Sexual side effects* are among the most troubling side effects that can occur with chronic, ongoing use of SSRI therapy and are reported in approximately a third of patients on SSRI therapy [5]. The most common reported problems are loss of libido, delayed orgasm or anorgasmia, erectile dysfunction (males), and lack of lubrication (females). Often, a careful history will determine that the complaints of erectile dysfunction or lack of lubrication are not primary issues per se but are the result of severe anorgasmia. There are numerous strategies that can be used in patients suffering from sexual side effects and a careful history regarding the nature of the actual side effects, their usual sexual habits, and their partner's (if there is one) knowledge of the situation. It should be noted that many patients state that the sexual side effects can remit over time, often taking many months or more; as a result, further intervention other than patience may not always be necessary. The addition of bupropion at a dose of 300 mg daily has been shown to reduce sexual side effects from SSRIs [1]. Buspirone can be used safely at doses between 20 and 60 mg daily and can help reverse sexual side effects [19]. If the patient does not wish to take a medication chronically in order to reverse sexual side effects, the use of cyproheptadine 4 mg orally 1–2 hours prior to sexual activity can reduce sexual side effects [24]. We recommend this be used no more than 3 times per week. Another method that can be used is the drug holiday method. We recommend that the patient's medication be stopped the day before planned sexual activity. On the day that sexual activity occurs, the person can delay their dose until afterward. The medication can then be resumed on a normal basis the following day; this results in only one total missed dose. Patients should not do this more than one time per week in order to minimize missed dosages. The drug holiday method is not recommended with fluoxetine (due to its long half-life) and caution should be used with paroxetine and venlafaxine due to their potent discontinuation syndrome (see below).
- *Movement disorders such as myoclonus* are defined as sudden, abrupt, shock-like involuntary movements caused by muscle contractions. Nocturnal jaw clenching may also occur. Usually, lowering the dose or switching meds can help, but these side effects may spontaneously remit as well [28].
- A *frontal lobe amotivational syndrome* can occur, characterized by apathy, affective blunting, and memory issues. Complaints of sedation may accompany this. (Note: excessive yawning is also a side effect of SSRIs and is not associated with fatigue.) This side effect may be more common in patients with comorbid Anxiety and OCD as it may occur at higher doses and may not improve with time as opposed to some other SSRI side effects [15]. The most common strategies to manage this include lowering the dose or switching agents. In our practice, we have had success using modafinil at usual therapeutic doses to counteract this side effect.

- Any of the SSRIs or SNRIs may lead to *weight gain*. This side effect may be associated with long-term use. Management of this side effect is usually conservative, with recommendations given around lifestyle changes such as appropriate diet and exercise.
- *Excessive sweating* is a common complaint. Conservative management works in most cases, which simply involves recommending the patient have a change of bed clothes available to change into in the middle of the night. While there is little data on pharmacological management of this side effects, benztropine at 0.5 mg nightly can be tried [1].
- *Hyponatremia* is a rare (0.5% per year incidence) problem that can occur with SSRIs or SNRIs; elderly, female, and patients using concomitant diuretics are in the highest risk category. This typically occurs within a few weeks of medication initiation or dose increase [14]. Symptoms typically include muscle cramps, fatigue, delirium, and seizures.
- *SSRI discontinuation syndrome* can occur with the abrupt discontinuation of many antidepressants, including the SSRIs (with the possible exception of fluoxetine due to its extended half-life) and the SNRIs, especially venlafaxine. While it does not demand medical intervention, the symptoms can be quite distressing and even disabling; dizziness, light-headedness, insomnia, fatigue, anxiety, headache, nausea, and sensory disturbances described as electric sensations in the head or limbs (colloquially known as "brain zaps") are reported most commonly [29]. While symptoms are acute, resolution can be achieved rapidly by reinstating the full dose of the medication. Very slow and extended tapers can ameliorate this problem in most patients. In the case of someone on a maximum dose of an SSRI, the taper period may last 6 months or longer to reduce the risk of discontinuation syndrome. This also has the side benefit of decreasing the risk of relapse, as slower tapers of medications can reduce the possibility of illness exacerbation after medications are stopped.
- *Serotonin syndrome* is a rare but serious medical condition that includes symptoms such as mental status changes, gastrointestinal symptoms, autonomic instability (tachycardia, hypertension, and hyperthermia), and neuromuscular abnormalities including myoclonus, hyperreflexia, hypertonicity, and rigidity; clinically, it presents very much like neuroleptic malignant syndrome [2, 3]. It has been most commonly associated with combinations of serotonergic agents but has been reported to occur with single agents. Treatment is usually supportive and includes discontinuation of the serotonergic agent; the addition of the 5-HT 2a antagonist cyproheptadine may also be of benefit [3].
- *Gastrointestinal bleeding* is a potential side effect of SSRI or SNRI use and may be exacerbated with the concomitant use of non-steroidal anti-inflammatory agents [14]. The use of medications to reduce the risk of GI bleeding may be warranted in high-risk patients.

2.4.1.3 Drug Interactions

Drug-drug interactions are also important considerations when choosing specific antidepressant pharmacotherapy. The action of the medication on the cytochrome P450 system is the most relevant piece of information when evaluating drug interactions with SSRIs or SNRIs, as many of the medications are potent inhibitors of various isoenzymes. Fluvoxamine is a significant inhibitor of the CYP1A2 isoenzyme, while paroxetine and fluoxetine are inhibitors of the CYP 2D6 isoenzyme. Sertraline, citalopram, and escitalopram are not potent inhibitors of the CYP450 enzyme system and may be considered preferred SSRIs in patients on multiple medications where drug-drug interactions are a concern [8]. Venlafaxine also has low or minimal impact on all of the p450 isoenzymes. See Table 2.6. Medications that are metabolized through the CYP450 system may have plasma levels increased if that specific isoenzyme is inhibited by an SSRI (or other CYP inhibitor). A list of common medications that are metabolized by specific isoenzymes are listed in Table 2.7. This is not meant to be a comprehensive list but to provide a guide to clinicians; consulting appropriate references on specific medications when prescribing is recommended when looking at potential drug-drug interactions. Other common isoenzyme inhibitors that can influence the plasma levels of OCD medications, as well as other medications, are listed in Table 2.8. Please see Table 1.13 in Chap. 1 which contains a comprehensive list of CYP inhibitors and inducers in order to facilitate better recognitions of potential drug-drug interactions.

Table 2.6 CYP450 inhibitory potential of SSRIs

CYP isoenzyme	Citalopram	Fluoxetine	Fluvoxamine	Paroxetine	Sertraline
CYP1A2	+/−	+	+++	+	+/−
CYP2C19	?	++	+++		+
CYP2D6	+	+++	+	+++	+
CYP3A4	?	++	++	+/−	+/−

Table adapted from [16]

Key: +/− unlikely;? unknown; + mild; ++ moderate; +++ substantial

Note: Venlafaxine has minimal inhibitory effects on the P450 isoenzymes

Table 2.7 Important substrates of CYP isoenzymes

1A2	2C19	2D6	3A4
Caffeine, theophylline, clozapine, clomipramine	Proton pump inhibitors, diazepam,	Many tricyclic antidepressants (TCAs), beta blockers, antiarrhythmic agents, atomoxetine, risperidone, risperidone, codeine, hydrocodone, oxycodone, dextromethorphan	Calcium channel blockers, erythromycin, alprazolam, midazolam, triazolam, statins (HMG-CoA reductase inhibitors), HIV protease inhibitors, ziprasidone

Table adapted from The Medical Letter on Drugs and Therapeutics [26]

Table 2.8 Other CYP isoenzyme inhibitors

1A2	2D6	3A4
Ciprofloxacin, cimetidine	Cimetidine	Erythromycin, amiodarone, grapefruit

Table adapted from The Medical Letter on Drugs and Therapeutics [26]

2.5 When to Refer

When a primary care physician decides to refer a patient out for specialty care is always dependent upon the training and the comfort level of the practitioner, much will depend on the resources available in the community. Because the first line of treatment for excessive anxiety secondary to any mental or psychiatric cause is CBT, referral to a therapist well versed in CBT for anxiety is always an appropriate first-line intervention. While the timing of when a referral to a psychiatrist occurs is up to the comfort level of the primary care physician in most respects, certain general rules apply.

In general, referral to mental health specialists should occur:

- When the patient requests specialized behavioral therapy for anxiety
- Failure of one or two SSRIs at maximum dose for 12–16 weeks
- Diagnostic uncertainty: if the clinician is having trouble making an accurate diagnosis and therefore unable to determine what the proper pharmacotherapy is.
- Patient becomes a high utilizer of primary care office or resources
- The PCP's own comfort level and experience

References

1. Borue X, Sharma M, Hudak R. Biological treatments for obsessive-compulsive and related disorders. J Obs Compuls Relat Disord. 2015;6:7–26.
2. Boyer EW, Shannon M. The serotonin syndrome. N Engl J Med. 2005;352(11):1112–20. https://doi.org/10.1056/NEJMra041867. Erratum in: N Engl J Med. 2007 Jun 7;356(23):2437. Erratum in: N Engl J Med. 2009 Oct 22;361(17):1714.
3. Caroff SN, Watson CB, Rosenberg H. Drug-induced hyperthermic syndromes in psychiatry. Clin Psychopharmacol Neurosci. 2021;19(1):1–11. https://doi.org/10.9758/cpn.2021.19.1.1. PMID: 33508784; PMCID: PMC7851465.
4. Chen MH, Tsai SJ. Treatment-resistant panic disorder: clinical significance, concept and management. Prog Neuro-Psychopharmacol Biol Psychiatry. 2016;70:219–26. https://doi.org/10.1016/j.pnpbp.2016.02.001. Epub 2016 Feb 3.
5. Clayton AH, Pradko JF, Croft HA, Montano CB, Leadbetter RA, Bolden-Watson C, Bass KI, Donahue RM, Jamerson BD, Metz A. Prevalence of sexual dysfunction among newer antidepressants. J Clin Psychiatry. 2002;63(4):357–66. https://doi.org/10.4088/jcp.v63n0414.
6. Diagnostic and Statistical Manuel of Mental Disorders Fifth Edition. American Psychiatric Association. 2013.
7. Furukawa TA, Watanabe N, Churchill R. Psychotherapy plus antidepressant for panic disorder with or without agoraphobia: systematic review. Br J Psychiatry. 2006;188:305–12. https://doi.org/10.1192/bjp.188.4.305.
8. Hemeryck A, Belpaire FM. Selective serotonin reuptake inhibitors and cytochrome P-450 mediated drug-drug interactions: an update. Curr Drug Metab. 2002;3(1):13–37. https://doi.org/10.2174/1389200023338017.

9. Horenstein A, Heimberg RG. Anxiety disorders and healthcare utilization: a systematic review. Clin Psychol Rev. 2020;81:101894. https://doi.org/10.1016/j.cpr.2020.101894. Epub 2020 Aug 6.
10. Hudak R, Jacob RG. Anxiety in the general medical setting. In: Ackerman KD, Dimartini AF, editors. Psychosomatic medicine. USA: Oxford University Press; 2015. p. 57–73.
11. Kessler RC, Chiu WT, Demler O, Merikangas KR, Walters EE. Prevalence, severity, and comorbidity of 12-month DSM-IV disorders in the National Comorbidity Survey Replication. Arch Gen Psychiatry. 2005;62(6):617–27. https://doi.org/10.1001/archpsyc.62.6.617. Erratum in: Arch Gen Psychiatry. 2005 Jul;62(7):709. Merikangas, Kathleen R [added]. PMID: 15939839; PMCID: PMC2847357.
12. Lader M. Benzodiazepine harm: how can it be reduced? Br J Clin Pharmacol. 2014;77(2):295–301. https://doi.org/10.1111/j.1365-2125.2012.04418.x. PMID: 22882333; PMCID: PMC4014015.
13. Meuret AE, Tunnell N, Roque A. Anxiety disorders and medical comorbidity: treatment implications. In: Kim YK, editor. Anxiety disorders. Advances in experimental medicine and biology, vol. 1191. Singapore: Springer; 2020. https://doi.org/10.1007/978-981-32-9705-0_15.
14. Moret C, Isaac M, Briley M. Problems associated with long-term treatment with selective serotonin reuptake inhibitors. J Psychopharmacol. 2009;23(8):967–74. https://doi.org/10.1177/0269881108093582. Epub 2008 Jul 17.
15. Murphy TK, Segarra A, Storch EA, Goodman WK. SSRI adverse events: how to monitor and manage. Int Rev Psychiatry. 2008;20(2):203–8. https://doi.org/10.1080/09540260801889211.
16. Page SA, Hudak R. Selective serotonin reuptake inhibitors in the treatment of obsessive-compulsive disorder. In: Hudak R, Dougherty DD, editors. Clinical obsessive compulsive disorders in adults and children. United Kingdom: Cambridge University Press; 2011.
17. Rickels K, Moeller HJ. Benzodiazepines in anxiety disorders: reassessment of usefulness and safety. World J Biol Psychiatry. 2019;20(7):514–8. https://doi.org/10.1080/15622975.2018.1500031. Epub 2018 Sep 25.
18. Rose GM, Tadi P. Social anxiety disorder. In: StatPearls [internet]. Treasure Island (FL): StatPearls Publishing; 2021.
19. Rosen RC, Lane RM, Menza M. Effects of SSRIs on sexual function: a critical review. J Clin Psychopharmacol. 1999;19(1):67–85. https://doi.org/10.1097/00004714-199902000-00013.
20. Roy-Byrne PP, Cowley DS. Course and outcome in panic disorder: a review of recent follow-up studies. Anxiety. 1994–1995;1(4):151–60. https://doi.org/10.1002/anxi.3070010402.
21. Roy-Byrne PP, Craske MG, Stein MB. Panic disorder. Lancet. 2006;368(9540):1023–32. https://doi.org/10.1016/S0140-6736(06)69418-X.
22. Sareen L, Stein M. A review of the epidemiology and approaches to the treatment of social anxiety disorder. Drugs. 2000;59(3):497–509. https://doi.org/10.2165/00003495-200059030-00007.
23. Samra CK, Abdijadid S. Specific Phobia. In: StatPearls [Internet]. Treasure Island (FL): StatPearls Publishing; 2021.
24. Schweitzer I, Maguire K, Ng C. Sexual side-effects of contemporary antidepressants: review. Aust N Z J Psychiatry. 2009;43(9):795–808. https://doi.org/10.1080/00048670903107575.
25. Stein MB, Goin MK, Pollack MH, et al. American Psychiatric Association. Practice guidelines for the treatment of patients with panic disorder. 2nd ed; 2010. https://psychiatryonline.org/guidelines.
26. The Medical Letter on Drugs and Therapeutics, September 21, 2020;62(1607):e152–153.
27. Thibaut F. Anxiety disorders: a review of current literature. Dialogues Clin Neurosci. 2017;19(2):87–8. https://doi.org/10.31887/DCNS.2017.19.2/fthibaut. PMID: 28867933; PMCID: PMC5573565.
28. Vandel P, Bonin B, Leveque E, Sechter D, Bizouard P. Tricyclic antidepressant-induced extrapyramidal side effects. Eur Neuropsychopharmacol. 1997;7(3):207–12. https://doi.org/10.1016/s0924-977x(97)00405-7.
29. Zajecka J, Tracy KA, Mitchell S. Discontinuation symptoms after treatment with serotonin reuptake inhibitors: a literature review. J Clin Psychiatry. 1997;58(7):291–7. https://doi.org/10.4088/jcp.v58n0702.

Chapter 3
Bipolar Disorder

A 35-year-old male, C.D., presents to your office for a first visit. He notes he has a history of "high blood pressure and high cholesterol." He is not currently taking medication as he didn't follow-up much with his last physician and so "ran out of refills." C.D. also reports a long history of depression and a remote history of alcohol use disorder. He notes that he is on disability due to depression. He relates that over the past couple of months, his mood has been "okay," but he doesn't experience much pleasure in life and has trouble staying motivated, including attending doctors' appointments. He explains that he doesn't have a lot of supports in his life as "I have burned a lot of bridges." He also reports chronic, mild issues with memory and attention. On further review, C.D. admits that he has been diagnosed as "bipolar" in the past though he is not sure he agrees with that diagnosis. He further admits that he was hospitalized at least three times in the past over his objection for "misunderstandings." While he appears a little uncomfortable in explaining this history, he does tell you that he was once hospitalized after he bought a car that he couldn't afford and drove to Atlantic City, where he gambled "for several days straight" and didn't sleep. He sadly adds that this episode directly precipitated his divorce. The patient then says, "I don't know, maybe I do get manic, but I think my ex-wife made a bigger deal out of it than she needed to." He does note once taking himself to the hospital as "I was so depressed, I was really, really thinking about killing myself." C.D. clarifies that he has been on "a lot" of medication in the past for bipolar disorder, including lithium, which he noted made him very thirsty and urinate a lot, and risperidone, which made him gain weight.

R. Hudak, J. M. Gannon, *Handbook of Psychiatric Disorders in Adults in the Primary Care Setting*, Current Clinical Practice,
https://doi.org/10.1007/978-3-030-98709-1_3

On exam, the patient is pleasant, casually dressed and makes good eye contact. He speaks softly and somewhat slowly, but in full, spontaneous sentences. He does look a little down but smiles appropriately with pleasantries. His speech tends to be a bit rambling at times, and he apologizes at one point for being longwinded. He denies any thoughts of death or suicidal thoughts. He smokes about a pack per day and is not interested in quitting. He has been sober from alcohol and all illicit substances for over 8 years. Currently, he is not very interested in medication treatment for his mood and is not engaged with a psychiatrist.

3.1 Introduction and Epidemiology

Bipolar disorder was first recognized by Jean-Pierre Falret as "folie circulaire" in the 1850s, though its history likely traces back hundreds if not thousands of years. At the turn of the twentieth century, the disorder was subsumed under the diagnosis of manic-depressive insanity due to the work of Emil Kraepelin [1] and then more recently still was reconceptualized and named bipolar disorder. Even in its early history, it was recognized as a mood disorder comprising distinct episodes of mania and depression lasting from several days to weeks. Bipolar disorder is often popularly associated with "extreme moods," which while generally accurate, belies the totality of its symptoms and profound effect on functioning. This oversimplification of a rather complex disorder also invites diagnostic confusion.

Call Out Box

Patients with other trauma-related and/or personality disorders will often seek help for mood lability or moodiness from primary care physicians. Of note, changes in mood will often be short in duration, lasting for minutes or hours rather than multiple days to weeks. Commonly, mood symptoms are associated with a defined stressor. Unfortunately, these patients may self-identify as having bipolar disorder due to popular misconceptions about the bipolar illness that even pervade medicine.

Despite some popular misconceptions, bipolar disorder is not common. Only 2% of the world's population meets diagnostic criteria for either bipolar I (1%) or bipolar II (1.1%) disorder [57], with equal prevalence among female and male patients. At the same time, misdiagnosis and delays in appropriate treatment in patients who do have bipolar disorder are also common [38, 39]. Patients with bipolar disorder often present as depressed, and so the diagnosis can be missed even by experienced psychiatrists. High levels of comorbid anxiety, substance use, and personality disorders can also cloud the diagnostic picture. Confounding this problem, people with bipolar disorder do not always have full insight into their symptoms or the impact these symptoms have on their quality of life. These individuals may actively avoid care and refuse offers of treatment. Given this complexity, bipolar disorder is unsurprisingly both over- and underdiagnosed [77].

C.D. currently presents as depressed and only has partial insight into having bipolar disorder. Like many patients with bipolar disorder, he also has a history of alcohol use disorder.

The course of bipolar disorder varies between patients and may change across a patient's lifetime. The average age of onset is 18 years of age [56], and multiple mood episodes can be expected over the ensuing decades [2]. While mood episodes themselves are highly treatable, they are quite likely to reoccur (Geddes and Miklowitz 2013). First episodes are equally likely to be depressed or manic, though most patients have predominately depressive episodes over the entire lifetime course of the illness [6]. Classically, patients with bipolar disorder experience complete remission between episodes. The median duration of mood episodes is around 13 weeks [70]; some patients will have depressive episodes followed immediately by manic episodes, some will have manic episodes immediately followed by depressive episodes, and others will have either manic or depressive episodes followed by periods of euthymia, i.e., normal mood. Rapid cycling can occur in some patients, where patients experience four or more discrete mood episodes a year. Still other patients will not have crisply delineated mood cycles. Many of these patients will not see complete remission of mood symptoms between episodes, though their symptoms will not meet full criteria for a mood episode. For example, some patients who have had distinct depressive and manic episodes may have chronically dysphoric mood between episodes and some difficulties with motivation but will not have any problems with sleep, appetite, or energy and experience no thoughts of death or suicide. Still other patients will have a continuous course of symptoms that may fluctuate, to some degree, but still meet criteria for a major mood disorder. In other words, these patients will experience prolonged episodes of depression or mania. These patients may also deteriorate over time, with worsening severity of symptoms.

C.D. alludes to having had multiple manic and depressive episodes. Moreover, he likely has subsyndromal depressive symptoms between episodes, which are not uncommon in bipolar disorders.

Risks for the development of bipolar disorder likely include genetic heritability, prenatal and perinatal insult, childhood deprivation, substance misuse, and extreme psychosocial stressors (Rowland et al. 2008). Importantly, bipolar disorder carries with it relatively high rates of morbidity and mortality. In a Swedish national cohort study of adults [19], bipolar men and women died 8 and 9 years earlier, respectively, than individuals without bipolar disorder. Causes of premature death included suicide; there were a tenfold risk for suicide among bipolar women and an eightfold risk for bipolar men when compared to risk of suicide in the general population. More commonly, premature death was linked to cardiovascular disease, diabetes, COPD, influenza, pneumonia, and unintentional injuries. Of note, patients with timely medical diagnosis of chronic disease had mortality rates that approached those of the general population, suggesting that good medical care could, at least in part, address early mortality in this population.

3.2 Diagnosis and Presentation

Bipolar I disorder is chiefly defined by the presence of mania. While most individuals with bipolar I disorder have experienced at least one major depressive episode, a depressive episode is not necessary to meet criteria for the diagnosis (see Table 3.1 below). Moreover, while people with bipolar I can also experience hypomanic episodes, the presence of hypomania is not required for the diagnosis. Individuals with bipolar II disorder, however, must have experienced at least one hypomanic and one major depressive episode to meet diagnostic criteria (see Table 3.1 below). Hypomania can be conceptualized as an attenuated form of mania. However, the commonly held idea that bipolar I disorder is more severe than bipolar II disorder is a misconception as many individuals with the latter disorder have severe, recurrent depressive episodes.

The differential for bipolar disorder is broad, but certain medical conditions can lead to depressive episodes and even mania. A good physical examination

Table 3.1 Criteria for bipolar I and II disorders

Bipolar I disorder	Bipolar II disorder
1. Criteria have been met for at least one manic episode (see table below) 2. Symptoms are not better accounted for by a schizophrenia spectrum illness 3. Symptoms must last at least for 1 week and be present most of the time OR Manic symptoms lead to hospitalization	1. Criteria have been met for at least one hypomanic episode and at least one major depressive episode. 2. There has never been a manic episode. 3. Symptoms are not better accounted for by a schizophrenia spectrum illness 4. Mood symptoms cause significant distress or functional impairment

Adapted from DSM 5 [22]

may reveal neurological deficits, and subsequent imaging could demonstrate a brain tumor or lesions associated with multiple sclerosis, both of which can cause mood dysfunction. Basic laboratories should be done to rule out thyroid disorders, which can be associated with depression and mania, as well as metabolic disturbances and anemias that can mimic depression in causing low mood and low energy.

Patients with mania are often described as feeling "on top of the world," though they can also present as quite irritable. Generally, patients with mania exhibit uncharacteristic amounts of energy and need (and get) much less sleep than usual. Manic patients often speak quickly and may be hard to follow, jumping from topic to topic, though on brief interviews, they can sometimes "hold it together" and so mask evidence of excessive thought production from the examiner. Classically, patients with mania will either be engaged in more projects and activities than usual (and frequently jump from project to project without completion) and/or are engaged in risky behaviors. Manic patients will not infrequently spend way beyond their budget and on items that they wouldn't normally buy, and sexual promiscuity and use of illicit substances is also common. Patients with hypomania are less likely to engage in high-risk activities. Mixed features of depression may cloud the diagnostic presentation somewhat; these can present in up 10–30% of manic episodes, are predictive of a more severe and disabling course, and are associated with a higher risk of completed suicide [76]. A summary and comparison of symptoms of mania and hypomania are detailed in Table 3.2.

C.D. notes a history of likely mania with distinct periods of impulsive spending, gambling, and decreased need for sleep. Mania can cause significant disruption in relationships due to the associated behaviors. C.D. admits that a manic episode preceded his divorce.

Bipolar patients with depressive episodes often present quite similarly to patients with major depressive disorder experiencing an active episode of depression (see Table 3.3 for a summary of diagnostic criteria). Bipolar depressed patients may present with low mood, anhedonia, and feelings of worthlessness as well as of disturbances of sleep and appetite. Patients will often complain of feeling tired and fatigued and describe sleep disturbances. Agitation may occur but, in the absence of mixed features, will not be associated with excessive energy. Suicidal ideation and suicidal behaviors are common. Of note, these symptoms rarely present in pure manic episodes.

Table 3.2 Criteria for mania and hypomania

<table>
<tr><td>Mania
Symptoms should present for at least 1 week and for the majority, if not all, of the time; if hospitalization is required, the duration requirement is not needed for diagnosis</td><td>Hypomania
Symptoms should be present for at least 4 days and for the majority, if not all, of the time</td></tr>
<tr><td colspan="2">The mood must be elated, expansive, or irritable and with marked increases in energy. Symptoms should be markedly different than what is "normal" for the patient.</td></tr>
<tr><td colspan="2">Three of the following (or four if the patient's mood is irritable) should be present (and not attributable to a medical conditions, medications, or substances of abuse):
Grandiosity or inflated self-esteem
Decreased need for sleep
Pressured speech and/or increased production of speech
"Racing thoughts" or excessive production of thoughts such that the train of thought can be very hard to follow, e.g. "flight of ideas"
Distractibility, i.e., difficulty maintaining focus
Increase in goal-directed behavior or psychomotor agitation. This can manifest as taking on new projects (and often not completing them) or purposeless, non-goal-oriented activity
Excessive involvement in activities that have a high potential for adverse consequences, e.g. being sexually promiscuous, spending excessive amounts of money, etc.</td></tr>
<tr><td>Mania
Presence of psychotic features, need for hospitalization, and/or marked social/occupational impairment</td><td>Hypomania
Not associated with marked social/occupational impairment, does not lead to hospitalization, and is not associated with psychotic features</td></tr>
<tr><td colspan="2">"With mixed features" is a specifier that can be given if three of the following are present during most days of the episode:
Dysphoria or depressed mood by subjective report or observations of others
Diminished interest or pleasure in activities by subjective report or observations of others
Psychomotor retardation nearly daily and observable by others
Fatigue or loss of energy nearly daily
Feelings of worthlessness or excessive/inappropriate guilt nearly daily
Recurrent thoughts of death, recurrent suicidal ideation without plan, suicide plan, or suicide attempt</td></tr>
</table>

Adapted from DSM 5 [22]

3.3 Bipolar Disorder in the Medical Setting

Primary care physicians and APPs working in primary care settings well appreciate that they are often the first (and sometimes only) point of contact within the medical community for patients with serious mental illness. Bipolar patients will often present to PCP offices complaining not only of mood symptoms, but given high anxiety and substance use disorder comorbidities, they will not uncommonly complain of anxiety symptoms or present with concerns suspicious for substance misuse or abuse. Given the complexity of bipolar disorder presentations, screening for bipolar disorder in patients with such complaints is generally recommended. Tools like the Mood Disorder Questionnaire [37] may be a helpful in guiding further questioning, though clinical correlation cannot be overemphasized. Obtaining collateral can also be invaluable, as patients may not always be reliable narrators.

Table 3.3 Criteria for a major depressive episode

Symptoms should be present for at least a period of 2 weeks, for most of the time, and should be markedly different than what is "normal" for the patient.
At least one of the symptoms must include depressed mood or loss of interest or pleasure (see below).
Five or more of the following must be present (and not attributable to medical conditions, medications, or substances of abuse): Depressed mood by subjective report or observations of others Markedly diminished interest or pleasure in activities by subjective report or observations of others Unintentional weight loss or weight gain or appetite changes Insomnia or hypersomnia nearly daily Psychomotor agitation or retardation nearly daily Fatigue or loss of energy nearly daily Feelings of worthlessness or excessive/inappropriate guilt nearly daily Decreased ability to think, concentrate, or make decisions by subjective report or observations of others Recurrent thoughts of death, recurrent suicidal ideation without plan, suicide plan, or suicide attempt
Symptoms cause significant distress and/or impairment in social/occupational functioning. Clinical judgment should be used when a patient is experiencing bereavement
"With mixed features" is a specifier than can be used if three of the following (or four if the patient's mood is irritable) are present during the majority of days: Elevated, expansive mood Grandiosity or inflated self-esteem Decreased need for sleep Pressured speech and/or increased production of speech "Racing thoughts" or excessive production of thoughts such that the train of thought can be very hard to follow, e.g. "flight of ideas" Increase in goal-directed behavior or psychomotor agitation Excessive involvement in activities that have a high potential for adverse consequences, e.g. being sexually promiscuous, spending excessive amounts of money, etc.

Adapted from DSM 5 [22]

Once a primary care clinician has a suspicion for bipolar disorder, the question then becomes, should the PCP begin treatment or refer out? It has been suggested that if a patient is stable but has a generally elevated risk to harm themselves or others, or has psychiatric comorbidities, they should be referred to a psychiatrist [20]. If a patient presents as manic, severely depressed, and/or acutely at risk of harming themselves or others, inpatient hospitalization may be needed. If the patient lacks capacity to consent or refuses hospitalization, local laws and customs around involuntary commitment proceedings should be followed. Otherwise, if psychiatric referral or consultation is not readily available in less complex cases, a PCP can attempt to initiate or continue treatment for acute mood episodes and/or for maintenance phases of the illness. Given that many patients with bipolar disorder have a lifelong course, quite elevated risks of suicide, significant functional impairment, and often benefit from psychotherapy, referral to mental health treatment where medication management, psychotherapeutic, and case management services are available is recommended for long-term management.

Patients with bipolar disorder, regardless of connection with behavioral health, still need to follow regularly with PCPs. Close follow-up is generally recommended. As noted above, patients with bipolar disorder often die younger than population controls and due to infectious, cardiometabolic, and pulmonary diseases. As with schizophrenia, there is evidence that medical conditions in individuals with bipolar disorder are underrecognized and undertreated [53]. Medical comorbidities only increase with age and duration of illness, making early intervention critical [71]. Underscoring the need for medical treatment is emerging evidence that those with significant medical illnesses may have a more severe illness course [27].

3.3.1 *Obesity and Cardiometabolic Concerns*

More than half of patients with bipolar disorder are overweight or obese, and metabolic syndrome may occur in up to one third of patients [25]. Rates of hypertension, hyperlipidemia, and smoking are two times higher [62], and rates of type 2 diabetes mellitus (T2DM) are three times higher, in bipolar patients than in the general population [11]. Moreover, patients with bipolar disorders have 5 times the risk of cardiac disease when compared to age, race, and sex-matched controls [30]. In fact, the leading cause of mortality in individuals with bipolar disorder is cardiac disease, accounting for 35–40% of deaths [59].

Obesity, diabetes, and hyperlipidemia are associated with therapeutic use of atypical antipsychotic medications for the treatment of bipolar disorder [24]. In fact, patients with bipolar disorder are equally likely as patients with schizophrenia to experience metabolic syndrome with atypical antipsychotics [17]. Non-antipsychotic mood stabilizers, like lithium and valproate, can also cause weight gain. However, medications alone are not likely to account for the risk of metabolic syndrome in this population. Increased mortality from cardiovascular disease among bipolar patients predates modern psychiatric treatment [75]. High rates of obesity have also been observed in medication-naïve bipolar patients [47]. Moreover, there may be common threads between the pathophysiology of bipolar disorders and diabetes mellitus type II, as well as possible interwoven genetic and epigenetic risk factors [11].

Mood states themselves, particularly depression, may drive behaviors that contribute to weight gain [25] and development of cardiometabolic disorders. Access to medical care is also negatively influenced by patient behaviors, as are poverty states associated with serious mental illness and negative attitudes of healthcare professionals toward patients with mental illness. Studies repeatedly demonstrate disparities in both health screening and disease interventions for individuals with serious mental illness, including those with bipolar disorder [62].

C.D. notes a history of hypertension and hyperlipidemia. He has had past exposure to medications that are associated with metabolic syndrome. Like many patients with bipolar disorder, he has not been adherent with recommended medical care. Reasons for this may include sequelae of chronically depressed mood, poverty-associated stressors, lack of social support, and stigma.

Given these collective concerns, it is imperative that the invested PCP consider patients with bipolar disorder at high risk for morbidity and mortality from cardiometabolic disorders and commit to rigorous, evidence-based screening and treatment. In addition to recommending lifestyle changes and dietary counseling, prescribing mood stabilizing mediations with less cardiometabolic risk where possible is recommended. Adjuvant treatment of antipsychotic medications with topiramate, metformin, and glucagon-like peptide-1 (GLP-1) agonists may also help patients lose weight (McElroy et al. 2021; [21]).

3.3.2 *Respiratory Disease*

Rates of smoking in the seriously mentally ill population remain as high as 60%, and patients with bipolar disorder who do smoke are often heavy smokers [36]. Smoking likely accounts for some of the elevated risk of cardiovascular disease in this population. Unsurprisingly, the incidence and prevalence of COPD is twice as common in patients with bipolar disorder [40], and lung cancer rates are four times higher, than in the general population [52]. The prevalence of asthma may also be more common [65]. Smoking cessation counseling and use of smoking cessation aides, including nicotine replacement therapies, bupropion, and varenicline [14, 36], are recommended. Lung cancer screening where clinically appropriate should be promoted [26].

3.3.3 *Renal Disease*

Patients with bipolar disorder are at an increased risk of renal disease, at least in part driven by high rates of DM2, HTN, and cardiovascular disease. Rates are even higher in patients with lithium exposure [41]. Lithium can cause renal damage in two ways: (1) through effecting tubular function via inhibition of antidiuretic hormone, leading to nephrogenic diabetes insipidus, and (2) interstitial nephritis leading to diminished renal filtering capacity. This latter effect can result in gradually decreasing estimated glomerular filtration rate (eGFR) and increasing serum creatinine on laboratory testing. It is associated with stage 1–3 chronic kidney disease [33]. Rarely, patients on lithium can develop end-stage renal disease.

Impaired urinary concentration secondary to tubular effects of lithium is quite common, affecting up to 40% of patient on lithium [72]. Some authors opine that up to 80% of patients on lithium have complaints related to tubular effects, including polydipsia, polyuria, and/or nocturia [6]. This can develop quite early with lithium use, and if the lithium is stopped, is often reversible. After years of treatment, however, nephrogenic diabetes insipidus is likely to be permanent. Medically urgent or emergent problems, however, generally only arise if the patient cannot drink enough water. In cases of water deprivation or dehydration, severe hypernatremia can occur. For most patients, though, the impact of lithium-induced nephrogenic diabetes insipidus is negligible and should only be treated if it becomes bothersome to the patient, like if it causes significant nocturia [33]. A first approach to side effect mitigation is to consolidate lithium to once daily dosing at the patient's bedtime. Dose reduction can also be helpful if clinically appropriate. Subsequent assessment and treatment is usually completed in conjunction with a nephrologist. Common evaluations include obtaining a 24-hour urine collection, urine and serum electrolytes, and a urine osmolarity [33]. Amiloride 5–10 mg given once per day can reduce thirst and polyuria. Thiazides are also sometimes used for lithium-induced nephrogenic diabetes insipidus, though potassium supplementation may then be required. Even more importantly, thiazides decrease lithium clearance, and dose decreases of up to 1/3 the pre-thiazide dose are generally needed to avoid toxic lithium levels [6]. Indomethacin can also be used in severe cases of nephrogenic diabetes insipidus [33], but the lithium dose should also be reduced to avoid supratherapeutic levels and/or toxicity.

C.D. notes past exposure to lithium and experiencing some degree of polydipsia and polyuria. For some patients, even mild symptoms of nephrogenic diabetes insipidus can impact adherence.

Recognition and prevention of interstitial nephritis with lithium is paramount. It has long been thought that episodes of lithium toxicity, in addition to duration of use, were most associated with later development of interstitial nephritis. In at least one study, however, episodes of lithium toxicity and duration of exposure were not associated with risk of chronic kidney disease, whereas younger age at lithium commencement, female gender, and lower baseline eGFR did increase risks [35]. While around 20% of patients on lithium develop renal insufficiency [33], the absolute risk of renal failure associated with lithium remains small and likely effects around 1% of patients [15, 33]. Generally, patients whose serum creatinine levels are above 1.6 [6] and/or whose eGRF has decreased to 30 or less should have their lithium discontinued after a gradual switch to another mood stabilizer. Stopping lithium should always be done in consultation with the patient, the patient's primary supports, and the patient's psychiatrist, though, as sometimes, the risks of clinical decompensation in difficult to treat bipolar disorder would suggest cautious continuation of lithium despite elevated risks of renal deterioration.

3.3.4 Thyroid and Parathyroid Disease

Thyroid dysfunction has long been associated with bipolar disorder. Thyroid disorders themselves can cause neuropsychiatric symptoms. Hyperthyroidism can lead to restlessness and mood lability, such as can be seen in mania, and hypothyroidism is well known to cause low mood and energy and can easily be misdiagnosed as major depressive disorder. Hyperthyroidism in bipolar disorder is relatively rare; when it occurs, it is often linked to lithium, which can rarely induce autoimmune-mediated thyrotoxicosis. Hypothyroidism is more common. In STEP-BD, 18% of patients had hypothyroidism [8]; the majority of these patients were women. While much of the excess burden of hypothyroidism in bipolar disorder can be attributed to lithium use, the presence of thyroperoxidase (TPO) antibodies is much higher in bipolar patients than in controls, independent of lithium exposure.

Thyroid dysfunction may also impact the clinical course of bipolar disorder. Subclinical or low normal thyroid function has been associated with difficult to treat bipolar depression [16]. Even today, T3 is sometimes used for treatment of nonresponsive depression, including in bipolar disorder. Moreover, thyroid dysfunction has long been associated with rapid cycling [18]. As such, regular screening for thyroid abnormalities in bipolar disorder is highly recommended. Treatment, even of subclinical hypothyroidism, may be of significant benefit in this population.

As previously noted, lithium has long been associated with thyroid dysfunction. Goiter can be seen in up to 50% of patients on long-term lithium [64]. Goiter associated with lithium is diffuse but nonobstructive and can sometimes be reduced with levothyroxine. About 20% of patients on lithium develop hypothyroidism, and its development is more common in women, older adults, and patients with elevated baseline TPO antibodies [6]. If hypothyroidism develops after a patient starts lithium, treatment with levothyroxine is recommended. Continuation of lithium, if clinically effective, is generally recommended. Many patients will no longer be hypothyroid if they stop lithium. Some, however, will; it is postulated that in these patients, lithium use exacerbated underlying hypothyroidism and/or intensified an autoimmune reaction leading to hypothyroidism.

Lithium has also been linked to increases in calcium and hyperparathyroidism. In one Swedish sample, 18% of patients on chronic lithium had frank hyperparathyroidism, and another 21% had hypercalcemia [55]. Symptoms of lithium-induced hyperparathyroidism may be similar to primary hyperparathyroidism, and fatigue, low mood, and memory concerns may be confused for depressive symptoms. Consultation with endocrinology and psychiatry is advised when a patient on lithium has signs/symptoms of hypercalcemia and/or hyperparathyroidism. While cessation of lithium may be corrective, in some chronic cases, hyperparathyroidism continues. The clinical risks of discontinuing lithium may also outweigh the risks of frank hyperparathyroidism. Treatment is the same as for primary hyperparathyroidism and may include calcimimetic therapies and/or surgical parathyroid adenoma removal.

3.4 Treatment of Bipolar Disorder

Like with most serious psychiatric disorders, a combination of medication management and psychotherapy is recommended for the treatment of bipolar disorder. Treatment is guided by the patient's psychiatric history, medical history, family history, risks of side effects, personal preferences, and current clinical presentation. Stabilization, prevention of mood relapse, and optimization of quality of life should be the overarching goal of treatment.

Treatment of bipolar disorder is primarily driven by current mood state as well as recent and remote mood episode history. When a patient is in an acute mood episode, medication treatment should target the primary polarity of that episode, i.e., mania/hypomania or depression. In early recovery, the focus of pharmacological treatment should be to help protect against relapse into the same polarity episode as well as against an immediate polarity switch. Maintenance treatment takes into account longer-term risk of relapse into mood episodes and episode polarity predominance for that particular patient [32].

3.4.1 Psychopharmacologic Treatment of Bipolar Mania

Mania can present as a psychiatric emergency. If a patient engages with their PCP and mania is suspected, psychiatric hospitalization should be considered. An understanding of local laws governing involuntary commitment qualifications and procedures is highly recommended, as not all manic patients will agree to voluntary psychiatric hospitalization. Patients who do not require hospitalization can be treated as outpatients but should be followed very closely and ideally, by a psychiatrist.

Generally, mania should be treated with antimanic agents, which include atypical antipsychotics, lithium, and some anticonvulsant medications. Stimulant medications and/or those with mood elevating properties should be withdrawn, and behavioral measures should be taken to help routinize schedules, reduce stress, and restore sleep. Atypical antipsychotics are often used as first-line agents for patients with psychotic mania and/or profound psychomotor agitation [48]. Short courses of benzodiazepines can be used in addition to antimanic agents for behavioral disturbances and lack of sleep. If the course of mania is protracted and/or is not responsive to medication, there is evidence supporting the use of electroconvulsive therapy (ECT) in mania.

The following table (see Table 3.4 below) includes first- and second-line treatments of mania as suggested by several major treatment guidelines. Combination therapies are generally employed when a patient is already on a medication that has been at least partially effective. A classic example of the use of combination therapy would be for a patient who had been stable on lithium at optimal blood levels but then became manic. In this case, another agent, for example, risperidone, could be added. Some newer agents, e.g., lurasidone and cariprazine, do not appear in older

Table 3.4 Evidence-based, psychopharmacologic treatments of bipolar mania

First-line treatments	Second-line treatments
Single agents	*Single agents*
Lithium (NICE; CPRBD; RANZ; CANMET)	Carbamazepine (CPRBD, CANMET)
Quetiapine (NICE; CPRBD; RANZ; CANMET)	Haloperidol (CPRBD)
Risperidone (NICE; CPRBD; RANZ; CANMET)	Olanzapine (CANMET)
Olanzapine (NICE; CPRBD; RANZ)	Ziprasidone (CANMET)
Valproate (CPRBD; RANZ; CANMET)	*Combination therapy*
Aripiprazole (CPRBD; RANZ; CANMET)	Olanzapine + lithium (CANMET)
Asenapine (RANZ; CANMET)	Olanzapine + valproate (CANMET)
Ziprasidone (CPRBD; RANZ)	Lithium + valproate (CANMET)
Haloperidol (NICE; RANZ)	
Paliperidone >6 mg daily (CANMET; RANZ (if other options fail or are not tolerated))	
Cariprazine (CANMET)	
Combination therapy	
Quetiapine + lithium (CANMET; CPRBD; RANZ (if other options fail or are not tolerated))	
Quetiapine + valproate (CANMET; CPRBD; RANZ (if other options fail or are not tolerated))	
Aripiprazole + lithium (CANMET; CPRBD; RANZ (if other options fail or are not tolerated))	
Aripiprazole + valproate (CANMET; CPRBD; RANZ (if other options fail or are not tolerated))	
Risperidone + lithium (CANMET; CPRBD; RANZ (if other options fail or are not tolerated))	
Risperidone + valproate (CANMET; CPRBD; RANZ (if other options fail or are not tolerated))	
Asenapine + lithium (CANMET; CPRBD; RANZ (if other options fail or are not tolerated))	
Asenapine + valproate (CANMET; CPRBD; RANZ (if other options fail or are not tolerated))	
Valproate + any second-generation antipsychotic (not clozapine) (CPRBD; RANZ (if other options fail or are not tolerated))	
Lithium + any second-generation antipsychotic (not clozapine) (CPRBD; RANZ (if other options fail or are not tolerated))	
Lithium + valproate (RANZ (if other options fail or are not tolerated))	
Carbamazepine (RANZ (if other options fail or are not tolerated))	

NICE: National Institute for Health and Care Excellence Guidelines -- Bipolar disorder, assessment and management [60]; CPRBD, Clinical Practice Recommendations for Bipolar Disorder [48]; RANZ, Royal Australian and New Zealand College of Psychiatrists clinical practice guidelines for mood disorders, bipolar disorder summary [49]; CANMET, Canadian Network for Mood and Anxiety Treatments (CANMAT) and International Society for Bipolar Disorders (ISBD) collaborative update of CANMAT guidelines for the management of patients with bipolar disorder [76]

treatment guidelines but are included in more recent versions. As they are not as well studied, they may not appear as highly recommended, but they are included in the table below. Third- and fourth-line treatments are not included here. Their use should be deferred to psychiatry. Such agents include clozapine, either as a stand-alone agent or treatment adjuvant. Clozapine is a Risk Evaluation and Mitigation

Strategy (REMS) regulated medication. More information on clozapine can be found in the chapter on Schizophrenia.

Most guidelines agree that first-line pharmacological treatments for mania include lithium, quetiapine, and risperidone. Valproate and Abilify are also generally considered first-line treatments. Combining lithium or valproate with atypical antipsychotics, particularly risperidone, aripiprazole, and quetiapine, would also be considered first-line mania treatments. Early evidence suggests that cariprazine and asenapine, either used as single agents or in combination with valproate or lithium, may also be first-line treatments. Olanzapine is often considered a first-line treatment, but given metabolic side effects of this medication, its use is not always recommended, either as a single agent or in combination with other mood stabilizing agents. Furthermore, in weighing both efficacy and the potential for side effect burden, use of carbamazepine, ziprasidone, and Haldol as first-line treatments for mania is less supported.

Recommended dosing of FDA-approved second-generation antipsychotics for mania are presented in Table 3.5. Dosing recommendations for lithium, valproate, and carbamazepine are reviewed later in the chapter. In general, antipsychotic dosing for mania approaches that of schizophrenia, especially when psychosis and behavioral agitation are present, though lower doses of medications should be trialed in patients who are older and/or who are at elevated risk of medication specific side effects. Proper dosing of medications should also take into account potential drug-drug interactions, renal/hepatic impairments where applicable, and other clinical parameters that can impact medication pharmacokinetics and pharmacodynamics.

Table 3.5 Antipsychotic dosing strategies for manic episodes

Agent	Daily initial dosing (mg)	Target dose (mg/day)/maximum daily dose (mg)
Quetiapine	100 (50 twice daily)	400–800/ 800
Risperidone	2–3	1–6/ 6
Olanzapine	10–15; 10 if added on to valproate or lithium	5–20 20
Aripiprazole	15; 10–15 if added to valproate or lithium	15 30
Asenapine (do not give with food or drink)	10–20 (5–10 mg twice daily); 10 (5 mg twice daily) if added to valproate or lithium	10–20 (given as 5–10 mg twice daily) 20 (given as 10 mg twice daily)
Ziprasidone (give with food)	80 (40 mg twice daily)	80–160 (given as 40–80 mg twice daily) 160 (given as 80 mg twice daily)
Cariprazine	1.5	3–6/6

Quetiapine [package insert] [66]; olanzapine [package insert] [63]; risperidone [package insert] [68]; cariprazine [package insert] [12]; aripiprazole [package insert] [3]; asenapine [package insert] [4]; ziprasidone [package insert] [78]

3.4.2 Treatment of Depression in Bipolar I Disorder

More commonly than in mania, and unlike in major depressive disorder or schizophrenia, combination treatment of bipolar depression is often necessary. Like in mania, though, monotherapy should be trialed first; a second agent can be added for partial response or for breakthrough symptoms. Antidepressants should generally be avoided as monotherapy in bipolar I disorder; they may be of benefit as add-on treatment for depression in some cases, though such management would ideally be done by a psychiatrist. Antidepressants should be avoided in individuals with a history of switching into mania with antidepressants, a history of rapid cycling, and/or who present with mixed features or agitation. A summary of evidence-based treatments of bipolar depression is shown below (see Table 3.6).

Table 3.6 Evidence-based, psychopharmacologic treatments of bipolar depression

First-line treatments	Second-line treatments
Single agents	*Single agents*
Quetiapine (NICE; CPRBP; RANZ; CANMET)	Valproate (CPRBP; CANMET)
Lamotrigine (NICE; CPRBP; RANZ; CANMET)	Cariprazine (CANMET)
Lithium (NICE; CPRBP; RANZ; CANMET)	
Olanzapine (NICE; CPRBP; RANZ)	*Combination therapy*
Lurasidone (RANZ; CANMET)	Risperidone + lithium (CPRBP)
Valproate (RANZ)	Risperidone + valproate (CPRBP)
	Lithium + valproate (CPRBP)
Combination therapy	Olanzapine + fluoxetine (CPRBP; CANMET)
Olanzapine + fluoxetine (NICE)	Lithium + lamotrigine (CPRBP)
Lithium + quetiapine (NICE; (RANZ (if other options fail or are not tolerated))	Adjuvant antidepressant (CPRBP; CANMET)
Lithium + olanzapine (NICE)	
Lithium + lamotrigine (NICE; (RANZ (if other options fail or are not tolerated); CANMET)	
Adjuvant antidepressant except with lamotrigine (RANZ (if other options fail or are not tolerated))	
Valproate + quetiapine (RANZ (if other options fail or are not tolerated))	
Quetiapine + lamotrigine (RANZ (if other options fail or are not tolerated); CANMET)	
Lurasidone + lithium (CANMET; RANZ (if other options fail or are not tolerated))	
Lurasidone + valproate (CANMET; RANZ (if other options fail or are not tolerated))	
Lithium + valproate (RANZ (if other options fail or are not tolerated))	
Adjuvant lamotrigine (CANMET)	

NICE, National Institute for Health and Care Excellence Guidelines -- Bipolar disorder, assessment and management [60]; CPRBD, Clinical Practice Recommendations for Bipolar Disorder [48]; RANZ, Royal Australian and New Zealand College of Psychiatrists clinical practice guidelines for mood disorders, bipolar disorder summary [49]; CANMET, Canadian Network for Mood and Anxiety Treatments (CANMAT) and International Society for Bipolar Disorders (ISBD) collaborative update of CANMAT guidelines for the management of patients with bipolar disorder [76]

Table 3.7 Antipsychotic dosing strategies for depressive episodes

Agent	Daily initial dosing (mg)	Target dose (mg/day)/maximum daily dose (mg)
Quetiapine	50 at bedtime	300/300
Olanzapine	Oral in combination with fluoxetine: Start at 5 of oral olanzapine and 20 of fluoxetine once daily	Olanzapine 6 to 12 and fluoxetine 25 to 50 Olanzapine 12 mg and fluoxetine 50 mg
Lurasidone	20	20–120/120

Quetiapine [package insert] [66]; olanzapine [package insert] [63]; lurasidone [package insert] [46]

As with mania, ECT is a safe and evidence-based option for bipolar depression in patients for whom medications are ineffective or cause intolerable side effects.

Like in the treatment of mania, lithium and quetiapine are first-line treatments, as is olanzapine, though the latter's use may be more limited given the risk of metabolic side effects. Lamotrigine is also effective as a first-line single agent, and like lithium, it is often used in combination therapy and as a first-line treatment approach. Some newer agents, e.g., lurasidone and cariprazine, do not appear in older guidelines but are included in more recent versions. Lurasidone especially is being increasingly recognized as a first-line treatment of bipolar depression. Valproate, while still used as a first-line treatment for bipolar depression, may not be as effective as other single agents though it is generally regarded as effective in combination therapy. The indication for risperidone in bipolar depression is more limited.

Recommended dosing of FDA-approved second-generation antipsychotics for bipolar depression is reviewed in the table below (see Table 3.7). Dosing recommendations for lithium, valproate, and lamotrigine are reviewed later in the chapter. In general, doses for bipolar depression are lower than those used for mania or schizophrenia. Still lower doses of medications may be indicated for patients who are older and/or who experience medication-related side effects. Proper dosing of medications should also consider potential drug-drug interactions, renal/hepatic impairments where applicable, and other clinical parameters that can impact pharmacokinetics and pharmacodynamics.

3.4.3 *Treatment of Euthymia +/– Residual Mood Symptoms (Maintenance Phase) in Bipolar I Disorder*

The maintenance phase of treatment starts about 6 months after a patient has recovered from an acute mood episode [49]. Maintenance treatment is focused on prophylaxis against future mood episodes. Some controversy remains about when in the course of the illness it is best to initiate maintenance treatment. Many psychiatrists will withdraw agents after full resolution of a first mood episode and wait until after the second known mood episode before initiating maintenance treatment. In the United States, however, maintenance treatment is often recommended after even one manic episode [32]. In general, maintenance treatment should be tailored to the patient's personal history of treatment response and/or the predominant polarity of their illness presentation, i.e., if they experience predominantly depressive or manic episodes. NICE guidelines specifically suggest maintaining the patient on the treatment that stabilized them during their most recent acute phase, which is a frequent clinical practice [60]. If the patient refuses to continue treatment effective during an acute mood episode, or if medication changes are needed due to side effects, other medications with good evidence for maintenance treatment can be initiated. Symptom, side effect, and adherence screening should be frequent, and treatments should be modified in accordance with findings. It is generally recommended to reduce medication burden during the maintenance phase to maximize patient adherence, minimize the risk of drug-drug interactions, and reduce the risk of serious medication side effects. Maintaining patients on single agents during the maintenance phase is a frequent goal, e.g., withdrawing quetiapine and continuing lithium on a now euthymic patient who had a severe depression 6 months ago. It may not always be possible to maintain patients on single agents, however, especially if the patient has inter-episode residual, difficult to treat mood symptoms, and/or a history of decompensation on single agents. If patients struggle with oral adherence to medications, long-acting injectable formulations of antipsychotics can be used in maintenance treatment. Table 3.8 summarizes several treatment guidelines to present first- and second-line agents useful for maintenance treatment of bipolar disorder.

A patient with a history of four depressive episodes and one manic episode may be said to have a predominant depressive polarity. Likewise, a patient with three episodes of mania and one episode of depression can be said to have a predominant manic polarity. Further questioning may help provide valuable information about C.D.'s course of illness and guide recommended treatment.

Many commonly used atypical antipsychotics are not FDA approved for the maintenance phase of bipolar disorder. Atypical antipsychotics that are approved have been included in Table 3.9. If the patient remains on these medications in the long term, doses can often be reduced over time. Dosing recommendations for lithium, valproate, lamotrigine, and carbamazepine are reviewed later in the chapter.

3.4.4 Treatment of Mixed States

Mixed features in bipolar disorder sometimes respond well to monotherapy; olanzapine, quetiapine, or valproate are considered first-line agents, as are combination therapy with olanzapine and valproate [49]. Lithium may not always adequately treat mixed features [6]; adjunctive antipsychotic agents can be helpful when the patient is already taking lithium or valproate [60]. Lamotrigine can be added to

Table 3.8 Evidence-based, psychopharmacologic treatments of bipolar depression

First line	Second line
Single agents Lithium (NICE; CPRBP; RANZ (manic dominant polarity); CANMET) Valproate (NICE; CPRBP; RANZ (manic dominant polarity); CANMET) Quetiapine (NICE (if previously effective in a manic or depressive episode); CPRBP; RANZ (for equal polarity); CANMET); Lamotrigine (CPRBP; RANZ (for primary depressive polarity); CANMET) Olanzapine (NICE; CPRBP; RANZ (if other treatments fail or are not tolerated)) Aripiprazole (CPRBP) Ziprasidone (CPRBP) Risperidone (CPRBP) Clozapine (CPRBP) Asenapine (CANMET) *Combination therapy* Lithium + valproate (NICE) Quetiapine + lithium (CANMET) Quetiapine + valproate (CANMET) Aripiprazole + valproate (CANMET) Aripiprazole + lithium (CANMET) Adjuvant olanzapine (RANZ (if other treatments fail or are not tolerated))	*Single agents* Olanzapine (CANMET) Risperidone (CANMET) Carbamazepine (CANMET) Paliperidone >6 mg (CANMET) *Combination therapy* Lurasidone + lithium (CANMET) Lurasidone + valproate (CANMET) Ziprasidone + lithium (CANMET) Ziprasidone + valproate (CANMET) Adjuvant risperidone (CANMET)

NICE, National Institute for Health and Care Excellence Guidelines -- Bipolar disorder, assessment and management [60]; CPRBD, Clinical Practice Recommendations for Bipolar Disorder [48]; RANZ, Royal Australian and New Zealand College of Psychiatrists clinical practice guidelines for mood disorders [49], bipolar disorder summary; CANMET, Canadian Network for Mood and Anxiety Treatments (CANMAT) and International Society for Bipolar Disorders (ISBD) collaborative update of CANMAT guidelines for the management of patients with bipolar disorder [76]

Table 3.9 Antipsychotic dosing strategies for the maintenance phase of bipolar disorder

Agent	Daily initial dosing (mg)	Target dose (mg/day)/maximum daily dose (mg)
Olanzapine	5–20	10–20/20
Ziprasidone + lithium or valproate	80 (40 twice daily)	80–160 (40–80 mg twice daily)/160 (80 mg twice daily)

monotherapy when mixed depressive features emerge, although given the slow titration of lamotrigine, this approach can sometimes be impractical [49].

3.4.5 *Treatment of Rapid Cycling*

Most guidelines suggest that the pharmacological management of rapid cycling bipolar disorders should not be approached differently than in patients with a lower prevalence of mood episodes [76]. Valproate, lithium, olanzapine, lamotrigine, quetiapine, and aripiprazole have all been studied in rapid cycling bipolar disorders [49]. There is some suggestion that combination treatment may be superior [76] to single agents. Lithium and valproate, lithium and carbamazepine, and lamotrigine used adjunctively to maintenance treatment are all conventional, combination therapy approaches. Of note, lithium may not be as effective in rapid cycling as it is in other forms of the disorder [6].

3.4.6 Treatment of Bipolar II Disorder

Treatment of hypomanic episodes can sometimes be supportive, involving minimal medication and focusing on reduction of stressors and implementing increased structure around sleep. However, disruptive symptoms are often treated pharmacologically and can involve single mood stabilizing agents prescribed at lower doses than would be used in mania. While randomized controlled trials of hypomania requiring medication treatment are limited, lithium, valproate, and atypical antipsychotics can be considered [76]. Evidence for optimal treatment of depression in bipolar II disorder is similarly more limited than for depression in bipolar I disorder. First-line strategies include quetiapine [49, 76] and lamotrigine [49]. Lithium may be considered second line [76]. Many experts believe that antidepressants may be safely used in monotherapy for acute bipolar II depression, though the evidence to support this practice, let alone its efficacy, is limited. As such, agents like sertraline and venlafaxine may be recommended as second-line treatments of depression in bipolar II disorder [76].

3.5 Lithium and Antiepileptic Medications Used as Evidence-Based Mood Stabilizers

In this section, we will explore some of the most commonly used agents in bipolar disorder, namely, lithium, valproate, carbamazepine, and lamotrigine. As noted above, atypical antipsychotics are commonly and effectively prescribed for the treatment of bipolar disorder, though they are associated with significant side effect burden. Many experts argue that lithium [28], and to a lesser extent valproate, are underutilized in the treatment of bipolar disorders given their strong clinical efficacy. More information on specific atypical antipsychotics medications, including potential side effects and drug interactions, can be found in the Schizophrenia chapter of this manual.

3.5.1 Lithium

Lithium has a long and fascinating history. Its utility in mood disorders was suspected as early as the late nineteenth century. Lithium's modern history began in the 1940s in Australia with the experimental work of the celebrated psychiatrist John Cade. Although clinical uptake of lithium was slow, it has, since the 1970s, emerged as the gold standard treatment of bipolar disorder. Lithium is a first-line treatment in acute mania, acute depression, and maintenance treatment. That said, lithium may work best in specific subpopulations of patients, including those with discrete mood episodes with typical symptoms, full inter-episode remissions, a family history of bipolar disorder and/or lithium response, and a lack of mood incongruent psychotic features [6].

While lithium is dispensed in a variety of preparations, e.g., lithium carbonate, lithium citrate, and lithium acetate, lithium carbonate is the most widely prescribed form. Both immediate-release and slow- or extended-release formulations of lithium carbonate are available. Changes in formulations of lithium are not recommended during treatment, as the formulations have different bioavailability. Extended release may be associated with fewer side effects for some patients. In addition, while some patients may better tolerate lithium twice daily, once daily dosing may be renally sparing (protecting mainly against tubular effects [45]). Given this, and as peak serum lithium levels are associated with fatigue, once daily dosing with extended-release lithium given before bedtime is widely recommended.

Thyroid, parathyroid, and renal dysfunction associated with lithium are described in the section above. Other (and generally more benign) side effects of lithium are summarized in Table 3.10 (see below) and include mild to moderate weight gain, fine tremor, fatigue, and gastrointestinal (GI) complaints. GI side effects can include decreased appetite, nausea, vomiting, and diarrhea. Both fatigue and GI side effects generally improve over time, and the latter can sometimes be improved by taking lithium with food, taking lithium in divided doses, or switching formulations of lithium. Sustained-release formulations may be better tolerated with nausea; diarrhea may improve with immediate-release formulations [29]. Severe GI side effects can lead to dehydration and lithium toxicity, so lithium levels should be closely monitored when these occur. Weight gain is generally addressed by exercise and dietary changes and deprescribing other medications with metabolic side effects if clinically appropriate. Tremor, which is generally fine, seen in the upper extremities, most pronounced against gravity, and indistinguishable from physiologic tremor, can sometimes be mitigated by dose reduction and elimination of caffeine [29]; in some patients, tremor may improve over time though it can also emerge with aging. If lithium-associated tremor is distressing to the patient, beta blockers can often be prescribed with good effect. Propranolol is most often used for this purpose and is generally effective at low doses (<120 mg daily). As course tremor is very common in lithium toxicity (and is often seen in body areas other than the upper extremities), lithium levels should be drawn if tremor emerges or worsens.

Table 3.10 Side effects of lithium and their treatment

Common side effects	Treatment approaches
Nocturia, polyuria, polydipsia	Switch to once daily dosing at bedtime ↓ Consider dose reduction (if clinically appropriate) ↓ Workup for nephrogenic diabetes insipidus (obtain 24 hour urine collection, urine and serum electrolytes, urine osmolality); consider referral to nephrology ↓ In collaboration with nephrology, start amiloride 5–10 mg per day
Hypothyroidism	Treat with levothyroxine
Fatigue	Switch dosing to once daily at bedtime. May improve with time
GI complaints	May improve with time. Take with food ↓ Take in divided doses ↓ Switch formulations (immediate release may help with diarrhea; extended release may help with nausea). Check trough level 5 days after switch
Tremor	Check level. May improve over time. Reduce caffeine and other substances that may cause tremor ↓ Reduce dose if clinically appropriate ↓ Start beta blocker

Lithium is generally started at 300 mg a day in the outpatient setting and at up to 900 mg on inpatient units, divided into two or three times daily dosing. It is then titrated every 5–7 days, informed by 12-hour trough serum lithium levels, to the therapeutic dose range. Lithium levels are necessary to both ensure clinical efficacy and to prevent lithium toxicity. Levels should always be checked 5 days after a dose change (to achieve steady state), at least every 3–6 months during maintenance treatment, and whenever there is clinical suspicion for toxicity or nonadherence. Steady-state doses are measured as 12-hour trough serum lithium levels and are generally directly proportional to dosing, such that if a patient's lithium dose was increased by a third, their serum blood level should increase by a third. Therapeutic lithium blood levels in acute depressive episodes are generally considered to be 0.8–1.0 mEq/L [76]; maintenance lithium levels have been known to fall in acute mania, requiring dose adjustments, and levels around 1.0 mEq/L are often needed to produce a therapeutic response. Many bipolar patients tolerate lower doses during maintenance treatment, with levels in the 0.6–0.75 mEq/L range [69]. If lithium is switched from twice daily dosing to once at night, evidence suggests that the dose can be reduced by 25% due to decreased renal clearance at night leading to 10–30% increased 12-hour trough concentrations [45].

Table 3.11 Labs, vitals, and histories needed for lithium

Investigations needed prior to starting lithium	Maintenance lithium
CBC Serum electrolytes Serum calcium Serum creatinine/BUN/eGFR Thyroid function tests Consider EKG, pregnancy tests Weight and BMI Personal and family medical history	12-hour trough serum lithium level at least 5 days after every dose change, every 3 months during the first year, and every 3 to 6 months ongoing Weight, BMI, serum electrolytes, calcium, creatinine, BUN, eGFR, and thyroid function tests at least every 6 months

Certain laboratory investigations, measurement of vitals, and medical histories are needed to start and maintain patients on lithium (see Table 3.11 below). Prior to starting lithium, obtaining a complete blood count (CBC) and serum electrolytes as well as serum calcium levels, creatinine, blood urea nitrogen (BUN), estimated glomerular filtration rate (eGFR), and thyroid function tests are recommended. Weight and body mass index (BMI) should also be obtained. Electrocardiograms (EKGs) should be considered, especially for patients with a personal or family history of cardiac disease. Pregnancy tests should be considered in individuals of childbearing potential. Baseline laboratory evaluations should generally be repeated at least every 6 months and more frequently in older or medically compromised patients. Weight should be taken at least annually.

Lithium toxicity is a medical emergency. While clinical manifestations are often quite pronounced when they appear acutely, toxicity can emerge more insidiously, especially in older adults. Symptoms of toxicity include course tremor, nausea and vomiting, diarrhea, lethargy, hyperreflexia, nystagmus, ataxia, and oliguria. It can also lead to decreased levels of consciousness, seizures, and coma.

While lithium toxicity is a risk with intentional overdose, many patients who develop toxicity are taking lithium as prescribed. Risk factors include dehydration (from exercise, hot weather, decreased oral intake, acute illness, etc.), impaired renal function (including nephrogenic diabetes insipidus), congestive heart failure, a reduced sodium diet, and drug-drug interactions. Generally, toxicity occurs at levels above 1.0 mEq/L but can sometimes present at lower levels, especially in older adults and medically compromised individuals. Mild symptoms often present between levels of 1.5 to 2.0 mEq/L; moderate intoxication with decreased levels of consciousness will appear at levels from 2.5–3.0 mEq/L. Levels above 3.0 mEq/L represent severe intoxication, where seizures and coma are most likely to occur [35]. Treatment of lithium toxicity includes hydration, serial monitoring of levels, bowl decontamination, and hemodialysis in select patients with levels above 2.5 mEq/L and in all patients with levels above 4.0 mEq/L [34].

Drug interactions can occur between lithium and many commonly prescribed and over-the-counter medications (see Table 3.12). Patients should be counseled extensively on the most common interactions and what medications to avoid when possible. If certain medications cannot be avoided, consultation with psychiatry is

Table 3.12 Drug interactions with lithium and mitigation strategies

Medications to avoid prescribing when a patient is taking lithium	If medication is medically necessary
Angiotensin-converting enzyme (ACE) inhibitors	Monitor lithium level. Lithium dose reduction may be needed with ACE initiation. Lithium dose increase may be required when medication is stopped
Angiotensin II receptor antagonists (ARBs)	Monitor lithium level. Lithium dose reduction may be needed with ARB initiation. Lithium dose increase may be required when medication is stopped
Methylxanthine (e.g., theophylline) and loop (e.g., furosemide), potassium-sparing (e.g., spironolactone), and other diuretics (excluding thiazide and thiazide-like diuretics)	May increase lithium levels with initiation; monitor lithium levels closely and change dose as needed
Thiazide and thiazide-like diuretics	Halve the dose of lithium with initiation; monitor levels frequently and increase/decrease lithium dose as necessary
Acetazolamide	Will likely increase lithium level substantially with initiation. Consider immediate lithium dose decreases with initiation and monitor lithium level closely
NSAIDs	Use, particularly chronic use, should be avoided. Lower lithium doses may be required

Adapted from [50]

highly recommended. In general, chronic non-steroidal anti-inflammatory drugs (NSAIDs) and diuretics should be avoided. If a diuretic must be used, amiloride is a safe option.

3.5.2 *Valproate*

There are multiple formulations of valproate on the market, including immediate release (Depakene), delayed release (Depakote, Depakote DR, and Depakote Sprinkle Capsules), and extended release (Depakote ER). The active ingredient in immediate release forms is valproic acid. Delayed release and extended release are the most frequently prescribed formulations as they are enteric coated and often better tolerated due to reduced risk of gastrointestinal upset. Delayed-release formulations contain both sodium valproate and valproic acid in a 1:1 ratio. Extended-release formulations contain the same bioactive ingredients as the delayed release but can be given once a day, whereas the delayed-release formulation is recommended to be given twice daily. Of note, Depakote ER is 10% to 20% less bioavailable than Depakote DR [23], so when switching between the two formulations, dose adjustments are often necessary.

Delayed-release valproate is generally started at 500 mg to 1000 mg a day. In mania, it is often initiated, in divided doses, at daily doses of up to 1500 mg [51].

Less commonly in mania, delayed-release valproate is loaded (in divided doses) based on the patient's weight; the formula used to calculate the total dose is 20 mg/kg/day. Generally, serum valproate levels should be checked every 2 days with this loading strategy. In mania, therapeutic delayed-release valproate doses generally range between 500 mg and 3000 mg total daily doses. In depression, lower doses of delayed-release valproate are used at initiation, i.e., 250 mg or 500 mg daily, and therapeutic doses generally range from 500 to 2000 mg daily.

Valproate dosing should be guided by clinical response rather than blood level, though therapeutic trough serum levels are generally thought to be between 50 and 100 mcg/mL. Levels of up to 125 mcg/mL or even higher, however, may be indicated for acute mania. Accurate serum blood levels can be obtained within 3–5 days of a dose change. Levels for delayed release and immediate release formulations, which are generally prescribed twice daily, should be obtained as a 12-hour trough level, i.e., 12 hours after the evening dose and before administration of the morning dose. Patients on extended-release formulations would ideally have levels taken about 24 hours after their last dose and right before the next dose is due. Obtaining accurate levels becomes complicated as most patients prefer to take Depakote ER at bedtime to mitigate sedation, and most laboratories are not open late hours. Levels obtained 12 hours after Depakote ER is taken can lead to levels up to 25% higher than they would be at 24 hours [67]. Asking patients to obtain their levels as late in the day as possible, ideally closer to 20 hours after last dose, will result in levels closer to true trough levels. Patients may also be encouraged to move up their dosing to earlier the day for a few days, as tolerated, to facilitate obtaining an accurate trough level.

Common but generally benign side effects of valproate include nausea, vomiting, diarrhea, sedation, tremor, weight gain, hair loss, and mild thrombocytopenia. Gastrointestinal symptoms are often transient, occurring upon first starting the medication and dissipating over time; if GI side effects are severe and accompanied by pain and/or loss of appetite, rare but potentially fatal hemorrhagic pancreatitis should be ruled out. Mild tremor in the absence of other symptoms of toxicity can often be treated by dose decrease or the addition of beta blockers like propranolol [51]. Weight gain can be particularly problematic with valproate as can hair loss. Treatment is often supportive, including diet and exercise for weight gain and biotin, zinc, and selenium for hair loss [42]. Thrombocytopenia may impact up to 18% of patients but is usually mild, may respond to dose decreases, and does not have a clear association with bleeding risks [9].

In addition to pancreatitis, other serious adverse events associated with valproate include hepatotoxicity. Cases of hepatocellular liver injury with jaundice have been reported, as have cases of hyperammonemia without liver enzyme elevation causing mental status change and even obtundation [44]. Importantly, up to 10–20% of patients experience asymptomatic and usually transient elevations in liver transaminases when starting valproate. Additionally, while valproate should generally be stopped if implicated in liver disease, in cases of mild hyperammonemia, lactulose or carnitine can sometimes be helpful [5] if discontinuation of valproate is non-optimal.

Valproate should generally be avoided in individuals who may become pregnant. If other treatments for bipolar disorder have been exhausted, valproate can be used, but effective contraception should be in place. Fetal risk with valproate exposure is high. Reported sequelae of fetal valproate exposure include major congenital malformations like spinal bifida, intellectual and cognitive disabilities, autism spectrum disorder and other developmental disorders, and attention deficit disorder [54].

Valproate toxicity is relatively rare but can occur both acutely and chronically. In acute cases, patients present with changes in mental status, hypernatremia, elevated liver transaminases, and/or hyperammonemia. In severe cases, patients can face cardiac or respiratory compromise. Chronic toxicity is more common in older individuals, in patients with hypoalbuminemia, and in patients on medications competing for protein binding. It can present subtly, with worsening tremor, progressive gait ataxia, and mild confusion. In cases where chronic toxicity is a risk, including in older adults and in patients with low serum albumin, routine monitoring of both total and free valproate levels, i.e., the fraction of valproate not bound to albumin, can be helpful.

Medications that elevate levels of glucuronosyltransferases, like phenytoin, carbamazepine, and phenobarbital, may increase the clearance of valproate. Given valproate's protein binding, levels of warfarin and phenytoin may need to be monitored when co-administered with valproate, as valproate can displace these medications and increase their levels. Finally, lamotrigine doses should also be reduced when co-administered with valproate, as valproate can increase lamotrigine levels and the risk of Steven-Johnson's syndrome.

Prior to starting valproate, a serum pregnancy test (if applicable), complete blood count, and complete metabolic profile (with liver function tests) should be ordered. These laboratory investigations should be repeated every 3 to 6 months thereafter. Weight and body mass index monitoring is also recommended.

3.5.3 *Carbamazepine*

Carbamazepine was the first anticonvulsant medication used to treat bipolar disorder, starting in the 1970s [13]. While it remains an evidence-based treatment for both manic episodes and maintenance treatment, carbamazepine is not commonly prescribed today due to its side effect profile and significant drug-drug interactions. Carbamazepine is an extremely potent enzyme inducer and even induces its own metabolism, usually occurring between 3 to 5 weeks of starting the medication.

Carbamazepine is usually started at total doses of 200–600 mg a day, divided into three to four times daily doses. As rapid titrations are not well tolerated by most patients, dose increases over 200 mg a day are not recommended. Generally, dose increases are done every 3 to 5 days, making it challenging to use in mania. Typical doses for acute mania range from 400 mg to 1600 mg, and blood levels between 8 and 12 mEq/ml are associated with efficacy in mania. Therapeutic blood levels in maintenance therapy have not been established [31], though average maintenance doses are around 1000 mg daily [38, 39]. All levels should be drawn as 12-hour trough levels and at least 5 days after a dose adjustment for accuracy.

Carbamazepine is often associated with significant side effect burden. Side effects include dizziness, ataxia, diplopia, fatigue, and nausea and are generally dose related. Severe hyponatremia can also occur, requiring urgent medical intervention. A benign rash can also be seen, though there is a small but significant risk of Stevens-Johnson syndrome and fatal toxic epidermal necrolysis with carbamazepine. Carbamazepine has also been associated with hepatotoxicity and several blood dyscrasias, ranging from mild leukopenia and thrombocytopenia to agranulocytosis (it is relatively contraindicated to give with clozapine due to agranulocytosis risk) and hemolytic anemia. Renal failure has also been reported. It is thus recommended that patients starting carbamazepine should have complete blood counts with differentials and liver function tests drawn before initiation, every 2 weeks during the first month of treatment, every 3 weeks over the next few months, and every 2 to 3 months thereafter [31]. Regular renal function tests and serum electrolytes may also be advisable [38, 39].

There are a multitude of clinically relevant drug interactions with carbamazepine. The use of drug interaction checkers is highly recommended. Significant decreases in carbamazepine levels can occur with concomitant acetazolamide, macrolide antibiotics, isoniazid, metronidazole, verapamil, diltiazem, and cimetidine. Carbamazepine can also significantly reduce levels of valproic acid, clonazepam, ethosuximide, lamotrigine, topiramate, and other antiepileptics as well as tricyclic antidepressants, several antipsychotics, steroid oral contraceptives, glucocorticoids, oral anticoagulants, cyclosporin, theophylline, and several chemotherapeutic agents and cardiovascular drugs. In summary, if a patient requires multiple medications, carbamazepine may be quite complicated to safely use.

3.5.4 Lamotrigine

Lamotrigine is an antiepileptic medication with strong efficacy for bipolar depression and for the maintenance phase of bipolar I and II disorders, particularly in patients with a primary depressive polarity. Generally, doses of 200 mg are targeted. Lamotrigine is often well tolerated in comparison to other mood stabilizers and does not have as many drug-drug interactions as other antiepileptic medications. It is not usually associated with weight gain or sexual dysfunction. The most common side effect of lamotrigine seems to be headache. Serious side effects are rare. The main challenge with lamotrigine is that due to a small but significant risk of Steven-Johnson's syndrome (SJS) or toxic epidermal necrosis (TEN), it must be titrated very slowly upon initiation and re-titrated if the patient does not take lamotrigine for 72 hours or greater at any time during treatment. Given these challenges, despite its tolerability and therapeutic efficacy, lamotrigine may not be the best treatment option in severe acute depression or for patients who are not highly adherent to oral medications.

SJS (TEN in its most severe form) is a severe skin rash, often accompanied by fever and flu-like symptoms, which involves the skin and mucous membranes. SJS rashes present as tender, purpuric, or hemorrhagic and do not blanche with pressure; classically, it involves the face, neck, and upper trunk. Signs of internal organ damage may appear on basic laboratories (complete blood count, liver function tests, and renal function tests) [10]. Within a few days of onset, skin blistering and peeling occurs and is very painful. This condition requires hospitalization, often within an intensive care unit. Mortality rates are high.

Fortunately, with lamotrigine, the incidence of serious rash requiring either hospitalization or meriting formal diagnosis with SJS or TEN appears to be less than 0.1% [7]. Most cases of SJS/TENs occur early during treatment, usually sometime after the first 5 days [10]. Serious rash most often occurs with rapid dose escalations and/or concurrent valproate administration [61]. Given this finding, it is highly recommended that standard dose titrations be adhered to, as described in Table 3.13.

The occurrence of benign rash with lamotrigine is not uncommon and occurred in nearly 10% of prospective trials [74]. Despite its relative rarity, given that untreated SJS could lead to devastating consequences, any patient on lamotrigine who develops a rash, especially in the first few months of treatment, should be advised to hold their next dose of lamotrigine and be seen for evaluation. Benign drug-related rashes are usually nonconfluent and nontender, will resolve within 2 weeks, are not accompanied by systemic symptoms (fever, malaise, lymphadenopathy, etc.), and will sparingly affect the face if at all [10]. Ideally, lamotrigine will be held for the duration of the rash. Alternatively, if the patient has achieved therapeutic levels, the dose can be reduced while the patient is closely observed. If the rash worsens or systemic symptoms develop, lamotrigine should be stopped, and further investigations begun. If the rash involves itching, it can be treated with antihistamines and/or topical steroids. Once the rash is resolved, lamotrigine can often be successfully rechallenged [61].

Lamotrigine interacts with other antiepileptic medications, including phenytoin, carbamazepine, oxcarbazepine, phenobarbital, and primidone, all of which may

Table 3.13 Dosing for lamotrigine starts

	Regular titration	In patients taking valproate	In patients taking carbamazepine (or phenytoin, primidone, etc.) and not on valproate
Weeks 1 and 2	25 mg daily	25 mg every other day	50 mg daily
Weeks 3 and 4	50 mg daily	25 mg daily	100 mg daily, in divided doses
Week 5	100 mg daily	50 mg daily	200 mg daily, in divided doses
Week 6	200 mg daily	100 mg daily	300 mg daily, in divided doses
Week 7	200 mg daily	100 mg daily	Up to 400 mg daily, in divided doses

Lamotrigine [package insert] [43]

increase its clearance. Conversely, valproate may significantly decrease lamotrigine's clearance. Given these interactions, alternate titration schedules should be followed if any of these medications are co-administered with lamotrigine, as reflected in the table above. Importantly, oral contraceptives may also decrease lamotrigine levels, so higher doses may be needed to maintain therapeutic efficacy. Certain protease inhibitors may also impact lamotrigine levels.

3.6 Psychosocial Treatment

Psychotherapy is a mainstay of treatment for bipolar I and II disorders. For most patients, medication management is the bedrock of successful treatment, but even the most effective medication regimen may not address all symptoms of the disorder let alone the accompanying functional impairment. Given this, combining psychotherapy and psychopharmacology is recommended for successful treatment of bipolar disorder [76]. While psychodynamic therapy has long been a treatment option for bipolar patients, given that bipolar patients often struggle with insight, many experts have opined that the efficacy of this treatment modality is limited in this population [73]. Over the course of recent decades, several novel psychotherapies have been devised and studied in bipolar disorder. Many of these therapies are symptoms focused and directive, encouraging medication adherence, providing psychoeducation, supporting family members, encouraging relapse prevention planning, and promoting healthy sleep cycles. Moreover, several of these modalities explore important connections between mood and cognitions and interpersonal relationships [73].

The most widely studied psychotherapies for bipolar disorder are summarized in Table 3.14. Many of these interventions can be offered in individual or group therapy or as a combination of both. While most evidence suggests that therapy is most helpful in the maintenance phase and/or in depressive episodes of bipolar disorder, therapy may be quite helpful in acute recovery from either mania or depressive episodes [58].

Ultimately, successful psychotherapy requires a positive therapeutic rapport between the therapist and the patient. While specialized therapies may not be available to all patients, a good therapist who can engender rapport, provide both psychoeducation and support, and promote problem-solving can be quite helpful to bipolar patients. As such, referral to psychotherapy is almost always recommended for patients with bipolar disorder, regardless of illness stage and availability of specialized treatment.

Table 3.14 Evidence-based psychotherapies for bipolar disorders

Therapy	Individual	Group	Focus
Psychoeducation	Yes	Yes	Teaches facts about the disorder to empower patients with information Focuses on medication adherence Empowers patients with relapse prevention strategies, e.g., teaches recognizing warning signs of an impending mood episode Promotes coping strategies around life stressors
Cognitive behavioral therapy	Yes	Yes	Helps patients recognize connections between thoughts, moods, and behaviors Uses structured tools to help patients change negative thoughts and behaviors Focuses on automatic negative thoughts and distorted thinking
Functional remediation	No	Yes	Focuses on remediation of cognitive deficits associated with bipolar disorder Uses group exercises to target memory, attention, concentration, executive function, etc.
Family-focused psychotherapy	Yes	Yes	Involves a patient and a family member or their choice (note: support does not have to be an actual family member) Focuses on providing psychoeducation about the illness to the patient and family Promotes problem solving and communication
Interpersonal social rhythm therapy	Yes	Yes	Combines psychoeducation with mood and activity tracking to promote regularity of routines (social rhythms), with a special focus on sleep Identifies and helps patients work through an interpersonal problem that impacts mood stability Recognizes and treats grieving over the loss of the "healthy" self
Integrated care management	Yes	Yes	Provides individual and group treatment combined with case management to promote treatment connection and communication between treating healthcare professionals Focuses on psychoeducation and illness management skills

Adapted from Swartz et al. [73]

3.7 Conclusions

Bipolar disorder may not be as common as popularly believed, though those with the disorder are often high utilizers of medical care. Like others with serious mental illness, bipolar patients experience high rates of morbidity and mortality due to poor access to mental health treatment, difficult to treat symptoms, and a high prevalence and undertreatment of common medical conditions. There are many effective medical and psychotherapeutic treatments for bipolar disorder. Though the pharmacological treatments require close monitoring and vigilance against serious side effects, much of this can be successfully managed by an astute PCP. Moreover, partnering with a psychiatrist, primary care clinicians are well equipped to provide preventative care and treatment of the many common medical conditions comorbid to this illness. A good PCP can, in fact, be a valuable patient ally for achieving a high quality of life despite the disorder's profound challenges.

References

1. Angst J, Sellaro R. Historical perspectives and natural history of bipolar disorder. Biol Psychiatry. 2000;48(6):445–57. https://doi.org/10.1016/s0006-3223(00)00909-4.
2. Angst J, Gamma A, Sellaro R, Lavori PW, Zhang H. Recurrence of bipolar disorders and major depression: a life-long perspective. Eur Arch Psychiatry Clin Neurosci. 2003;253(5):236–40.
3. Aripiprazole [package insert]. Tokyo, Japan: Otsuka Pharmaceutical Co., Ltd.; 2014.
4. Asenapine [package insert]. Irvine, CA: Merck Sharp & Dohme B. V.; used by Allergan under license; 2017.
5. Baddour E, Tewksbury A, Stauner N. Valproic acid-induced hyperammonemia: incidence, clinical significance, and treatment management. Ment Health Clin. 2018;8(2):73–7. https://doi.org/10.9740/mhc.2018.03.073. PMID: 29955549; PMCID: PMC6007737.
6. Bauer M, Gitlin M. The essential guide to lithium treatment. Switzerland: Springer; 2016.
7. Bowden CL, Asnis GM, Ginsberg LD, Bentley B, Leadbetter R, White R. Safety and tolerability of lamotrigine for bipolar disorder. Drug Saf. 2004;27(3):173–84. https://doi.org/10.2165/00002018-200427030-00002.
8. Bowden CL, Perlis RH, Thase ME, Ketter TA, Ostacher MM, Calabrese JR, Reilly-Harrington NA, Gonzalez JM, Singh V, Nierenberg AA, Sachs GS. Aims and results of the NIMH systematic treatment enhancement program for bipolar disorder (STEP-BD). CNS Neurosci Ther. 2012;18(3):243–9. https://doi.org/10.1111/j.1755-5949.2011.00257.x. Epub 2011 Jun 7. PMID: 22070541; PMCID: PMC6493527.
9. Buoli M, Serati M, Botturi A, Altamura AC. The risk of thrombocytopenia during valproic acid therapy: a critical summary of available clinical data. Drugs R D. 2018;18(1):1–5. https://doi.org/10.1007/s40268-017-0224-6. PMID: 29260458; PMCID: PMC5833908.
10. Calabrese JR, Sullivan JR, Bowden CL, Suppes T, Goldberg JF, Sachs GS, Shelton MD, Goodwin FK, Frye MA, Kusumakar V. Rash in multicenter trials of lamotrigine in mood disorders: clinical relevance and management. J Clin Psychiatry. 2002;63(11):1012–9. https://doi.org/10.4088/jcp.v63n1110. PMID: 1244481.
11. Calkin CV, Gardner DM, Ransom T, Alda M. The relationship between bipolar disorder and type 2 diabetes: more than just co-morbid disorders. Ann Med. 2013;45(2):171–81. https://doi.org/10.3109/07853890.2012.687835. Epub 2012 May 24
12. Cariprazine [package insert]. Parsippany, NJ: Actavis Pharma, Inc; 2015.
13. Chen CH, Lin SK. Carbamazepine treatment of bipolar disorder: a retrospective evaluation of naturalistic long-term outcomes. BMC Psychiatry. 2012;12:47. https://doi.org/10.1186/1471-244X-12-47. PMID: 22620289; PMCID: PMC3410809.
14. Chengappa KN, Perkins KA, Brar JS, Schlicht PJ, Turkin SR, Hetrick ML, Levine MD, George TP. Varenicline for smoking cessation in bipolar disorder: a randomized, double-blind, placebo-controlled study. J Clin Psychiatry. 2014;75(7):765–72. https://doi.org/10.4088/JCP.13m08756.
15. Close H, Reilly J, Mason JM, Kripalani M, Wilson D, Main J, Hungin AP. Renal failure in lithium-treated bipolar disorder: a retrospective cohort study. PLoS One. 2014;9(3):e90169. https://doi.org/10.1371/journal.pone.0090169. PMID: 24670976; PMCID: PMC3966731.

16. Cole DP, Thase ME, Mallinger AG, Soares JC, Luther JF, Kupfer DJ, Frank E. Slower treatment response in bipolar depression predicted by lower pretreatment thyroid function. Am J Psychiatry. 2002;159(1):116–21. https://doi.org/10.1176/appi.ajp.159.1.116.
17. Correll CU, Frederickson AM, Kane JM, Manu P. Equally increased risk for metabolic syndrome in patients with bipolar disorder and schizophrenia treated with second-generation antipsychotics. Bipolar Disord. 2008;10(7):788–97. https://doi.org/10.1111/j.1399-5618.2008.00625.x.
18. Cowdry RW, Wehr TA, Zis AP, Goodwin FK. Thyroid abnormalities associated with rapid-cycling bipolar illness. Arch Gen Psychiatry. 1983;40(4):414–20. https://doi.org/10.1001/archpsyc.1983.01790040068010.
19. Crump C, Sundquist K, Winkleby MA, Sundquist J. Comorbidities and mortality in bipolar disorder: a Swedish national cohort study. JAMA Psychiat. 2013;70(9):931–9. https://doi.org/10.1001/jamapsychiatry.2013.1394.
20. Culpepper L. The diagnosis and treatment of bipolar disorder: decision-making in primary care. Prim Care Companion CNS Disord. 2014;16(3):PCC.13r01609. https://doi.org/10.4088/PCC.13r01609. Epub 2014 Jun 19. PMID: 25317368; PMCID: PMC4195640.
21. Cuomo A, Bolognesi S, Goracci A, Ciuoli C, Beccarini Crescenzi B, Maina G, Rosso G, Facchi E, Maccora C, Giordano N, Verdino V, Fagiolini A. Feasibility, adherence and efficacy of liraglutide treatment in a sample of individuals with mood disorders and obesity. Front Psychiatry. 2019;9:784. https://doi.org/10.3389/fpsyt.2018.00784. PMID: 30728788; PMCID: PMC6351474.
22. Diagnostic and Statistical Manual of Mental Disorders: DSM-5. 5th ed., American Psychiatric Association; 2013.
23. Dutta S, Reed RC. Divalproex to divalproex extended release conversion. Clin Drug Investig. 2004;24(9):495–508. https://doi.org/10.2165/00044011-200424090-00001.
24. Elmslie JL, Silverstone JT, Mann JI, Williams SM, Romans SE. Prevalence of overweight and obesity in bipolar patients. J Clin Psychiatry. 2000;61(3):179–84. https://doi.org/10.4088/jcp.v61n0306.
25. Fagiolini A, Frank E, Houck PR, Mallinger AG, Swartz HA, Buysse DJ, Ombao H, Kupfer DJ. Prevalence of obesity and weight change during treatment in patients with bipolar I disorder. J Clin Psychiatry. 2002;63(6):528–33. https://doi.org/10.4088/jcp.v63n0611.
26. Flores EJ, Park ER, Irwin KE. Improving lung cancer screening access for individuals with serious mental illness. J Am Coll Radiol. 2019;16(4 Pt B):596–600. https://doi.org/10.1016/j.jacr.2018.12.045. PMID: 30947893; PMCID: PMC6536304.
27. Forty L, Ulanova A, Jones L, Jones I, Gordon-Smith K, Fraser C, Farmer A, McGuffin P, Lewis CM, Hosang GM, Rivera M, Craddock N. Comorbid medical illness in bipolar disorder. Br J Psychiatry. 2014;205(6):465–72. https://doi.org/10.1192/bjp.bp.114.152249. Epub 2014. PMID: 25359927; PMCID: PMC4248234.
28. Gannon JM. Three recommendations for addressing the ongoing lithium underutilization crisis in bipolar disorder. Bipolar Disord. 2021;23(1):84–5. https://doi.org/10.1111/bdi.12914. Epub 2020 Apr 28.
29. Gitlin M. Lithium side effects and toxicity: prevalence and management strategies. Int J Bipolar Disord. 2016;4(1):27. https://doi.org/10.1186/s40345-016-0068-y. Epub 2016 Dec 17. PMID: 27900734; PMCID: PMC5164879.
30. Goldstein BI, Fagiolini A, Houck P, Kupfer DJ. Cardiovascular disease and hypertension among adults with bipolar I disorder in the United States. Bipolar Disord. 2009;11:657–62.
31. Goodwin FK, Jamison KR. Manic-depressive illness: bipolar disorders and recurrent depression. New York, NY: Oxford University Press; 2007.
32. Grunze H, Vieta E, Goodwin GM, Bowden C, Licht RW, Möller HJ, Kasper S, WFSBP Task Force on Treatment Guidelines for Bipolar Disorders. The World Federation of Societies of Biological Psychiatry (WFSBP) guidelines for the biological treatment of bipolar disorders: update 2012 on the long-term treatment of bipolar disorder. World J Biol Psychiatry. 2013;14(3):154–219. https://doi.org/10.3109/15622975.2013.770551.

33. Gupta S, Kripalani M, Khastgir U, Reilly J. Management of the renal adverse effects of lithium. Advances in Psychiatric Treatment. Cambridge University Press. 2013;19(6):457–66. https://doi.org/10.1192/apt.bp.112.010306.
34. Haussmann R, Bauer M, von Bonin S, Grof P, Lewitzka U. Treatment of lithium intoxication: facing the need for evidence. Int J Bipolar Disord. 2015;3(1):23. https://doi.org/10.1186/s40345-015-0040-2. Epub 2015 Oct 22. PMID: 26493348; PMCID: PMC4615994.
35. Hayes JF, Osborn DPJ, Francis E, Ambler G, Tomlinson LA, Boman M, Wong ICK, Geddes JR, Dalman C, Lewis G. Prediction of individuals at high risk of chronic kidney disease during treatment with lithium for bipolar disorder. BMC Med. 2021;19(1):99. https://doi.org/10.1186/s12916-021-01964-z. PMID: 33906644; PMCID: PMC8080385.
36. Heffner JL, Strawn JR, DelBello MP, Strakowski SM, Anthenelli RM. The co-occurrence of cigarette smoking and bipolar disorder: phenomenology and treatment considerations. Bipolar Disord. 2011;13(5–6):439–53. https://doi.org/10.1111/j.1399-5618.2011.00943.x. PMID: 22017214; PMCID: PMC3729285.
37. Hirschfeld RMA, Williams JBW, Spitzer RL, et al. Development and validation of a screening instrument for bipolar spectrum disorder: the Mood Disorder Questionnaire. Am J Psychiatry. 2000;157(11):1873–5.
38. Hirschfeld RM, Lewis L, Vornik LA. Perceptions and impact of bipolar disorder: how far have we really come? Results of the national depressive and manic-depressive association 2000 survey of individuals with bipolar disorder. J Clin Psychiatry. 2003b;64(2):161–74.
39. Hirschfeld R, Bowden CL, Gitlin MJ, Keck PE, Suppes T, Thase ME, Wagner KD, Perlis RH. Practice guideline for the treatment of patients with bipolar disorder (revision). Focus. 2003a;1(1):64–110.
40. Hsu JH, Chien IC, Lin CH. Increased risk of chronic obstructive pulmonary disease in patients with bipolar disorder: A population-based study. J Affect Disord. 2017;220:43–8. https://doi.org/10.1016/j.jad.2017.05.049. Epub 2017 May 31.
41. Iwagami M, Mansfield KE, Hayes JF, Walters K, Osborn DP, Smeeth L, Nitsch D, Tomlinson LA. Severe mental illness and chronic kidney disease: a cross-sectional study in the United Kingdom. Clin Epidemiol. 2018;10:421–9. https://doi.org/10.2147/CLEP.S154841. PMID: 29713199; PMCID: PMC5907783.
42. Jain S. Valproate-induced hair loss: What to tell patients. Curr Psychol. 2011;10(11):62.
43. Lamotrigine [package insert]. Research Triangle Park, NC: GlaxoSmithKline; 2009.
44. LiverTox: Clinical and Research Information on Drug-Induced Liver Injury [Internet]. Bethesda (MD): National Institute of Diabetes and Digestive and Kidney Diseases; 2012. Valproate. [Updated 2020 Jul 31].
45. Ljubicic D, Letica-Crepulja M, Vitezic D, Bistrovic IL, Ljubicic R. Lithium treatments: single and multiple daily dosing. Can J Psychiatr. 2008;53(5):323–31. https://doi.org/10.1177/070674370805300507.
46. Lurasidone [package insert]. Chuo-ku, Osaka, Japan: Dainippon Sumitomo Pharma Co. Ltd.; 2013.
47. Maina G, Salvi V, Vitalucci A, D'Ambrosio V, Bogetto F. Prevalence and correlates of overweight in drug-naïve patients with bipolar disorder. J Affect Disord. 2008;110(1–2):149–55. https://doi.org/10.1016/j.jad.2007.12.233. Epub 2008 Jan 29.
48. Malhi GS, Adams D, Lampe L, Paton M, O'Connor N, Newton LA, Walter G, Taylor A, Porter R, Mulder RT, Berk M, Northern Sydney Central Coast Mental Health Drug & Alcohol; NSW Health Clinical Redesign Program; CADE Clinic. University of Sydney Clinical practice recommendations for bipolar disorder. Acta Psychiatr Scand Suppl. 2009;439:27–46. https://doi.org/10.1111/j.1600-0447.2009.01383.x.
49. Malhi GS, Bassett D, Boyce P, Bryant R, Fitzgerald PB, Fritz K, Hopwood M, Lyndon B, Mulder R, Murray G, Porter R, Singh AB. Royal Australian and New Zealand College of Psychiatrists clinical practice guidelines for mood disorders. Aust N Z J Psychiatry. 2015;49(12):1087–206. https://doi.org/10.1177/0004867415617657.

50. Malhi GS, Bell E, Outhred T, Berk M. Lithium therapy and its interactions. Aust Prescr. 2020;43(3):91–3. https://doi.org/10.18773/austprescr.2020.024. Epub 2020 Jun 2. Erratum in: Aust Prescr. 2020 Aug;43(4):141. PMID: 32675910; PMCID: PMC7358048.
51. McElroy SL, Keck PE Jr, Pope HG Jr, Hudson JI. Valproate in the treatment of bipolar disorder: literature review and clinical guidelines. J Clin Psychopharmacol. 1992;12(1 Suppl):42S–52S. https://doi.org/10.1097/00004714-199202001-00007.
52. McGinty EE, Zhang Y, Guallar E, Ford DE, Steinwachs D, Dixon LB, Keating NL, Daumit GL. Cancer incidence in a sample of Maryland residents with serious mental illness. Psychiatr Serv. 2012;63(7):714–7. https://doi.org/10.1176/appi.ps.201100169. PMID: 22752037; PMCID: PMC3878874.
53. Mcintyre Roger S, Soczynska JK, Beyer JL, Woldeyohannes HO, Law CWY, Miranda A, Konarski JZ, Kennedy SH. Medical comorbidity in bipolar disorder: reprioritizing unmet needs. Curr Opinion Psychiatry. 2007;20(4):406. https://doi.org/10.1097/YCO.0b013e3281938102.
54. Meador KJ. Fetal valproate exposure and attention-deficit/hyperactivity disorder. JAMA Netw Open. 2019;2(1):e186603. https://doi.org/10.1001/jamanetworkopen.2018.6603.
55. Meehan AD, Humble MB, Yazarloo P, Järhult J, Wallin G. The prevalence of lithium-associated hyperparathyroidism in a large Swedish population attending psychiatric outpatient units. J Clin Psychopharmacol. 2015;35(3):279–85. https://doi.org/10.1097/JCP.0000000000000303.
56. Merikangas KR, Akiskal HS, Angst J, Greenberg PE, Hirschfeld RMA, Petukhova M, Kessler RC. Lifetime and 12-month prevalence of bipolar spectrum disorder in the National Comorbidity Survey Replication. Arch Gen Psychiatry. 2007;64(5):543–52.
57. Merikangas KR, Jin R, He JP, Kessler RC, Lee S, Sampson NA, Viana MC, Andrade LH, Hu C, Karam EG, Ladea M, Medina-Mora ME, Ono Y, Posada-Villa J, Sagar R, Wells JE, Zarkov Z. Prevalence and correlates of bipolar spectrum disorder in the world mental health survey initiative. Arch Gen Psychiatry. 2011;68(3):241–51. https://doi.org/10.1001/archgenpsychiatry.2011.12. PMID: 21383262; PMCID: PMC3486639.
58. Miklowitz DJ, Efthimiou O, Furukawa TA, Scott J, McLaren R, Geddes JR, Cipriani A. Adjunctive psychotherapy for bipolar disorder: a systematic review and component network meta-analysis. JAMA Psychiat. 2021;78(2):141–50.
59. Miller C, Bauer MS. Excess mortality in bipolar disorders. Curr Psychiatry Rep. 2014;16(11):499. https://doi.org/10.1007/s11920-014-0499-z.
60. National Collaborating Centre for Mental Health (UK). Bipolar disorder: The NICE guideline on the assessment and management of bipolar disorder in adults, children and young people in primary and secondary care. London: The British Psychological Society and The Royal College of Psychiatrists; 2014.
61. Ng F, Hallam K, Lucas N, Berk M. The role of lamotrigine in the management of bipolar disorder. Neuropsychiatr Dis Treat. 2007;3(4):463–74. PMID: 19300575; PMCID: PMC2655087.
62. Nielsen RE, Kugathasan P, Straszek S, Jensen SE, Licht RW. Why are somatic diseases in bipolar disorder insufficiently treated? Int J Bipolar Disord. 2019;7(1):12. https://doi.org/10.1186/s40345-019-0147-y. PMID: 31055668; PMCID: PMC6500513.
63. Olanzapine [package insert]. Indianapolis, IN: Eli Lilly and Company; 2009.
64. Perrild H, Hegedüs L, Baastrup PC, Kayser L, Kastberg S. Thyroid function and ultrasonically determined thyroid size in patients receiving long-term lithium treatment. Am J Psychiatry. 1990;147(11):1518–21. https://doi.org/10.1176/ajp.147.11.1518.
65. Perugi G, Quaranta G, Belletti S, Casalini F, Mosti N, Toni C, Dell'Osso L. General medical conditions in 347 bipolar disorder patients: clinical correlates of metabolic and autoimmune-allergic diseases. J Affect Disord. 2015;170:95–103.
66. Quetiapine [package insert]. Wilmington, DE: AstraZeneca Pharmaceuticals LP; 2013.
67. Reed RC, Dutta S. Does it really matter when a blood sample for valproic acid concentration is taken following once-daily administration of divalproex-ER? Ther Drug Monit. 2006;28(3):413–8. https://doi.org/10.1097/01.ftd.0000211814.12311.3f.
68. Risperidone [package insert]. Titusville, NJ: Ortho-McNeil-Janssen Pharmaceuticals, Inc; 2009.

69. Severus WE, Kleindienst N, Seemüller F, Frangou S, Möller HJ, Greil W. What is the optimal serum lithium level in the long-term treatment of bipolar disorder--a review? Bipolar Disord. 2008;10(2):231–7. https://doi.org/10.1111/j.1399-5618.2007.00475.x.
70. Solomon DA, Leon AC, Coryell WH, Endicott J, Li C, Fiedorowicz JG, Boyken L, Keller MB. Longitudinal course of bipolar I disorder: duration of mood episodes. Arch Gen Psychiatry. 2010;67(4):339–47. https://doi.org/10.1001/archgenpsychiatry.2010.15. PMID: 20368510; PMCID: PMC3677763.
71. Soreca I, Fagiolini A, Frank E, Houck PR, Thompson WK, Kupfer DJ. Relationship of general medical burden, duration of illness and age in patients with bipolar I disorder. J Psychiatr Res. 2008;42(11):956–61. https://doi.org/10.1016/j.jpsychires.2007.10.009. Epub 2008 Feb 20.
72. Stone KA. Lithium-induced nephrogenic diabetes insipidus. J Am Board Fam Pract. 1999;12(1):43–7. https://doi.org/10.3122/15572625-12-1-43.
73. Swartz HA, Swanson J. Psychotherapy for bipolar disorder in adults: a review of the evidence. Focus (Am Psychiatr Publ). 2014;12(3):251–66. https://doi.org/10.1176/appi.focus.12.3.251. PMID: 26279641; PMCID: PMC4536930.
74. Wang XQ, Xiong J, Xu WH, Yu SY, Huang XS, Zhang JT, Tian CL, Huang DH, Jia WQ, Lang SY. Risk of a lamotrigine-related skin rash: current meta-analysis and postmarketing cohort analysis. Seizure. 2015;25:52–61. https://doi.org/10.1016/j.seizure.2014.12.001; Epub 2014 Dec 23.
75. Weiner M, Warren L, Fiedorowicz JG. Cardiovascular morbidity and mortality in bipolar disorder. Ann Clin Psychiatry. 2011;23(1):40–7. PMID: 21318195; PMCID: PMC3190964.
76. Yatham LN, Kennedy SH, Parikh SV, Schaffer A, Beaulieu S, Alda M, O'Donovan C, Macqueen G, McIntyre RS, Sharma V, Ravindran A, Young LT, Milev R, Bond DJ, Frey BN, Goldstein BI, Lafer B, Birmaher B, Ha K, Nolen WA, Berk M. Canadian Network for Mood and Anxiety Treatments (CANMAT) and International Society for Bipolar Disorders (ISBD) collaborative update of CANMAT guidelines for the management of patients with bipolar disorder: update 2013. Bipolar Disord. 2013;15(1):1–44.
77. Zimmerman M, Ruggero CJ, Chelminski I, Young D. Is bipolar disorder overdiagnosed? J Clin Psychiatry. 2008;69(6):935–40. https://doi.org/10.4088/jcp.v69n0608. PMID: 18466044.
78. Ziprasidone [package insert]. New York, NY: Pfizer; 2014.

Chapter 4
Schizophrenia

A 60-year-old patient, A.B., presents to your clinic for an initial visit. He has a history of schizophrenia, and his medical history is otherwise unknown. Rooming staff tells you that the patient was brought in by his new group home; prior to his moving there a month ago, he had been homeless. Vitals are reported as unremarkable except for blood pressure of 145/90 and a body mass index of 30. You review the patient's medication list and see that the patient is on nightly risperidone 4 mg prescribed by a local psychiatrist, Dr. G. When you enter the room, you note that the patient is wearing several layers of clothing, inappropriate for the warm weather, and smells of stale cigarette smoke. He does not make good eye contact when you introduce yourself. He appears distracted at times though is fully oriented on questioning. He is generally cooperative but with an occasional irritable edge. He stands from a chair and walks over to the exam table without any difficulty, though you do notice a very slight resting tremor in his right hand when he is seated. His speech is minimal and slow. He says his mood is good, and he denies any anxiety, but he is minimally expressive. During your physical exam, he mumbles to himself several times. You ultimately ask if he is hearing anything other than the sound of your voice. He denies this but then rather abruptly announces that he refuses to "let the FBI interfere," a statement that he cannot or will not explain when you seek clarification. In reviewing his medication, he tells you that he takes risperidone for sleep, though he denies having any issues with sleep. He says he sees a "Dr. G" for medication and meets regularly with a nice lady named Mandy who is "teaching [me] how to relax." He also denies any drug and alcohol use but admits to smoking 1 pack per day and states that he is not interested in quitting.

R. Hudak, J. M. Gannon, *Handbook of Psychiatric Disorders in Adults in the Primary Care Setting*, Current Clinical Practice,
https://doi.org/10.1007/978-3-030-98709-1_4

4.1 What Is Schizophrenia?

4.1.1 Introduction and Epidemiology

Schizophrenia is a psychiatric disorder that has captured the public imagination for well over a century. Psychosis, the hallmark of this disorder, has punctuated human history for far longer. While most medical professionals understand that people with schizophrenia do not spend their lives in gothic asylums, few are aware that many people with schizophrenia can live with minimal symptoms and achieve traditional markers of "success," including having a career, living independently, sustaining long-term romantic relationships, and raising children. As such, A.B.'s case, while prototypical for schizophrenia, is not as common a presentation to mental health clinics as one may think. In this chapter, we hope to provide a more realistic and nuanced depiction of schizophrenia and its treatment. While destigmatizing the illness is a lofty goal, we hope that reading the next few pages will empower primary care physicians (PCPs) and advanced practice providers (APPs) working in primary care with the knowledge necessary to comfortably address this population's healthcare needs. Working hand in hand with psychiatrists and trained behavioral health staff, whenever possible, is critical to providing whole person care to this population.

While worldwide, the lifetime prevalence of schizophrenia is only around 0.7%, this disorder remains one of the leading causes of disability across the globe. Higher and lower incidences of schizophrenia [54] have been found in certain regions of the world, but diagnostic heterogeneity likely influences these findings. Schizophrenia is generally thought to be equally common in men and women, though men may be more likely to have a severe course and a younger age of onset [42]. Men are most likely to develop schizophrenia in their late teens and early 20s, whereas women develop schizophrenia primarily in their late 20s and into their early 30s and have a second peak of onset in their mid to late 40s [37]. While it was once thought that, in the United States, schizophrenia was more common in African Americans, this is now considered to be a byproduct of racial bias impacting diagnosis.

Heritability likely plays some role in the development of schizophrenia, but heritability risks should not be overstated. If one of a pair of monozygotic twins is diagnosed with schizophrenia, the risk of schizophrenia manifesting in the other twin is only around 50% [31]. Other putative risk factors are broad and include being single, being born to migrant parents, being fathered by a man of advanced paternal age, living in an urban environment, living in poverty, surviving childhood trauma, and birth month (rates of schizophrenia are higher in those born in winter and early spring) [13]. Specific maternal health factors are also commonly associated with an increased risk of schizophrenia and include preeclampsia, maternal infection (particularly if occurring during second trimester and from influenza, rubella, poliomyelitis, or toxoplasmosis), severe stress, and obstetrical complications [13]. Finally, substance use during adolescence, especially heavy use of high potency, THC-containing marijuana, has also been associated with the development of schizophrenia [23].

The prognosis, response to treatment, and natural course of schizophrenia spectrum disorders can widely vary between patients [73], so much so that many clinicians opine that there must be multiple "schizophrenias" that we have not yet defined. With treatment, some patients have as few as one or two acute episodes of psychosis over their lifetime, while others may have multiple episodes requiring multiple periods of intensive intervention, including inpatient hospitalizations. Acute episodes can last days to weeks to months. Between acute episodes, which are commonly defined as a marked increase in positive psychotic symptoms requiring aggressive psychiatric intervention, some patients will have minimal to no symptoms. Still others will have significant psychotic symptoms at their baseline (during the "maintenance" phase of treatment). Some patients will completely recover after acute episodes; others will lose functionality with each episode. Still other patients will have minimal positive symptoms but have profound negative symptoms that have an episodic, chronic but stable, or chronic and gradually worsening course. Until the era when reliable biomarkers can be identified to not only confirm diagnosis but guide treatment selection and predict treatment response, careful diagnosis by interview and patient-centered treatment selection guided by the available evidence base as well as patient preference remains the standard of care.

While a strong, therapeutic relationship with healthcare team members and informed natural supports can help promote treatment engagement, patients with schizophrenia sometimes lack insight into either having an illness or the benefits of treatment. This lack of insight can greatly impede a patient's recovery. While patients with schizophrenia may not always appreciate a need for treatment, forced treatment is usually not an option outside of a locked mental health facility. Moreover, involuntary admission criteria to these facilities generally require substantive risk to the patient's life or that of others, though the nuances of this varies from region to region. Patients who broadly lack capacity to make decisions in multiple life domains may qualify for guardianship or conservatorship, based on regional law; even in patients with a legal guardian or conservator, however, compelling mental health treatment is legally complex and ethically fraught. While many treatment barriers exist in schizophrenia, a patient's own refusal to engage in care is one of the most difficult for loved ones and caregivers to understand. Combined with an all-too-common lack of readily available behavioral health and community resources for individuals with serious mental illness, lack of mental healthcare utilization is thought to heavily contribute to relatively high rates of homelessness [28], unemployment [65], and incarceration [62] in this population.

While there is an elevated risk of violence associated with schizophrenia, mental illness is linked with only an estimated 4% of the violence that occurs in the population at large [76]. In addition, most acts of violence committed by people with schizophrenia will be against caregivers rather than strangers. Elevated risk for violence in schizophrenia is associated with general violence risk factors; these include male gender, nonadherence with psychiatric treatment, comorbid antisocial personality disorder, and substance misuse. In one study, when patients with comorbid substance abuse disorders were excluded, the rates of having committed a violent offense among people with schizophrenia was 8.5% compared to 5.3% in the general population [26]. Moreover, individuals with schizophrenia are at much greater risk of being victims, rather than perpetrators, of violent crime. Given this finding, trauma-informed care in this population can be very helpful.

4.2 Schizophrenia in the Medical Setting

4.2.1 Primary Care

PCPs and primary care teams play a critical role in the lives of people with schizophrenia. Early identification of the disorder is essential, and many PCPs will find themselves referring people with psychotic symptoms to psychiatry, including at first onset of symptoms. Longer duration of untreated psychosis after the first emergence of symptoms has been associated with poorer outcomes [1], so timely referral to psychiatry, especially where specialized early course treatments are available, is critical. Lack of behavioral health resources, let alone high-quality psychiatric care, can be a significant barrier to initial referral and to ongoing care, leaving PCPs with the rather daunting prospect of assuming the role of primary treater. In all but the most stable patients with schizophrenia, however, psychiatric engagement is highly recommended.

While patients with schizophrenia may struggle with consistently accessing psychiatric care, engagement with medical care is also fraught. While about 5% of patients with schizophrenia die from suicide (most commonly early in the course of illness) [57], and while mortality rates from accidents and injuries are high in this population, most of the excess mortality associated with schizophrenia is attributable to common medical conditions [16], including cardiovascular, respiratory, and infectious diseases. Malignancies like lung cancer are also a common cause of death. The prevalence of tobacco dependency in schizophrenia is quite elevated [79], and individuals with schizophrenia who do smoke are often heavy smokers. Smoking, along with high rates of metabolic syndrome, likely accounts for the majority of the up to 15–25 year decreased lifespan in individuals with schizophrenia spectrum disorder [77].

Given these findings, individuals with schizophrenia spectrum disorders clearly require excellent PCPs who will champion preventative care, provide ongoing care of commonly comorbid medical illness, and work with psychiatric teams on screening for and treating potential medication side effects. Unfortunately, health disparities are common in this population, driven by multiple factors, including stigma by clinicians, a fragmented healthcare system, poverty, and illness-related factors. Individuals with schizophrenia are less likely to receive appropriate routine health screening, even when they appropriately present for care [43, 50], and they do not consistently receive standard of care wellness counseling [11]. There is also compelling evidence that patients with schizophrenia do not receive adequate workup of presenting complaints [21, 39], monitoring and treatment of comorbid medical disorders [30, 41, 53], or treatment for life-threatening conditions [40].

A number of guidelines have been proposed for screening for metabolic syndrome associated with atypical antipsychotics (also called second-generation antipsychotics (SGAs)) frequently prescribed for the disorder. A review of these tools suggests that a patient's personal medical history be taken at baseline (just prior to antipsychotic initiation) and that weight/waist circumference/BMI, blood pressure, and serum fasting glucose and lipids be obtained at baseline and at 6 weeks, at 12 weeks, and at least yearly after antipsychotic initiation. Counseling on healthy lifestyles should also be given alongside those screenings [14]; this is especially critical as patients with schizophrenia are thought to be more sedentary [70] and often eat nutritionally poorer diets [19]. These guidelines dovetail with those established by the American Psychiatric Association, the American Diabetes Association (ADA), the American Psychiatric Association (APA), the American Association of Clinical Endocrinologists (AACE), and the North American Association for the Study of Obesity (NAASO) in 2004 for routine metabolic screening with SGAs [2]. It is these specific guidelines, illustrated in Table 4.1, that are generally considered the standard of care in monitoring individuals taking atypical antipsychotics.

A.B. is on risperidone, has a mildly elevated blood pressure, and is obese. Collaboration with others may help in gathering further medical history. Obtaining fasting lipids and a hemoglobin A1c is indicated based on his being prescribed risperidone. Subsequent discussions with the patient's psychiatrist on continued use of risperidone in lieu of more metabolically neutral antipsychotics may be helpful. Evidence-based treatment of untreated medical conditions is indicated.

Table 4.1 Metabolic monitoring for prescribing second-generation antipsychotics (SGAs). Personal and family medical history should include a specific review of obesity, diabetes, hypertension, and cardiovascular disease

	Baseline	1 month	2 months	3 months	6 months	9 months	Annually
Personal and family medical history	x			x			x
Weight	x	x	x	x	x	x	x
Waist circumference	x			x			x
Blood pressure	x			x			x
Fasting glucose/ hemoglobin A1c	x			x			x
Fasting lipid profile	x			x			x

Adapted from ADA et al. [2]

Avoiding the use of medications associated with high cardiometabolic risk, and attempting medication switches to more neutral medication if the patient is at risk for, or is developing, metabolic syndrome, is a best clinical practice. That said, such switches may not always be clinically appropriate, particularly if the patient is at high risk for severe psychotic decompensation and has already undergone multiple treatment trials that were not effective and/or caused other, even less tolerable side effects. While some metabolic effects may be dose related, i.e., mitigated by dose reduction, this isn't always clear. As noted above, patients with schizophrenia often lead sedentary lifestyles and have poor diets, and specific symptoms of the illness (like negative symptoms and lack of insight into need for medical treatment) can also interfere with healthcare follow-up. As such, effective, evidence-based behavioral therapies for weight loss in schizophrenia [6, 12] have been developed to help activate patients to improve their diet and increase physical activity. While these specific interventions may not be readily accessible to patients and their caregivers in a community setting, more general, high-quality, patient-centered dietary counseling and physical training can be quite helpful to patients with schizophrenia. Antipsychotic-associated weight gain may also be mitigated by topiramate and metformin; these medications have also demonstrated efficacy in promoting weight loss in patients on SGAs [35, 48]. Further research is needed into routine use of glucagon-like peptide agonists for antipsychotic-associated weight gain, although early studies have shown promise [68].

In addition to metabolic disturbances, patients prescribed antipsychotic medications may struggle with other medication side effects that can benefit from active PCP management. Anticholinergic burden with antipsychotics is often high, which can lead to memory impairment, dry mouth, constipation, blurred vision, urinary retention, and tachycardia [46]. When patients are prescribed highly anticholinergic antipsychotics (see tables below), avoiding prescribing anticholinergic medications used for medical indications, e.g., oxybutynin for incontinence, is recommended. Obtaining orthostatic vitals and screening for orthostatic hypotension in patients complaining of light-headedness, dizziness, or falls is also recommended for patients prescribed antipsychotics with significant effects at alpha receptors (e.g., clozapine, quetiapine, iloperidone). Care should be taken when prescribing antihypertensives in patients on such medications. Sometimes, dividing the dose of the antipsychotic medication can be helpful for orthostatic symptoms, as well as can decreasing the dose or switching to a different antipsychotic when feasible. Behavioral management strategies, including the use of support stockings and increasing fluid and dietary salt intake, are often helpful. If those strategies are not effective, prescribing fludrocortisone is recommended.

As noted above, rates of tobacco dependence are also extremely high in this population, with prevalence rates around 60% worldwide [15]. Tobacco use screening, tobacco use counseling, and tobacco abuse treatment are all done quite successfully by both psychiatrists and PCPs. While many patients with schizophrenia are heavy smokers and may struggle to quit, they can and do benefit from smoking cessation treatments, with good evidence for the use of bupropion [75] and at least moderate evidence for varenicline [24, 75]. Research is still lacking in establishing effective behavioral interventions to supplement these medication treatments [75].

As was done in A.B.'s case, screening for tobacco use is always indicated. Tobacco cessation counseling should also be completed at every visit. Complete cessation should be a goal for all patients.

Finally, while sexual dysfunction may occur in schizophrenia secondary to symptoms of the disorder itself, sexual side effects are common with many antipsychotics. This may be due to effects on serotonergic and adrenergic receptors. Prolactin elevation is also common with certain antipsychotics. This neurotransmitter activity can lead to decreased labido, erectile dysfunction, and anorgasmia. Ejaculatory disturbance, including retrograde ejaculation, has also been reported. Risk of osteoporosis and breast and endometrial cancer with prolactin elevation has occasionally been raised as an academic concern. However, no clear evidence has linked antipsychotic-induced hyperprolactinemia to these serious medical sequelae. For the treatment of sexual side effects, dose reduction of the antipsychotic can be attempted if otherwise clinically appropriate in stable patients. In the case of hyperprolactinemia, causes beyond medication side effects should be ruled out. Once workup has been completed, and antipsychotic dose reduction has failed or is contraindicated, addition of dopamine agonists, like bromocriptine or low-dose aripiprazole, can be trialed.

4.2.2 When to Refer

Sometimes, treatment of antipsychotic side effects benefits from the input of specialists. While initial workup by psychiatry and primary care is always recommended, and can sometimes negate the need for referral, the following specialties can be helpful in providing treatment recommendations in specific circumstances.

4.2.2.1 Neurology

Antipsychotic-induced movement disorders that can be loosely classified as extrapyramidal symptoms (EPS) are an often overlooked yet common side effect of antipsychotic medication. EPS is often noted by careful PCPs on physical examination. EPS more often presents with certain older or "first-generation antipsychotics" (FGAs), which may be chosen to treat patients with financial limitations (as they are often inexpensive), due to patient preference, and as they have much lower metabolic risks than do SGAs. Symptoms often emerge early in treatment; if symptoms occur after at least 3 months of exposure (or after 1 month of exposure in patients over 60), they are considered "late" or "tardive" symptoms. While tardive EPS may unfortunately persist after medication is stopped, sudden antipsychotic withdrawal or patient self-discontinuation can also result in EPS emergence or worsening and so should be avoided. Withdrawal EPS symptoms can often be addressed by restarting the agent, and if needed, slowly withdrawing it over the course of months; functional relief may also occur with judicious use of benzodiazepines in the case of dyskinesias.

The most alarming of the acute EPS, classically occurring within hours to a few days of initial antipsychotic exposure, are acute dystonias. Dystonias are spams of single muscles or muscle groups and can also be seen in other parts of the face (leading to grimacing, spasmodic blinking, etc.) or in the tongue, neck (e.g., torticollis), limbs, or trunk. The most well-known of the acute dystonias is oculogyric crisis, where patients experience the frightening sensation of their eyes spasmodically deviating, usually laterally or vertically. Patients in occulogyric crisis often call their PCPs in alarm or present to medical emergency rooms and urgent care centers. Occulogyric crises are generally painful and accompanied by lateral neck flexion, involuntary mouth opening, tongue protrusion, drooling, and difficulty speaking. Another type of severe, but often tardive, dystonia is opisthotonos, which includes severe arching of the neck and back. Dystonias most often occur in younger patients exposed to high potency, high-dose dopamine blocking antipsychotics. Acute dystonias often resolve with oral or intramuscular diphenhydramine or benztropine; tardive dystonias sometimes also respond to anticholinergic treatment, though botulinum toxin therapy for isolated muscle groups and dopamine depleting agents have also been used. Tardive dystonias can be quite disabling.

Parkinsonism is a classic type of EPS that generally presents early in treatment but can also emerge with dose changes and changes in drug metabolism during chronic treatment. The existence of strictly tardive, drug-induced Parkinsonism is debatable. Antipsychotic-associated Parkinsonism is generally indistinguishable from Parkinson's disease, with its classic, low frequency, high amplitude resting tremor. Bradykinesia and akinesia, cogwheel rigidity, masked faces, and shuffling gait may also be present. These symptoms will often diminish with dose reduction of the antipsychotic, addition of anticholinergic medication like benztropine, and time on medication.

A.B. has a slight resting tremor. Further evaluation may reveal mild cogwheeling. If not bothersome, this would not necessarily require intervention.

Akathisia is a particularly challenging form of EPS that also emerges early in treatment and can be quite disturbing for patients; it has even been linked to patient suicide. Akathisia is characterized by a feeling of internal restlessness and a need to move. It can be misdiagnosed as psychotic agitation or anxiety. Treatment for akathisia can be achieved by removal of the offending agent; benzodiazepines and non-cardioselective beta blockers like propranolol can also be helpful.

Tardive dyskinesia (TD) is the most classic of the tardive, antipsychotic-induced movement disorders and is characterized by repetitive, rhythmic, and occasionally purposeful seeming movements, e.g., may present as piano playing-like finger movements. TD can wax and wane in severity over time. Mild cases may be barely noticeable; severe cases can be quite disabling. Most commonly seen in the oral-buccal area and in the hands, tardive dyskinesia can also manifest as foot tapping or other rhythmic movements in the toes, trunk writhing, shrugging movements of the shoulders, and eye blinking. The incidence of TD is generally thought to be around 20% of patients on antipsychotics chronically [8]; the incidence increases with age and is most commonly linked to use of high potency, high-dose D2 blocking agents. It may be more common in women as well as in those with primary mood disorders, in smokers, and in patients with diabetes. African American patients and those with cognitive disorders or traumatic brain injuries may also be at higher risk. Tardive dyskinesia can sometimes be suppressed by increasing antipsychotic doses, though this is not a recommended treatment as symptoms will likely re-emerge over time and with increased severity. Discontinuing medications and/or switching to lower potency medications and/or SGAs (particularly clozapine) should generally be attempted with the emergence of TD and with some immediacy, as TD is sometimes reversible in early stages. Abrupt discontinuations are not recommended as withdrawal TD can emerge and lead to further complications. If dose reductions or medication switches are ineffective or clinically inadvisable, use of VMAT2 inhibitors is a reasonable approach. Examination for TD should be done every 6 months for patients on antipsychotic medications to monitor for TD or its progression; the Abnormal Involuntary Movement Scale (AIMS) is most used for this purpose.

Likely related to EPS and/or catatonia is the rarely seen but oft feared neuroleptic malignant syndrome (NMS). NMS is most frequently encountered within 72 hours of exposure to (or withdrawal from) high potency, D2 blocking FGAs and presents with the classic triad of fever, muscle rigidity, and sympathetic nervous system lability (e.g., tachycardia and/or hypertension). It may also present with markedly elevated CPK, increased respiratory rate, and altered mental status. While this condition can be deadly without treatment, it is important to rule out other etiologies that can mimic this condition, including malignant hyperthermia, heat stroke, alcohol or benzodiazepine withdrawal, anticholinergic syndrome, and central nervous system infections. NMS is quite rare, with an estimated incidence between 0.1% and 0.2% [67] in patients prescribed antipsychotics. NMS risk may be effectively mitigated by using lowest effective doses of antipsychotics and slower titrations of antipsychotics. If a patient has NMS, the antipsychotic should be discontinued and supportive treatment initiated. If the condition persists, benzodiazepines, dantrolene, bromocriptine, and ECT have all been reported as potentially effective treatments [38].

Seizures have also been associated with antipsychotics, particularly clozapine. High blood levels and rapid titrations of clozapine are likely risk factors for clozapine associated seizures. Tonic-clonic seizures are most often reported, though other seizure types may occur. Myoclonus can sometimes be a harbinger of frank seizure activity. Consultation with neurology is highly recommended when seizures are suspected. If antipsychotic therapy is to continue, lowering the dose of the medication and initiating anticonvulsant therapy may be indicated.

4.2.2.2 Cardiology

Many antipsychotic medications are associated with specific cardiac risks. The most well appreciated of these is QTc prolongation, which is associated with the ventricular tachyarrhythmia torsades de pointes. Of note, while the Bazett formula is still widely used to calculate QTc from electrocardiograms (ECGs), both the Fridericia and Framingham formulas are recommended for this purpose, as they may more accurately correct for heart rate and improve prediction of mortality risk [38]. While the quality of studies examining risk of QTc prolongation associated with antipsychotic medications varies widely, certain medications like pimozide should be used with caution. Routine screening with ECGs is not recommended, excepting before starting certain medications (e.g., chlorpromazine, iloperidone, pimozide, ziprasidone) or with significant dose changes with these medications, concerns for drug-drug interactions or renal/hepatic impairment, or change in patient cardiac history. Psychiatrists frequently consider a QTc interval > 500 msec as a threshold for concern, but the evidence supporting this approach is limited. When prescribing QTc prolonging antipsychotics, care should be used to limit the use of other QTc prolonging medications.

Other cardiac risks of antipsychotic medications include tachycardia, which can be seen with orthostatic hypotension, or can be due to anticholinergic side effects or direct medication effect. Clozapine especially is associated with tachycardia; while this is often a benign finding with clozapine, other causes of tachycardia should be ruled out (especially myocarditis) and an ECG obtained. Myocarditis and cardiomyopathy have both been reported with clozapine. Rates are overall very low, likely below 0.3% [38]. Myocarditis is most common in the first 6 months of treatment with clozapine, whereas cardiomyopathy tends to occur later. Patients prescribed clozapine and presenting with a combination of symptoms including shortness of breath, fatigue, chest pain, fever, palpitations, edema, and/or tachycardia merit urgent evaluation. Obtaining an ECG, C-reactive protein, and troponin (I and T subtypes) is indicated, as is consultation with cardiology [38]. When a patient has benign, medication-induced tachycardia, beta blockers can be prescribed, if not medically contraindicated and if the patient is symptomatic and has a resting pulse above 120 bpm.

4.2.2.3 Hematology

Severe neutropenia can occur with clozapine. Clozapine prescribing necessitates regular absolute neutrophil count monitoring as per Food and Drug Administration (FDA) Risk Evaluation and Mitigation Strategy (REMS) guidelines. The REMS also requires patient education on reporting of any signs of infection, particularly with clozapine initiation. The overall risk of neutropenia with clozapine, however, appears to be quite low, with an estimated incidence of 0.9% of clozapine-treated patients; of these patients, the fatality rate was 2.1% [52]. Notably, neutropenia and other dyscrasias have also been reported with multiple other antipsychotics. Consultation with hematology can be helpful if drug-induced blood dyscrasia is suspected.

4.3 Diagnosis and Symptoms of Schizophrenia

Schizophrenia spectrum disorders are a group of illnesses that include schizophrenia, schizoaffective disorder, and delusional disorder as well as psychotic disorders that are more time limited. While each of these disorders have different diagnostic criteria, they are often treated very similarly, and all include the presence of one or more of the following: delusions, hallucinations, disorganized thinking (as manifested in speech), grossly disorganized or abnormal behavior (including catatonia), and negative symptoms. The first four of these symptoms are generally regarded as "positive" or "psychotic" symptoms (see Table 4.2).

Table 4.2 Core positive (psychotic) symptoms of schizophrenia spectrum disorders

Hallucinations: Perceptual disturbances occurring in the absence of external stimuli.
Auditory hallucinations: The most common type of hallucination. Can have positive, neutral, or negative qualities and varying levels of importance to patients. Often take the form of "voices," which can sound human, alien, or mechanical. Single words, phrases, whole sentences, and/or conversations may be reported by patients. Command auditory hallucinations are important to screen for, as is the patient's intent to act on them as well as is the patient's ability to ignore/resist commands.
Visual hallucinations are the second most commonly occurring hallucination in schizophrenia and are generally not the sole hallucination type present. Classically crisp, seen during the day (and not just at night), and can include parts of, or full, objects.
Tactile, olfactory, and gustatory hallucinations are less common but often underrecognized. Tactile hallucinations can include sensations of being stabbed, burned, or shocked or being spiritually or physically invaded. Gustatory and olfactory hallucinations can include unpleasant smells and tastes.

(continued)

Table 4.2 (continued)

Delusions: Fixed, false beliefs that do not change when evidence contradicting their validity is presented. Most people with schizophrenia experience delusions at some point in their illness. Delusions often develop over time, starting with "ideas of reference," where seemingly random events or objects encountered in the environment hold specific meaning for the patient. Most delusions are highly salient and when strongly held, drive other cognitions and even behaviors. Types of delusions include: Persecutory delusions: The belief that one is being persecuted, attacked, or harmed in some way by individuals or groups. Grandiose delusions: The belief that one has special powers or is wealthy, talented, and/or famous. Jealous delusions: The belief that one's romantic partner is unfaithful. Erotomanic delusions: The belief that one is in a romantic relationship with a high status, often famous individual. Somatic delusions: The belief that there is something wrong with one's bodily functions. Religious delusions: Usually contain grandiose and/or persecutory elements that are religious in nature. Delusions of control: The belief that one's mind or body is being controlled by an external entity. Can lead to passivity phenomena, including feeling that one's mind is being read, or that thoughts are being inserted or withdrawn from one's head or broadcast to others. Delusions of sin or guilt: The belief that one has committed a terrible offense and/or is the direct cause of a bad outcome. Nihilistic delusions: The belief that one does not exist, part of one's body doesn't exist or has died, others don't exist, others have been replaced, and/or the world has ended or is ending. Related delusions include Capgras delusions, or the belief that a familiar person has been replaced by another, and Cotard's syndrome, where the sufferer believes that they are fully or partly dead or are missing organs. Mixed delusions: a combination of delusional types above.
Disorganized speech: Considered secondary to "thought disorder." Classically, patients will be difficult to follow during interviews. Illogical speech: Occurs when the patient speaks in loosely connected sentences or parts of sentences (e.g., loosening of associations), or when the patient is seemingly unable to complete a train of thought (e.g., derailment, tangentiality). Incoherent speech: Words will be left out of sentences, words will be "approximated" (substituted for others in sometimes bizarre ways), and neologisms (made up words) will be used.
Disorganized behavior: Odd or purposeless behavior that can present as intermittently agitated or silly and interferes with activities of daily living Catatonic behavior: An extreme form of disorganized behavior seen within catatonia. Catatonia can be associated with several psychiatric and/or medical disorders, including schizophrenia, and includes a series of symptoms such as mutism, maintaining odd postures, stupor, grimacing, mimicking others' speech and/or movement, odd and repetitive movements, agitation, and others

Diagnostic and Statistical Manual of Mental Disorders: DSM 5 [22]; Marcsisin et al. [49]

Clinical Tip
Medical causes of hallucinations must always be ruled out before attributing them to a psychiatric disorder. Visual hallucinations are frequently seen in delirium caused by both medical illness and substance withdrawal or intoxication. In the absence of delirium, hallucinations and delusions can both be seen secondary to substance/medication and specific medical illnesses. Tactile hallucinations, e.g., "formication," or the feeling of bugs crawling on the skin, is especially common in substance withdrawal. Olfactory hallucinations can occur in seizure auras. As such, a time course of when the psychotic symptoms occurred in relation to substance/medication use and/or medical illness is critical.

Negative symptoms can be defined as an absence of normal thoughts, behaviors, and feelings and can include anhedonia (a lack of pleasure/enjoyment in activities), passivity, social withdrawal, and affective flattening on the mental status exam, e.g., blunted or flat affect. They are often associated with poor outcomes. Cognitive symptoms often present in schizophrenia spectrum disorders though are not included as diagnostic criteria in DSM 5 (Diagnostic and Statistical Manual of Mental Disorders: DSM-5). These are often nonspecific and overlap with positive and negative symptoms but include difficulties with complex decision making (executive function), deficits in memory, disorders of verbal fluency, and social cognitive deficits. Also not included in diagnostic criteria for the disorder, but commonly seen in many individuals (some chronically and perhaps most in acute stages of illness), is a lack of insight into having a psychotic illness. Patients who lack insight may reject part or all of their diagnosis and refuse some or all treatment.

A.B.'s mumbling to himself may represent, "responding to internal stimuli," which can be an indicator of auditory hallucinations. A.B. may have other positive symptoms, including persecutory or grandiose delusions, as illustrated by his referring to being involved with the FBI. A.B.'s disheveled appearance may also be influenced by delusional beliefs that influence his choice in clothing. However, this is more likely due to negative symptoms, behavioral disorganization, and/or cognitive impairment.

Clinical Tip
While most treatments of schizophrenia have focused on positive symptoms, negative symptoms and cognitive symptoms have the greatest morbidity and impact on functioning.

Schizophrenia is the most common diagnosis in the schizophrenia spectrum and other psychotic disorders family of diagnoses. To meet diagnostic criteria for schizophrenia, at least two positive symptoms or one positive symptom and negative symptoms, must be present for at least a month (or less with treatment). All told, symptoms, at least in their attenuated form, must occur for a total of 6 months. Like with all psychiatric diagnoses, major areas of functioning must also be adversely affected.

Schizoaffective disorder differs only from schizophrenia in that, in addition to meeting criteria for schizophrenia, the patient must also meet mood episode criteria for the majority of the total duration of illness. Psychotic symptoms must also be present for at least 2 weeks in the absence of mood symptoms. Schizoaffective disorder is commonly considered a gray area between schizophrenia and major mood disorders. It may be more meaningful, however, to think of schizoaffective disorder as schizophrenia with a superimposed major mood disorder. Mood episodes could be either manic or depressive. If manic episodes are part of the presentation, the patient would be diagnosed as having schizoaffective disorder, bipolar type. If only major depressive episodes are present, the patient would be diagnosed with schizoaffective disorder, depressed type. Negative and cognitive symptoms may be somewhat less common than in schizophrenia.

Patients with delusional disorders present with predominant delusions for at least 1 month or longer. Hallucinations can be present but are always related to the delusional theme and are not prominent. The patient's functioning is often not significantly impaired, nor is the patient's behavior particularly bizarre. Many patients with delusional disorder will preferentially present to primary care for attention, especially if their delusions are somatic in nature. Delusional parasitosis, for example, is much more frequently treated by PCPs and dermatologists than psychiatrists.

Brief psychotic disorders may include hallucinations, delusions, and disorganized speech, but they last less than a month. Schizophreniform disorder presents similarly but lasts for at least a month but not more than six. Many, but not all, patients meeting schizophreniform disorder criteria will progress to schizophrenia.

Ideally, a patient will be diagnosed with a schizophrenia spectrum disorder by a psychiatrist. If the diagnosis is not clear, this can sometimes take several visits. Neuropsychiatric testing may be helpful for confirming the diagnosis in some cases but is seldom necessary. A thorough medical workup for medical illness and/or drug use that can cause psychotic symptoms and/or confound diagnostic efforts, completed by, or in conjunction with, a primary care physician, is ideal. Referral to subsequent specialists may be helpful in certain cases. In later-onset psychosis, dementia must absolutely be ruled out. The often-treatable anti-N-methyl-d-aspartate (NMDA) receptor encephalitis is gaining increasing attention as potential mimic of schizophrenia, but neurosyphilis, Huntington's disease, and Wilson's disease remain the important rule-out diagnoses in patients of all ages when history and/or physical exam is suspicious for neuropsychiatric disease. Where psychotic symptoms wax and wane, delirium must be at the top of the differential; delirium can be due to a variety of medical illnesses and disorders, including lupus. Certain seizure disorders can also rarely cause episodic psychosis, as can the classic board exam zebra, intermittent porphyria. A standard evaluation for schizophrenia will include a medical and family medical history, vital signs, a complete blood count and blood chemistries, TSH, fasting lipids and glucose, hemoglobin A1c, and a urine drug screen [38]. Such laboratory evaluations can help identify other causes of psychosis (e.g., hyperthyroidism, hypercalcemia, drug-induced psychoses), identify a need for further medical workup and specific prescribing considerations (e.g., elevated liver enzymes), and provide a baseline comparator for monitoring while the patient is on antipsychotic medications. When the patient has focal neurological signs or symptoms (headaches with or without other symptoms of increased intracranial pressure, weakness, rapid progression of memory loss over a few months, personality change, etc.), possible recent seizures, or later age of psychotic symptom onset, brain imaging is recommended. Otherwise, the yield of routine brain imaging in the setting of possible schizophrenia appears to be very low, other than to perhaps reassure the patient and family. Similarly, EEGs should only be ordered when seizures or a deliriogenic process is potentially present. Of note, treatment for acute psychosis should only rarely be deferred, even if the cause is unknown.

Individuals who have sustained serious head injuries, and those with specific developmental disorders (e.g., 22q11.2 deletion), may also be more likely to develop schizophrenia, but psychotic or psychotic-like symptoms can also be directly caused by these neuropsychiatric conditions and preclude a diagnosis of schizophrenia. Likewise, while substance use disorders are very common in individuals with schizophrenia spectrum illnesses, intoxication and withdrawal can also cause psychotic symptoms. In the case of substance-induced psychotic disorders, these can persist for some weeks after the removal of the offending substance. Finally, especially in the case of schizoaffective disorder, it is important to distinguish schizophrenia spectrum disorders from bipolar disorder, complicated trauma with dissociative symptoms, and borderline personality disorder. In this latter disorder, hallucinations are quite common. In such cases of diagnostic ambiguity, diagnostic clarification with a psychiatrist with experience in this area is critical.

Patients with schizophrenia spectrum disorders are frequently diagnosed with comorbid mental disorders. Episodic depression in schizophrenia, particularly post psychotic episodes, is very common. Anxiety disorders are also exceedingly common, as is obsessive-compulsive disorder. Given high rates of victimization, unsurprisingly, posttraumatic stress disorder comorbidity is also common. Recognition and treatment of these comorbid conditions is recommended to help ensure best outcomes.

4.4 Treatment

4.4.1 Pharmacotherapy

Antipsychotics are generally required to treat the acute episodes of psychosis and during maintenance treatment. The goal of treatment during acute episodes is to eliminate psychotic symptoms (or at least reduce them to the patient's pre-exacerbation baseline level of symptoms) and return the patient to their previous level of functioning. Most patients who have schizophrenia will need some degree of ongoing treatment, usually involving antipsychotic medication, to promote an optimal level of functioning between acute episodes as well as to prevent relapse into an acute episode. This constitutes maintenance treatment. During acute episodes, doses of most medications can be rather rapidly titrated to therapeutic doses, as tolerated by the patient. Additional dose increases should be made more slowly to monitor for side effect emergence and to allow medication to reach steady-state blood levels between increases. The full clinical effect of antipsychotics may not be seen for at least 4–6 weeks, though if a 20% reduction of psychotic symptoms is not seen by about 2 weeks, the medication is not likely to be efficacious for the patient and a switch to an alternate agent should be considered [66]. Medication trials are taken in a step wise fashion, as summarized in Fig. 4.1 below (Fig. 4.1). Medications can usually be given once daily, especially once the patient is clinically stable and in the maintenance phase of treatment. Maintenance treatment with the lowest effective doses of antipsychotics is recommended to prevent relapse while mitigating side effect burden; sometimes, medication doses necessary to treat acute symptoms can be very gradually lowered once the patient has been stable for a few months.

More information would be required to determine if A.B. is acutely psychotic or if he is presenting at his psychiatric baseline. If the patient is treatment adherent, increases in risperidone may be helpful to address ongoing symptoms, especially if the patient is acutely psychotic. Increased vigilance around side effect monitoring (especially for worsening EPS) would be required with this approach. If this patient's symptoms are chronic, other medication trials could be attempted for reduction of positive symptoms. This is best done when a good history of previous medication trials with treatment response and side effects is available.

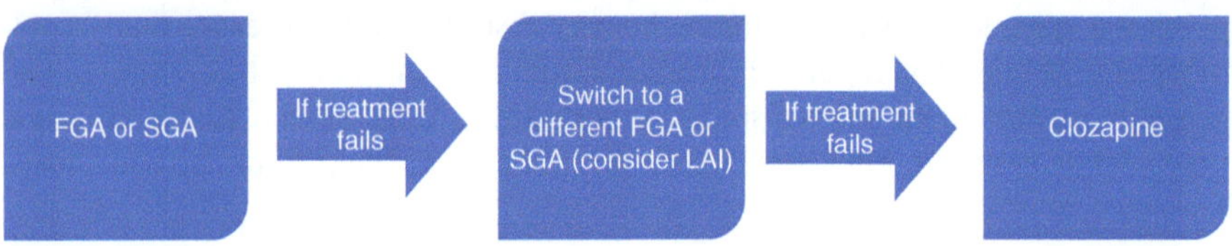

Fig. 4.1 Standard, step wise approach to treating acute, psychotic symptoms of schizophrenia. Patients should be titrated to a therapeutic dose of a First Generation Antipsychotic (FGA) or a Second Generation Antipsychotic (SGA), preferably of their choice and in consideration of side effect profile, druging interactions, cost, and other patient specific factors. If the patient does not respond by 4–6 weeks, a switch to a different FGA or SGA should be attempted. A Long-Acting Injectable (LAI) formulation should be considered if adherence in in question and/or based on patient preference. After two antipsychotic treatement failures, clozapine should be considered. If patients do not have adequate response to clozapine, or refuse or are ineligible for clozapine, antipychotic polypharmacy, ECT, and adjuvant medication trials with Lithium, AEDs, and other medications are sometimes attempted [38]

First episode schizophrenia is the initial 2–5 years after illness onset, usually occurring in the late teens or in the 20s. Specialized, federally funded programs for individuals in their first episode of schizophrenia are available throughout the United States and involve "coordinated specialty care" by a team of psychiatrists, therapists, and other specialists to provide medication management, therapy, family psychoeducation, and vocational and educational support tailored to the needs of the individual. Similar programs exist internationally. In general, antipsychotics should be started at low doses, as this population often responds rapidly and with good affect [72] and is more prone to experiencing side effects.

Antipsychotics have 60–70% efficacy in the treatment of acute psychosis and, excepting in treatment resistant schizophrenia, have equivalent efficacy rates. In general, antipsychotics only treat positive symptoms; they rarely have an impact on negative and cognitive symptoms. Use and choice of antipsychotics should be driven by a patient's history of medication trials and treatment response, patient preference, and potential side effect burden. Risks of metabolic syndrome and EPS are often considered trade-offs, with older, "first-generation antipsychotics" (FGAs) carrying a higher risk of acute and tardive EPS and newer, "second-generation antipsychotics" (SGAs) presenting with higher risks of weight gain, hypercholesterolemia, and diabetes mellitus 2. Other serious side effects, including orthostasis and QTc prolongation, should also be considered in prescribing antipsychotic medications, as should potentially serious side effects due to anticholinergic burden (e.g., severe constipation and delirium), sedation, and prolactin elevation. Even less medically significant side effects should be considered, as they can be quite bothersome to patients and so impact treatment adherence. While lack of insight is a major driver of medication nonadherence in schizophrenia, so too are side effects. As such, it is very important to routinely screen for and aggressively manage side effects to both help promote adherence and quality of life for patients.

Treatment-resistant schizophrenia can be defined as an inadequate clinical response to two trials of antipsychotic medications, prescribed at optimal doses and over an adequate duration, and with documented mediation adherence. Treatment resistance affects over 30% of people with schizophrenia [60]. Clozapine is the gold standard treatment for treatment-resistant schizophrenia and has the only FDA approval for this indication.

Patients with comorbid psychiatric illnesses, including anxiety disorders and obsessive-compulsive disorder, benefit from treatment of these illnesses, including with medications like antidepressants. Treatment of mood episodes is strongly recommended, and mood stabilizers and antidepressants are considered standard adjuvants to antipsychotics in patients with schizoaffective disorder. Treatment of psychosis itself with more than one antipsychotic or adjuvant lithium, anticonvulsants, and benzodiazepines is common, though the evidence for this approach is limited [38]. When a patient has been stable for a significant time period (6 months to a year or more), especially when clinical effectiveness of the medication regimen is in question and/or side effects have emerged, individual adjuvant medications can be very gradually tapered, sometimes to complete discontinuation. Such a taper is perhaps best done by a psychiatrist and over the course of up to several months, as careful monitoring for emergence of acute symptoms is necessary. A thorough review of the patient's history and response to medication trials is also recommended, as risks of deprescribing may outweigh potential benefit, especially in patients with multiple psychotic episodes, unclear illness comorbidity, and a complicated treatment course.

Antipsychotic medications are usually administered in oral capsule or tablet form, though some come in intramuscular injections for acute agitation and/or psychosis. Some antipsychotics also can be conveniently dispensed as long-acting injectable formulations that can be given every few weeks to months, depending on the formulation. These medications are often prescribed based on patient preference and are highly encouraged for patients who have difficulty remembering to take their oral medications and/or have issues with intermittent impaired insight leading to adherence issues. A summary of antipsychotics and their different formulations, dosing considerations, common side effects and relative risks of these side effects, metabolism, and potential interactions/need for medication adjustments are summarized in the tables below.

Clinical Tip

Long-acting injectable antipsychotics have been shown to reduce hospitalizations and mortality associated with schizophrenia [38]. They are generally administered in psychiatrists' offices and/or at pharmacies (depending on state regulations). In the event that a patient misses a dose, retitration at lower doses and initiation of oral medication may be needed. Specialty consultation is recommended.

4.4.1.1 First-Generation Antipsychotic Medications

FGAs are usually classified by their potency at the dopamine 2 receptor and in comparison to chlorpromazine, the first antipsychotic. Higher potency FGAs require lower doses to achieve comparable therapeutic effects. They also carry higher risks of EPS but lower risks of sedation and orthostasis. Risk of QTc prolongation is variable among FGAs. Like with all medications, drug interactions, including interactions with commonly prescribed medications that may cause competitive inhibition and increase blood levels, should be monitored. Details including potency, dosing and dosing considerations, potential side effects, and metabolism/major drug interactions are included in Table 4.3.

Table 4.3 Commonly prescribed FGAs

Medication/ potency	Dosing and dosing considerations	Potential SEs	Metabolism/ major interactions
Haloperidol (Haldol)/high	Tablet: 0.5, 1, 2, 5, 10, 20 mg Oral solution: 2 mg/mL Initial oral: 0.5–5 mg BID or TID (totaling 1–15 mg/day) depending on symptom severity Usual oral dose: 5–20 mg/day Max oral dose: 100 mg/day Immediate release injectable (haloperidol lactate): 5 mg/mL (1 mL, 10 mL); usually given as 2–5 mg IM every 4–8 hours Max immediate release injectable dose: 20 mg *Long-acting injectable:* Name: Haloperidol decanoate Initial dose: With loading strategy (no oral haloperidol overlap)—Consider IM loading dose of 20× oral haloperidol. For individuals naive to Haldol Decanoate and/or if IM dose >100 mg, consider giving 100 mg IM at initiation and the remainder 3–7 days later. Discontinue oral haloperidol at first injection Without loading strategy—consider an IM dose of 10× oral haloperidol with continued oral haloperidol for 3–4 months Maintenance dose: 10× oral haloperidol dose every 4 weeks Maximum dose: 450 mg every 4 weeks Renal impairment: No recommendations Hepatic impairment: No recommendations	High: EPS (acute and tardive), prolactin elevation, QTC prolongation (when given IV) Moderate: QTC prolongation (when given orally), weight gain Low: hypercholesterolemia, glucose abnormalities, orthostasis, sedation	CYP 2D6 (major), CYP 3A4 (major), CYP 1A2 (minor)/avoid combining with nilotinib

(continued)

Table 4.3 (continued)

Medication/ potency	Dosing and dosing considerations	Potential SEs	Metabolism/ major interactions
Fluphenazine (Prolixin)/high	Tablet: 1, 2.5, 5, 10 mg Oral elixir: 2.5 mg/mL Oral solution: 5 mg/mL Initial oral: 2.5–10 mg/day, divided dosing, every 6–8 hours Usual oral dose: 6–20 mg/day Max oral dose: 40 mg/day Immediate release injectable: 2.5 mg/mL, dose at 33–50% of oral dose Max immediate release injectable dose: 10 mg *Long-acting injectable:* Name: Prolixin Decanoate Initial dose: 1.25× the stable oral fluphenazine dose. Oral fluphenazine should be continued at full dose for 1 week after the first injection and then at half the dose for 2 weeks Maintenance dose: 6.25 mg–25 mg typically given every 2–4 weeks. Oral equivalence 1.25× the oral dose when injected every 3 weeks Maximum dose: 100 mg Renal impairment: Use with caution (non-dialyzable) Hepatic impairment: Use with caution	High: EPS (acute and tardive), prolactin elevation Moderate: weight gain Low: glucose abnormalities, hypercholesterolemia, orthostasis, sedation, QTc prolongation	CYP 2D6 (major)/may need to lower dose when prescribed with strong CYP 2D6 inhibitors (e.g., paroxetine, fluoxetine, bupropion, quinidine) to avoid side effects
Pimozide (Orap)/high Not FDA approved for schizophrenia but used off-label and to treat delusional disorders, especially delusional parasitosis	Tablet: 1–2 mg Initial: 0.5–2 mg/day Usual dose: 2–4 mg/day Max dose: 10 mg/day Renal: No specific recommendations Hepatic: Consider dose reduction in severe insufficiency	High: EPS (acute and tardive) Moderate: QTc prolongation Low: weight gain, glucose abnormalities, hypercholesterolemia, sedation, anticholinergic side effects, orthostatic hypotension	CYP 3A4 (major), CYP 1A2 (minor)/ avoid concomitant use of CYP1A2 or CYP3A4 inducers or inhibitors. Perform CYP2D6 genotyping if doses greater than 4 mg/day are used; in poor CYP2D6 metabolizers, do not give more than 4 mg/day and do not increase dose earlier than 14 days from start. Use with other QTc prolongating agents is contraindicated. Avoid use with fluvoxamine, clarithromycin (lower antipsychotic dose if must use), and ketoconazole

Table 4.3 (continued)

Medication/ potency	Dosing and dosing considerations	Potential SEs	Metabolism/ major interactions
Loxapine (Loxitane)/mid Adasuve requires an FDA risk evaluation and mitigation strategy (REMS) program because of potential for bronchospasm	Capsule: 5, 10, 25, 50 mg Initial oral: 20 mg/day Usual dose: 60–100 mg/day Max oral dose: 250 mg/day Oral inhalation formulation (Adasuve, an aerosol powder, breath-activated): 10 mg Max oral inhalation: 10 mg/day Renal: No specific recommendations Hepatic: No specific recommendations	Moderate: EPS (acute and tardive), prolactin elevation, sedation, anticholinergic side effects, orthostatic hypotension Low: weight gain, glucose abnormalities, hypercholesterolemia, QTc prolongation	CYP 1A2, CYP 2D6, CYP 3A4/ increase monitoring with CNS depressants; combination with metoclopramide is contraindicated
Perphenazine (Trilafon)/mid	Tablet: 2, 4, 8, 16 mg Initial: 8–16 mg/day Usual dose: 8–32 mg/day Max dose: 64 mg/day Renal: No specific recommendations Hepatic: Consider dose reduction	Moderate: weight gain, EPS (acute and tardive), prolactin elevation, sedation, anticholinergic side effects Low: glucose abnormalities, hyperlipidemia, QTc prolongation	CYP 2D6/ CYP2D6 poor metabolizers will have higher blood concentrations. Known interaction with ziprasidone
Chlorpromazine (Thorazine)/low	Tablet: 10, 25, 50, 100, 200 mg Initial: 25–100 mg/day Usual dose: 200–800 mg/day Max dose: 1000–2000 mg/day Immediate release injectable: 25 mg/mL; give at much lower dose than oral Max immediate release injectable dose: 200 mg/day Renal impairment: No specific recommendations Hepatic impairment: Consider dose reduction	High: anticholinergic side effects, sedation, EPS (tardive), QTc prolongation, orthostatic hypotension Moderate: EPS (acute), glucose abnormalities, weight gain Low: prolactin elevation, hyperlipidemia	CYP 2D6 (major), CYP 1A2 (minor), CYP 3A4 (minor)/may need to decrease if concomitantly prescribed propranolol or tamoxifen (avoid co-administration with tamoxifen when possible) administration with other QTc prolonging agents (e.g., thioridazine, pimozide, ziprasidone) is contraindicated. Avoid excessive sun exposure and wear sunscreen

Keepers et al. [38]; Haloperidol [package insert] [32]; Fluphenazine [package insert] [29]; Pimozide [package insert] [59]; Loxapine [package insert] [44]; Perphenazine [package insert] [58]; Chlorpromazine [package insert] [74]; Marcsisin et al. [49]

4.4.1.2 Second-Generation Antipsychotics

SGAs have a different pharmacological profile than FGAs, blocking 5HT receptors in addition to D2. Some, like aripiprazole, will also partially agonize the D2 blocker or, like clozapine, quetiapine, aripiprazole, and ziprasidone, partially agonize 5HT1A. Some of these medications may also more rapidly dissociate from the D2 receptor than FGAs. These pharmacological properties make it less likely that patients will experience acute or tardive EPS, though EPS is still not rare, especially with risperidone and paliperidone. Akathisia risk is also not uncommon with certain SGAs, particularly aripiprazole. Given the potent D2 blocking associated with risperidone and paliperidone, prolactin elevation is also not infrequently seen with these medications.

Metabolic side effects are much more common with SGAs than FGAs. Generally, the risk of weight gain is considered highest with clozapine, though the risk with olanzapine is nearly equivalent. Risk of weight gain with quetiapine, in turn, is slightly lower, followed by risperidone and then iloperidone. Cariprazine has also been sometimes associated with weight gain. Weight gain is considered less common with asenapine, aripiprazole, brexpiprazole, lurasidone, ziprasidone, and lumateperone. Cholesterol elevation appears most likely to occur with clozapine, olanzapine, and quetiapine; glucose elevations are most common with clozapine and olanzapine.

Details including dosing and dosing considerations, potential side effects, and metabolism/major drug interactions for SGAs are summarized in Table 4.4.

Table 4.4 Commonly prescribed SGAs

Medication	Dosing and dosing considerations	Potential SEs	Metabolism/major interactions
Aripiprazole (Abilify)	Tablet: 2, 5, 10, 15, 20, 30 mg Tablet, disintegrating: 10, 15 mg Tablet with ingestible event marker (Mycite): 2, 5, 10, 15, 20, 30 mg. Do not split or crush Solution: 1 mg/mL (150 mL). If tablet dose is 30 mg, use 25 mg oral solution Initial: 10–15 mg/day Usual range: 10–15 mg/day Max dose: 30 mg/day *Long-acting injectables:* Name: Aripiprazole monohydrate (Maintena) Initial dose: 400 mg; continue oral aripiprazole for 2 weeks Maintenance dose: 400 mg monthly Maximum dose: 400 mg monthly Name: Aripiprazole lauroxil (Aristada) Initial dose: Give one injection of initio (675 mg) with a single oral dose of 30 mg of aripiprazole AND chosen maintenance dose of Aristada OR give chosen maintenance dose of Aristada and 21 days of oral aripiprazole Maintenance dose (oral equivalence): 441 mg (10 mg/d) monthly; 662 mg monthly, 882 mg every 6 weeks, or 1064 mg every 8 weeks (15 mg/d); 882 mg monthly (20 mg/d or higher) Maximum dose: 882 mg monthly Renal impairment: No specific recommendations Hepatic impairment: No specific recommendations	Moderate: akathisia Low: weight gain, glucose abnormalities, hyperlipidemia, parkinsonism, dystonia, tardive dyskinesia, prolactin elevation, sedation, anticholinergic symptoms, orthostatic hypotension	CYP 2D6, 3A4/ adjust dose if a poor CYP2D6 metabolizer or with concomitant use of a CYP3A4 inhibitor (e.g., decrease dose with strong inhibitors like ketoconazole, clarithromycin, verapamil), CYP3A4 inducer (e.g., increase dose with strong inducers like phenobarbital, phenytoin, rifamycin), or CYP2D6 inhibitor (e.g., decrease dose with paroxetine, fluoxetine, bupropion, quinidine)

Table 4.4 (continued)

Medication	Dosing and dosing considerations	Potential SEs	Metabolism/major interactions
Asenapine (Saphris)	Tablet, sublingual: 2.5, 5, 10 mg (instructions for patients: do not split, crush, or swallow; place under tongue and allow to dissolve completely. Do not eat food or drink for at least 10 minutes) Initial: 10 mg/day Usual dose: 20 mg/day Max dose: 20 mg/day Transdermal system (Secuado): 3.8 mg/24 hours (= 5 mg bid sublingual tab), 5.7 mg/24 hours, 7.6 mg/24 hours (= 10 mg bid sublingual tab) Initial: 3.8 mg/24 hrs Usual dose: 3.8–7.6 mg/24 hrs Max dose: 7.6 mg/24 hrs Renal impairment: No specific recommendations Hepatic impairment: Use not recommended in severe impairment	Moderate: weight gain, glucose abnormalities, hyperlipidemia, akathisia, dystonia, tardive dyskinesia, prolactin elevation, sedation, orthostatic hypotension, QTc Prolongation Low: Parkinsonism, dystonia, anticholinergic symptoms	Glucuronidation by UGT1A4 and CYP 1A2/ consider dose adjustment in smokers and with concomitant use of CYP1A2 inhibitors (e.g.,. decrease dose of asenapine with fluvoxamine, ciprofloxacin, and primaquine). Avoid combining with paroxetine when possible
Brexpiprazole (Rexulti)	Tablet: 0.25, 0.5, 1, 2, 3, 4 mg Initial: 1 mg/day Usual dose: 2–4 mg/day Max dose: 4 mg/day Renal impairment: maximum recommended dosage is 2 mg in moderate, severe, or end-stage renal impairment (CrCL <60 mL/min) Hepatic impairment: maximum recommended dose is 3 mg in moderate to severe hepatic impairment (Child-Pugh score ≥ 7)	Moderate: hyperlipidemia, akathisia, sedation Low: weight gain, glucose abnormalities, parkinsonism, dystonia, tardive dyskinesia, prolactin elevation, anticholinergic symptoms, orthostatic hypotension	CYP 2D6, 3A4/ have dose if patient on strong CYP2D6 or CYP 3A4 inhibitors. Quarter dose if patient on a combination of strong/moderate CYP2D6 (or if patient a poor CYP2D6 metabolizer) and CYP3A4 inhibitors. Double the usual dose if patient on a strong CYP3A4 inducer
Cariprazine (Vraylar)	Tablet, sublingual: 2.5, 5, 10 mg Initial: 10 mg/day Usual dose: 20 mg/day Max dose: 20 mg/day Renal impairment: no dosage adjustment required in patients with mild to moderate (CrCL ≥30 mL/minute) impairment. Use is not recommended in patients with severe renal impairment (CrCL <30 mL/minute) Hepatic impairment: Use not recommended in severe impairment (Child-Pugh score between 10 and 15)	Moderate: weight gain, akathisia, dystonia, sedation, anticholinergic symptoms Low: glucose abnormalities, hyperlipidemia, parkinsonism, dystonia, tardive dyskinesia, prolactin elevation, anticholinergic, orthostatic hypotension	CYP 3A4/have dose with strong CYP3A4 inhibitors. Not recommended with CYP3A4 inducers

(continued)

Table 4.4 (continued)

Medication	Dosing and dosing considerations	Potential SEs	Metabolism/major interactions
Clozapine (Clozaril, FazaClo, Versacloz) Prescribers must enroll in and complete REMS education at www.clozapinerems.com before prescribing. Pharmacies must also be enrolled. Requires following absolute neutrophil counts (ANCs) at regular intervals dictated by time on treatment. Treatment interruptions of more than 30 days reset monitoring frequencies	Tablet: 25, 50, 100, 200 mg Tablet, disintegrating: 12.5, 25, 100, 150, 200 mg Oral suspension: 50 mg/mL (100 mL) Initial: 12.5–25 mg; do not increase by more than 25–50 mg/day for first two weeks. Do not increase by more than 100 mg twice a week thereafter Usual dose: 300–450 mg. Treatment interruptions of 48 hours or more require retitration Max dose: 900 mg Renal impairment: No specific recommendations Hepatic impairment: No specific recommendations	High: weight gain, glucose abnormalities, hyperlipidemia, sedation, anticholinergic symptoms, orthostatic hypotension Moderate: akathisia, QTc prolongation Low: parkinsonism, dystonia, tardive dyskinesia, prolactin elevation	CYP 1A2 (major), 3A4, 2D5, 2C19 (minor)/adjust dose with concomitant use of strong CYP1A2 inhibitors and inducers and with strong CYP3A4 inducers. Smoking reduces clozapine levels via CYP1A2 induction. Use caution in combining with CNS depressants
Iloperidone (Fanapt)	Tablet: 1, 2, 4, 6, 8, 10, 12 mg Initial: 2 mg/day. Titrate slowly with no more than 4 mg/day increases in dose. Retitrate if treatment interrupted for more than 3 days Usual dose: 12–24 mg/day Max dose: 24 mg/day Renal impairment: No adjustments necessary Hepatic impairment: not recommended in severe impairment	High: orthostatic hypotension Moderate: weight gain, glucose abnormalities, akathisia, prolactin elevation, sedation Low: hyperlipidemia, parkinsonism, dystonia, tardive dyskinesia, anticholinergic, QTc prolongation	CYP 2D6, 3A4 (major)/adjust dose with concomitant use of strong CYP2D6 or CYP3A4 inhibitors and halve dose 50% in CYP2D6 poor metabolizers

Table 4.4 (continued)

Medication	Dosing and dosing considerations	Potential SEs	Metabolism/major interactions
Lumateperone (Caplyta)	Capsule: 42 mg (instructions for patients: take with food) Initial: 42 mg/day Usual dose: 42 mg/day Max dose: 42 mg/day Renal impairment: no recommended adjustments Hepatic impairment: avoid use in patients with moderate or severe hepatic impairment (Child-Pugh B or C)	Moderate: akathisia Low: weight gain, glucose abnormalities, hyperlipidemia, parkinsonism, dystonia, prolactin elevation, sedation, anticholinergic symptoms, orthostatic hypotension	CYP 3A4/avoid concomitant use CYP 3A4 inducers and strong or moderate CYP 3A4 inhibitors
Lurasidone (Latuda)	Tablet: 20, 40, 60, 80, 120 mg (instructions for patients: take with food of ≥ 350 calories) Initial: 40 mg Usual dose: 40–120 mg Max dose: 160 mg Renal impairment: In moderate to severe impairment (CrCL <50 mL/min), use a lower initial dose (20 mg/day) and a max of 80 mg/day Hepatic impairment: in moderate to severe impairment (Child-Pugh score ≥ 7), use an initial dose of 20 mg/day. In moderate impairment, use a max dose of 80 mg/day. In severe impairment, use a max dose of 40 mg/day	Moderate: glucose abnormalities, hyperlipidemia, parkinsonism, dystonia, tardive dyskinesia, sedation Low: weight gain, dystonia, tardive dyskinesia, prolactin elevation, anticholinergic symptoms, orthostatic hypotension	CYP 3A4/adjust dose for concomitant use of moderate to strong CYP3A4 inhibitors or inducers. Avoid with strong CYP3A4 inhibitors when possible

(continued)

Table 4.4 (continued)

Medication	Dosing and dosing considerations	Potential SEs	Metabolism/major interactions
Olanzapine (Zyprexa)	Tablet: 2.5, 5, 7.5, 10, 15, 20 mg Tablet, disintegrating: 5, 10, 15, 20 mg (can be swallowed with or without liquid) Short-acting IM powder for solution: 10 mg/2 mL Initial oral: 5–10 mg/day Usual oral dose: 10–20 mg/day Max oral dose: 20 mg (often used up to 30 mg; 60 mg has been reported in the literature) Usual immediate release injectable dose: 2.5–10 mg. 1.5× greater half-life than oral in the elderly Max immediate release injectable dose: 30 mg/day. About 40% oral dose removed by first-pass metabolism; IM not affected by first-pass metabolism *Long-acting injectable:* Name: Relprevv (this is a REMS medication requiring registration, patient education, reporting, and patient monitoring) Initial dose (oral equivalence)—continue oral olanzapine for 8 weeks. Give 210 mg every 2 weeks or 405 mg every 4 weeks (10 mg/day); 300 mg every 2 weeks (15 mg/day or 20 mg/day) Maintenance dose (oral equivalence): 150 mg every 2 weeks or 300 mg every 4 weeks (10 mg/day); 210 mg every 2 weeks or 405 mg every 4 weeks (15 mg/day); 300 mg every 2 weeks (20 mg/day) Maximum dose: 300 mg every 2 weeks Renal impairment: lower oral initial dose of 5 mg/day should be considered Hepatic impairment: no adjustment necessary for mild/moderate impairment	High: weight gain, glucose abnormalities, hyperlipidemia, sedation Moderate: akathisia, parkinsonism, prolactin elevation, anticholinergic symptoms, orthostatic hypotension, QTc prolongation Low: dystonia, tardive dyskinesia	CYP 1A2 (major), CYP 3A4 (minor), and glucuronidation/administration with CYP 1A2 inducers may require increase in olanzapine dose. Use with CNS depressants should be avoided when possible. Increased monitoring may be required if administered with antihypertensives. Smokers may require a 30% greater daily dose than nonsmokers because of CYP1A2 induction. Women may need lower daily doses. Concomitant use of IM olanzapine with IM benzodiazepines is not recommended due to risk of cardiorespiratory suppression

Table 4.4 (continued)

Medication	Dosing and dosing considerations	Potential SEs	Metabolism/major interactions
Paliperidone (Invega)	Tablet, extended release: 1.5, 3, 6, 9 mg (instructions for patients: do not split or crush) Initial: 6 mg; increase by no more than 3 mg/day every 5 days Usual dose: 3–12 mg Max dose: 12 mg *Long-acting injectable:* Name: Invega Sustenna Initial dose: 234 mg on day 1 and 156 mg 1 week later Maintenance dose beginning at week 5 (oral equivalence): 39–78 mg monthly (3 mg); 117 mg monthly (6 mg); 156 mg monthly (9 mg); 234 mg monthly (12 mg) Maximum dose: 234 mg/month Name: Invega Trinza Initial dose: After the patient has been stable on Sustenna for 4 months, start at maintenance dose Maintenance dose (equivalence to monthly Sustenna): 273 mg every 3 months (78 mg); 410 mg every 3 months (117 mg); 546 mg every 3 months (156 mg); 819 mg every 3 months (234 mg) Maximum dose: 819 mg every 3 months Name: Invega Hafyera Administer INVEGA Initial dose: when the next once-a-month (after at least 4 Sustenna injections have been given) or every 3-month (after at least 1 Trinza injection has been given) paliperidone palmitate LAI is due, start at maintenance dose Maintenance dose (equivalence to monthly Sustenna): 1092 mg (156 mg) every 6 months; 1560 mg (234 mg) every 6 months Renal impairment: for CrCL 50–79 mL/min, use a lower initial oral dose of 3 mg and a max dose of 6 mg. For CrCL 10–49 mL/min, use a lower initial oral dose of 1.5 mg and max of 3 mg a day. Use not recommended in CrCL <10 ml/min Hepatic impairment: No adjustment necessary for mild/moderate impairment	High: prolactin elevation Moderate: weight gain, akathisia, parkinsonism, dystonia, tardive dyskinesia, orthostatic hypotension Low: glucose abnormalities, hyperlipidemia, dystonia, sedation, anticholinergic symptoms, QTc prolongation	Primarily renal excretion/ combining with other QTc prolonging agents may require decreasing paliperidone dose. Not recommended with preexisting severe gastrointestinal narrowing disorders. Tablet shell is expelled in the stool

(continued)

Table 4.4 (continued)

Medication	Dosing and dosing considerations	Potential SEs	Metabolism/major interactions
Quetiapine (Seroquel)	Tablet, immediate release: 25, 50, 100, 200, 300, 400 mg Tablet, extended release: 50, 150, 200, 300, 400 mg Initial, immediate release: 50 mg Initial, extended release: 300 mg. (instructions for patients: take without food or with <300 calories) Usual dose: 400–800 mg. For immediate release, to be given in divided dosing (though commonly given once per day). Retitrate for gap in treatment of more than 1 week Max dose: 800 mg Renal impairment: no specific recommendations Hepatic impairments: start at lower doses (IR tablets 25 mg/day; ER tablets 50 mg/day) and increase gradually (IR tablets 25–50 mg/day; ER tablets 50 mg/day)	High: hyperlipidemia, sedation Moderate: weight gain, glucose abnormalities, anticholinergic symptoms, orthostatic hypotension, QTc prolongation Low: akathisia, parkinsonism, dystonia, tardive dyskinesia, prolactin elevation	CYP 3A4 (major), CYP 2D6 (minor)/avoid and/or monitor closely if prescribing with CNS depressants. Monitor when combining with antihypertensives. If giving with CYP 3A4 inducers, quetiapine dose may need to be increased. If administered with CYP 3A4 inhibitors, dose may need to be decreased
Risperidone (Risperdal)	Tablet: 0.25, 0.5, 1, 2, 3, 4 mg Tablet, disintegrating: 0.25, 0.5, 1, 2, 3, 4 mg (do not crush or split; contains phenylalanine) Oral solution: 1 mg/mL (30 mL) (check labeling for compatible liquids) Initial: 2 mg Usual dose: 2–8 mg Max dose: 8 mg (though doses up to 16 mg/day have been used in clinical trials) *Long-acting injectable:* Name: Consta (*intramuscular*) Initial dose: Give maintenance dose with oral risperidone for 3 weeks Maintenance dose (oral risperidone equivalent): 25 mg every 2 weeks (if 3 mg daily or less); 37.5 mg every 2 weeks (if greater 4–5 mg daily); 50 mg every 2 weeks (if over 5 mg daily) Maximum dose: 50 mg every 2 weeks Name: Perseris (extended-release *subcutaneous* injectable suspension) Initial dose: If patient can tolerate 3 mg or more oral risperidone daily, start maintenance dose Maintenance dose (oral equivalence): 90 mg monthly (3 mg); 120 mg (4 mg) Maximum dose: 120 mg monthly Renal impairment: For CrCL <30 mL/min, start oral at lower doses (0.5 mg bid) and titrate slowly (0.5 mg or less twice daily and not more than once a week) Hepatic impairment: do not use with severe hepatic impairment (Child-Pugh class C)	High: prolactin elevation Moderate: weight gain, glucose abnormalities, akathisia, parkinsonism, dystonia, tardive dyskinesia, prolactin elevation, sedation, orthostatic hypotension, QTc prolongation Low: hyperlipidemia, dystonia, anticholinergic symptoms	CYP 2D6 (major), CYP 3A4 (minor)/may need to decrease antipsychotic dose if giving with moderate to strong CYP 2D6 inhibitors. If given with antihypertensives, may need to decrease dose

Table 4.4 (continued)

Medication	Dosing and dosing considerations	Potential SEs	Metabolism/major interactions
Ziprasidone (Geodon)	Capsule: 20, 40, 60, 80 mg (instructions for patients: take with food, >500 calories) Solution reconstituted, IM: 20 Initial oral: 40 mg Usual oral dose: 80–160 mg; dose adjustments should be made not more than once every 48 hours Usual IM dose: 20 mg/day Max oral dose: 320 mg Max IM dose: 40 mg/day Renal impairment: In mild or moderate impairment, no dose adjustment is necessary Hepatic impairment: in mild or moderate impairment, no dose adjustment is necessary	Moderate: akathisia, sedation, orthostatic hypotension Low: weight gain, glucose abnormalities, hyperlipidemia, parkinsonism, dystonia, tardive dyskinesia, anticholinergic symptoms, QTc prolongation	Aldehyde oxidase (major), CYP 3A4 (minor), CYP 1A2 (minor)/ administration with carbamazepine may require increased dose of ziprasidone. Administration with ketoconazole may require decreased dose of ziprasidone. Administration with QTc prolonging agents is contraindicated

Keepers et al. [38]; Aripiprazole [package insert] [3]; Asenapine [package insert] [4]; Brexpiprazole [package insert] [7]; Cariprazine [package insert] [9]; Clozapine [package insert] [10]; Iloperidone [package insert] [34]; Lumateperone [package insert] [45]; Lurasidone [package insert] [47]; Olanzapine [package insert] [55]; Paliperidone [package insert] [56]; Quetiapine [package insert] [61]; Risperidone [package insert] [63]; Ziprasidone [package insert] [80]; Marcsisin et al. [49]

4.4.2 Psychosocial Treatments

The overarching goal of psychiatric treatment of schizophrenia spectrum disorders, as with other serious mental illnesses, is to help facilitate "recovery." Here, recovery does not always mean a complete remission of symptoms. Recovery is a process whereby people with mental illness find hope and meaning in their lives. It focuses on coping, resilience, and making and meeting highly personalized and strength-based goals, often in social, educational, housing, and vocational domains [71]. Psychosocial treatments are critical in recovery and can include modalities like traditional talk therapies, psychiatric rehabilitation approaches, as well as structured living environments. Many of these treatments also target core symptoms of the disorder, including those not adequately addressed by pharmacologic approaches (e.g., cognitive and negative symptoms). Some evidence-based psychosocial approaches will be outlined below.

4.4.2.1 Psychiatric Rehabilitation

Psychiatric rehabilitation was born in the wake of deinstitutionalization, a period when patients who had lived for years if not decades in psychiatric institutions were suddenly released into the community after sometimes abrupt hospital closure. Community "re-integration" became an important focus of treatment. The modern form of psychiatric rehab was largely disseminated from academic centers, informed by the clubhouse movement, and supported by patients themselves. Today, psychiatric rehabilitation can be found integrated into larger systems of care or as a standalone program. In general, the focus of "psych rehab" is on mental health recovery through several domains, including skill building and maintenance in housing, basic living skills, social skills, vocational, educational, financial, and legal domains. Psych rehab programs are centered on instilling hope and empowering people with serious mental illness (often called clients, consumers, or members in this context) in their recovery, with a particular focus on teaching wellness strategies and promoting social connectedness and support.

4.4.2.2 Case Management

Patients with serious mental illness often interact with multiple agencies providing medical and behavioral health support. In doing so, patients often have to navigate complex systems to obtain housing, vocational support, disability payments, and insurance coverage. Doing so can be exceedingly challenging—more so if the patient experiences cognitive processing challenges, negative symptoms, distrust stemming from paranoia, or comorbid anxiety. Case management can help ensure that a patient is successfully engaging with services and in a coordinated way conducive to the patient's self-identified goals. Some case managers can meet with patients in patients' homes, places of employment, or other community settings. Depending on the agency providing the service, and patient needs, some case managers are able to provide intensive services, meeting with patients multiple times a week, while others may only interact with patients on a more limited basis. Some case managers offer more specialty services, for example, to patients with forensic or substance dependency challenges. Case management services in which the caseloads are small and whereby the patients are seen frequently has been shown to reduce lengths of psychiatric hospitalization and increase patient retention in care [18].

4.4.2.3 Assertive Community Treatment

Generally considered the most intensive level of services that patients can receive outside of a hospital setting, Assertive Community Treatment (ACT) was formulated to provide support to people with schizophrenia in transitioning from long-term hospitalization to community living [69]. ACT is composed of a multidisciplinary team, including psychiatrists, nurses, therapists, vocational specialists, forensics specialists, substance dependence specialists, peer counselors, and other behavioral health professionals, who provide services 24 hours a day, 7 days a week. This level of care has been repeatedly shown to reduce hospitalization, increase housing stability and independent living, and promote employment [51], though fidelity to the model is important to ensure good outcomes. As the model is often labor and cost intensive, and the caseloads relatively small, to qualify for ACT, patients must often meet specific criteria beyond their diagnosis, including high service utilization, history of incarceration, and/or homelessness.

4.4.2.4 Supported/Supportive Housing

Patients with schizophrenia live in a variety of settings, ideally informed by patient preference and level of support needed to maximize functional outcomes and promote psychiatric stability. Many patients can live independently in private housing, either alone or in a family setting, with minimal professional support. Other patients benefit from supported housing, where patients live independently but with support from agencies that provide flexible levels of services based on patient need. Such programs may include support with meal preparation, house cleaning, budgeting, and patient self-medication administration (e.g., helping fill pillboxes, providing fill reminders, etc.). Some supported housing agencies may offer rent assistance or facilitate with government-subsidized housing programs (e.g., Section 8 Housing Voucher Program). These programs often have a high level of retention and have been shown to reduce patient hospitalization [64]; among chronically homeless populations, including those with serious mental illness, they have been found to reduce homelessness and promote housing stability [5].

A.B. is fortunately in supported housing after a history of homelessness. His housing supports have helped link him to psychiatric services. They also provide meals, transportation, and administer his medications. On further discussion, supportive housing staff tell you that they frequently attempt to engage him in community and recreational activities (e.g., playing Bingo, painting, going on outings, etc.).

4.4.2.5 Residential Care Facilities

Many patients with schizophrenia have psychiatric and/or medical needs that benefit from a higher level of support than that which can be provided in independent housing. These patients may be said to require residential care. Definitions of what constitutes a residential care facility, however, are quite broad and extend to facilities that provide little more than room and board to those that more formally support medication administration and various activities of daily living. These facilities can be run by governmental, nonprofit, and even for-profit organizations, though all generally require state licensure. Types of residential care facilities can include adult residential facilities, community care homes, group homes, domiciliary homes, personal care homes, adult foster homes, and others [27]. Some offer transitional programs with goals of helping the patient successfully transition into independent living; others provide more permanent support. Some residential care facilities cater to special populations, like women with children, older adults, individuals with substance abuse disorders, or registered sex offenders. Of note, residential care facilities do not include nursing homes, which provide a level of medical support that these facilities cannot provide.

4.4.2.6 Psychotherapy

Psychotherapy is a cornerstone of treatment of nearly all mental health conditions, including schizophrenia. Ideally, in the treatment of schizophrenia, a good therapist will demonstrate unconditional positive regard for the patient, offering empathy and supportive listening. This can be particularly helpful as patients with schizophrenia often feel isolated from others and distressed by their symptoms.

A.B. is receiving psychotherapy. He enjoys a positive rapport with this therapist. While he cannot communicate what exact modality of therapy his therapist has engaged him in, by his description, it might be a form of supportive or personal therapy.

There are several types of psychotherapy that can be used in the treatment of patients with schizophrenia. Supportive therapy is often considered as usual care in schizophrenia. From the psychodynamic tradition, supportive therapy focuses on the relationship between the therapist and patient and may examine use of defenses and transference reactions to help the patient better understand maladaptive behaviors. Personal therapy adapts supportive therapy and incorporates patient psychoeducation and stress reduction techniques specific to the patient's stage of illness [33]. Other evidence-based practices include family psychoeducation, social skills training, supported employment, cognitive remediation, and cognitive behavioral therapy for psychosis, among others.

Family psychoeducation was developed by Carol Anderson and Gerard E. Hogarty in the 1970s, a time when families were often excluded from a patient's treatment yet expected to care for the patient when they weren't in a hospital. Family psychoeducation was thus devised to maximize a family's strengths and provide education to empower the family to create a supportive, low-stress domestic environment conducive to patient recovery. Multiple studies support the use of this treatment to reduce risk of psychotic relapse; it may also improve patient functioning and family well-being [20].

In social skills training, social cognitive challenges of schizophrenia are addressed, often through a series of modules using modeling and role-playing devised to improve performance in social situations ranging from basic conversation to job interviews. Given that at least 80% of people with serious mental illness, including schizophrenia, are unemployed [17], employment support is often necessary. Supported employment is focused solely on a patient's attaining and keeping a job. Most modern approaches to supported employment focus on rapid attainment of competitive employment as well as on job retention.

In therapies incorporating cognitive remediation, like cognitive enhancement therapy (CET), cognitive deficits are targeted, often using pencil and paper or computerized tasks. Different exercises are completed in a drill and practice approach and focus on different cognitive domains reflective of the rather broad and nonspecific nature of cognitive impairment in schizophrenia. CET also incorporates social skills training to address social cognitive impairments. Studies consistently demonstrate that cognitive remediation results in moderate effect size improvement in overall cognitive functioning in patients [78]; furthermore, it may prevent brain loss in early course illness [25].

Cognitive behavioral therapy for psychosis is a newer approach to the treatment of schizophrenia that focuses mostly on positive symptoms. Hallucinations and delusions are individually addressed via explicit formulations whereby the patient and the therapist seek a shared understanding of the cognitive basis of these symptoms. The symptoms are framed as products of distorted thinking and underlying cognitive biases. Treatment approaches include reality testing and dialogue to explore the symptoms further. Relaxation techniques and coping skills are also incorporated into treatment. The National Health Service in the United Kingdom has adopted CBTp as a standard practice, and multiple trials have demonstrated that it has at least modest benefits for both positive and negative symptoms [36].

4.5 Summary

Patients with schizophrenia represent a small percentage of people living in our communities, but they are often encountered by PCPs due to unmet medical and psychiatric needs. Despite frequently high service utilization, patients with schizophrenia are often undertreated. While referral to psychiatry is indicated in all but perhaps the most stable patient with schizophrenia, in extreme circumstances, PCPs can and do become the de facto psychiatrist for these seriously mentally ill patients. While most medical professionals agree that this is not ideal, the ability of the PCP to provide potentially lifesaving services should not be underestimated. When a patient is engaged with a psychiatrist, primary care teams can shift focus to the too often neglected medical care of these patients, identifying and treating comorbid medical illness, working with psychiatrists to address medication-related side effects, promoting health and wellness activities, and serving as patient advocates for much needed support services.

References

1. Addington J, Van Mastrigt S, Addington D. Duration of untreated psychosis: impact on 2-year outcome. Psychol Med. 2004;34(2):277–84. https://doi.org/10.1017/s0033291703001156. PMID: 14982133.
2. American Diabetes Association, American Psychiatric Association, American Association of Clinical Endocrinologists, North American Association for the Study of Obesity. Consensus

development conference on antipsychotic drugs and obesity and diabetes. Diabetes Care. 2004;27(2):596–601. https://doi.org/10.2337/diacare.27.2.596. PMID: 14747245.
3. Aripiprazole [package insert]. Tokyo, Japan: Otsuka Pharmaceutical Co, Ltd; 2014.
4. Asenapine [package insert]. Irvine, CA: Merck Sharp & Dohme B. V.; used by Allergan under license; 2017.
5. Aubry T, Bloch G, Brcic V, Saad A, Magwood O, Abdalla T, Alkhateeb Q, Xie E, Mathew C, Hannigan T, Costello C, Thavorn K, Stergiopoulos V, Tugwell P, Pottie K. Effectiveness of permanent supportive housing and income assistance interventions for homeless individuals in high-income countries: a systematic review. Lancet Public Health. 2020;5(6):e342–60. https://doi.org/10.1016/s2468-2667(20)30055-4.
6. Brar JS, Ganguli R, Pandina G, Turkoz I, Berry S, Mahmoud R. Effects of behavioral therapy on weight loss in overweight and obese patients with schizophrenia or schizoaffective disorder. J Clin Psychiatry. 2005;66(2):205–12. https://doi.org/10.4088/jcp.v66n0208. PMID: 15705006.
7. Brexpiprazole [package insert]. Tokyo, Japan: Otsuka Pharmaceutical Co., Ltd., 2017.
8. Carbon M, Kane JM, Leucht S, Correll CU. Tardive dyskinesia risk with first- and second-generation antipsychotics in comparative randomized controlled trials: a meta-analysis. World Psychiatry. 2018;17(3):330–40. https://doi.org/10.1002/wps.20579. PMID: 30192088; PMCID: PMC6127753.
9. Cariprazine [package insert]. Parsippany, NJ: Actavis Pharma, Inc; 2015.
10. Clozapine [package insert]. East Hanover, NJ: Novartis Pharmaceuticals Corporation; 2017.
11. Crawford MJ, Jayakumar S, Lemmey SJ, Zalewska K, Patel MX, Cooper SJ, Shiers D. Assessment and treatment of physical health problems among people with schizophrenia: national cross-sectional study. Br J Psychiatry. 2014;205(6):473–7. https://doi.org/10.1192/bjp.bp.113.142521. Epub 2014 Oct 16. PMID: 25323141.
12. Daumit GL, Dickerson FB, Wang NY, Dalcin A, Jerome GJ, Anderson CA, Young DR, Frick KD, Yu A, Gennusa JV 3rd, Oefinger M, Crum RM, Charleston J, Casagrande SS, Guallar E, Goldberg RW, Campbell LM, Appel LJ. A behavioral weight-loss intervention in persons with serious mental illness. N Engl J Med. 2013;368(17):1594–602. https://doi.org/10.1056/NEJMoa1214530. Epub 2013 Mar 21. PMID: 23517118; PMCID: PMC3743095.
13. Davis J, Eyre H, Jacka FN, Dodd S, Dean O, McEwen S, Debnath M, McGrath J, Maes M, Amminger P, McGorry PD, Pantelis C, Berk M. A review of vulnerability and risks for schizophrenia: beyond the two hit hypothesis. Neurosci Biobehav Rev. 2016;65:185–94. https://doi.org/10.1016/j.neubiorev.2016.03.017. Epub 2016 Apr 9. PMID: 27073049; PMCID: PMC4876729.
14. De Hert M, Vancampfort D, Correll CU, Mercken V, Peuskens J, Sweers K, van Winkel R, Mitchell AJ. Guidelines for screening and monitoring of cardiometabolic risk in schizophrenia: systematic evaluation. Br J Psychiatry. 2011;199(2):99–105. https://doi.org/10.1192/bjp.bp.110.084665. PMID: 21804146.
15. de Leon J, Diaz FJ. A meta-analysis of worldwide studies demonstrates an association between schizophrenia and tobacco smoking behaviors. Schizophr Res. 2005;76(2–3):135–57. https://doi.org/10.1016/j.schres.2005.02.010. PMID: 15949648.
16. De Mooij LD, Kikkert M, Theunissen J, Beekman ATF, de Haan L, Duurkoop PWRA, Van HL, Dekker JJM. Dying too soon: excess mortality in severe mental illness. Front Psych. 2019;10:855. https://doi.org/10.3389/fpsyt.2019.00855. PMID: 31920734; PMCID: PMC6918821.
17. Diehl S, Douglas D, Gay K, Hart J. Road to recovery: employment and mental illness. Arlington: National Alliance on Mental Illness; 2014.
18. Dieterich M, Irving CB, Park B, Marshall M. Intensive case management for severe mental illness. Cochrane Database Syst Rev. 2010;10:CD007906. https://doi.org/10.1002/14651858.CD007906.pub2. Update in: Cochrane Database Syst Rev. 2017 Jan 06;1:CD007906. PMID: 20927766; PMCID: PMC4233116.
19. Dipasquale S, Pariante CM, Dazzan P, Aguglia E, McGuire P, Mondelli V. The dietary pattern of patients with schizophrenia: a systematic review. J Psychiatr Res. 2013;47(2):197–207. https://doi.org/10.1016/j.jpsychires.2012.10.005. Epub 2012 Nov 12. PMID: 23153955.

20. Dixon L, Adams C, Lucksted A. Update on family psychoeducation for schizophrenia. Schizophr Bull. 2000;26(1):5–20. https://doi.org/10.1093/oxfordjournals.schbul.a033446. PMID: 10755667.
21. Druss BG, Bradford DW, Rosenheck RA, Radford MJ, Krumholz HM. Mental disorders and use of cardiovascular procedures after myocardial infarction. JAMA. 2000;283(4):506–11. https://doi.org/10.1001/jama.283.4.506. PMID: 10659877.
22. Diagnostic and Statistical Manual of Mental Disorders: DSM 5. 5th ed., American Psychiatric Association; 2013.
23. D'Souza DC, Radhakrishnan R, Sherif M, Cortes-Briones J, Cahill J, Gupta S, Skosnik PD, Ranganathan M. Cannabinoids and psychosis. Curr Pharm Des. 2016;22(42):6380–91. https://doi.org/10.2174/1381612822666160826105628. PMID: 27568729.
24. Dutra SJ, Stoeckel LE, Carlini SV, Pizzagalli DA, Evins AE. Varenicline as a smoking cessation aid in schizophrenia: effects on smoking behavior and reward sensitivity. Psychopharmacology. 2012;219(1):25–34. https://doi.org/10.1007/s00213-011-2373-6.
25. Eack SM, Hogarty GE, Cho RY, Prasad KM, Greenwald DP, Hogarty SS, Keshavan MS. Neuroprotective effects of cognitive enhancement therapy against gray matter loss in early schizophrenia: results from a 2-year randomized controlled trial. Arch Gen Psychiatry. 2010;67(7):674–82. https://doi.org/10.1001/archgenpsychiatry.2010.63. Epub 2010 May 3. PMID: 20439824; PMCID: PMC3741671.
26. Fazel S, Långström N, Hjern A, Grann M, Lichtenstein P. Schizophrenia, substance abuse, and violent crime. JAMA. 2009;301(19):2016–23. https://doi.org/10.1001/jama.2009.675.
27. Fleishman M. The problem: how many patients live in residential care facilities? Psychiatr Serv. 2004;55(6):620–2. https://doi.org/10.1176/appi.ps.55.6.620. PMID: 15175457.
28. Folsom DP, Hawthorne W, Lindamer L, Gilmer T, Bailey A, Golshan S, Garcia P, Unützer J, Hough R, Jeste DV. Prevalence and risk factors for homelessness and utilization of mental health services among 10,340 patients with serious mental illness in a large public mental health system. Am J Psychiatry. 2005;162(2):370–6. https://doi.org/10.1176/appi.ajp.162.2.370. PMID: 15677603.
29. Fluphenazine [package insert]. Irvine, CA: Gensia Laboratories, Ltd; 1996.
30. Frayne SM, Halanych JH, Miller DR, et al. Disparities in diabetes care: impact of mental illness. Arch Intern Med. 2005;165:2631–8.
31. Gottesman II. Schizophrenia genesis: the origin of madness. New York: Freeman; 1991.
32. Haloperidol [package insert]. Titusville, NJ: Janssen Pharmaceuticals, Inc.; 2017.
33. Hogarty GE. Personal therapy for schizophrenia and related disorders: a guide to individualized treatment. New York: Guilford; 2002. 338 pages
34. Iloperidone [package insert]. Washington, DC: Vanda Pharmaceuticals Inc.; 2016.
35. Jarskog LF, Hamer RM, Catellier DJ, Stewart DD, Lavange L, Ray N, Golden LH, Lieberman JA, Stroup TS; METS Investigators. Metformin for weight loss and metabolic control in overweight outpatients with schizophrenia and schizoaffective disorder. Am J Psychiatry. 2013;170(9):1032–40. https://doi.org/10.1176/appi.ajp.2013.12010127. PMID: 23846733; PMCID: PMC3874085.
36. Jauhar S, McKenna PJ, Radua J, Fung E, Salvador R, Laws KR. Cognitive-behavioural therapy for the symptoms of schizophrenia: systematic review and meta-analysis with examination of potential bias. Br J Psychiatry. 2014;204(1):20–9. https://doi.org/10.1192/bjp.bp.112.116285. PMID: 24385461.
37. Jones PB. Adult mental health disorders and their age at onset. Br J Psychiatry Suppl. 2013;54:s5–10. https://doi.org/10.1192/bjp.bp.112.119164. PMID: 23288502.
38. Keepers GA, Fochtmann LJ, Anzia JM, Benjamin S, Lyness JM, Mojtabai R, Servis M, Walaszek A, Buckley P, Lenzenweger MF, Young AS, Degenhardt A, Hong SH. (Systematic review). The American Psychiatric Association practice guideline for the treatment of patients with schizophrenia. Am J Psychiatry. 2020;177(9):868–72. https://doi.org/10.1176/appi.ajp.2020.177901. PMID: 32867516.

39. Kisely S, Smith M, Lawrence D, Cox M, Campbell LA, Maaten S. Inequitable access for mentally ill patients to some medically necessary procedures. CMAJ. 2007;176(6):779–84. https://doi.org/10.1503/cmaj.060482. PMID: 17353530; PMCID: PMC1808525.
40. Kisely S, Crowe E, Lawrence D. Cancer-related mortality in people with mental illness. JAMA Psychiat. 2013;70:209–17.
41. Laursen TM, Mortensen PB, MacCabe JH, Cohen D, Gasse C. Cardiovascular drug use and mortality in patients with schizophrenia or bipolar disorder: a Danish population-based study. Psychol Med. 2014;44(8):1625–37. https://doi.org/10.1017/S003329171300216X. Epub 2013 Nov 18. PMID: 24246137.
42. Li R, Ma X, Wang G, Yang J, Wang C. Why sex differences in schizophrenia? J Transl Neurosci (Beijing). 2016;1(1):37–42. PMID: 29152382; PMCID: PMC5688947.
43. Lord O, Malone D, Mitchell AJ. Receipt of preventive medical care and medical screening for patients with mental illness: a comparative analysis. Gen Hosp Psychiatry. 2010;32(5):519–43. https://doi.org/10.1016/j.genhosppsych.2010.04.004. Epub 2010 Aug 5. PMID: 20851274.
44. Loxapine [package insert]. Corona, CA: Watson Pharmaceuticals; 2017.
45. Lumateperone [package insert]. New York, NY: Intra-Cellular Therapies, Inc.; 2019.
46. Lupu AM, MacCamy KL, Gannon JM, Brar JS, Chengappa KR. Less is more: deprescribing anticholinergic medications in persons with severe mental illness. Ann Clin Psychiatry. 2021;33(1):e1–e13. https://doi.org/10.12788/acp.0019. Epub ahead of print. PMID: 33529289.
47. Lurasidone [package insert]. Chuo-ku, Osaka, Japan: Dainippon Sumitomo Pharma Co. Ltd.; 2013.
48. Maayan L, Vakhrusheva J, Correll CU. Effectiveness of medications used to attenuate antipsychotic-related weight gain and metabolic abnormalities: a systematic review and meta-analysis. Neuropsychopharmacology. 2010;35(7):1520–30. https://doi.org/10.1038/npp.2010.21. Epub 2010 Mar 24. PMID: 20336059; PMCID: PMC3055458.
49. Marcsisin MJ, Rosenstock JB, Gannon JM, editors. Schizophrenia and related disorders. Oxford University Press; 2017.
50. Mitchell AJ, Pereira IE, Yadegarfar M, Pepereke S, Mugadza V, Stubbs B. Breast cancer screening in women with mental illness: comparative meta-analysis of mammography uptake. Br J Psychiatry. 2014;205(6):428–35. https://doi.org/10.1192/bjp.bp.114.147629. PMID: 25452600.
51. McDonagh MS, Dana T, Selph S, Devine EB, Cantor A, Bougatsos C, Blazina I, Grusing S, Fu R, Kopelovich SL, Monroe-DeVita M, Haupt DW. Treatments for schizophrenia in adults: a systematic review [Internet]. Rockville: Agency for Healthcare Research and Quality (US); 2017 Oct. Report No.: 17(18)-EHC031-EF. PMID: 29537779.
52. Myles N, Myles H, Xia S, Large M, Kisely S, Galletly C, Bird R, Siskind D. Meta-analysis examining the epidemiology of clozapine-associated neutropenia. Acta Psychiatr Scand. 2018;138(2):101–9. https://doi.org/10.1111/acps.12898. Epub 2018 May 21. PMID: 29786829.
53. Nasrallah HA, Meyer JM, Goff DC, McEvoy JP, Davis SM, Stroup TS, Lieberman JA. Low rates of treatment for hypertension, dyslipidemia and diabetes in schizophrenia: data from the CATIE schizophrenia trial sample at baseline. Schizophr Res. 2006;86(1–3):15–22. https://doi.org/10.1016/j.schres.2006.06.026. Epub 2006 Aug 1. PMID: 16884895.
54. Nimgaonkar VL, Fujiwara TM, Dutta M, Wood J, Gentry K, Maendel S, Morgan K, Eaton J. Low prevalence of psychoses among the Hutterites, an isolated religious community. Am J Psychiatry. 2000;157(7):1065–70. https://doi.org/10.1176/appi.ajp.157.7.1065. PMID: 10873912.
55. Olanzapine [package insert]. Indianapolis, IN: Eli Lilly and Company; 2009.
56. Paliperidone [package insert]. Titusville, NJ: Janssen Pharmaceuticals, Inc.; 2009.
57. Palmer BA, Pankratz VS, Bostwick JM. The lifetime risk of suicide in schizophrenia: a reexamination. Arch Gen Psychiatry. 2005;62(3):247–53. https://doi.org/10.1001/archpsyc.62.3.247.
58. Perphenazine. [package insert]. Princeton, NJ: Sandoz Inc.

59. Pimozide. [package insert]. Sellersville, PA: Gate Pharmaceuticals, Div. of Teva Pharmaceuticals.
60. Potkin SG, Kane JM, Correll CU, Lindenmayer JP, Agid O, Marder SR, Olfson M, Howes OD. The neurobiology of treatment-resistant schizophrenia: paths to antipsychotic resistance and a roadmap for future research. NPJ Schizophr. 2020;6(1):1. https://doi.org/10.1038/s41537-019-0090-z. PMID: 31911624; PMCID: PMC6946650.
61. Quetiapine [package insert]. Wilmington, DE: AstraZeneca Pharmaceuticals LP; 2013.
62. Ramsay CE, Goulding SM, Broussard B, Cristofaro SL, Abedi GR, Compton MT. Prevalence and psychosocial correlates of prior incarcerations in an urban, predominantly African-American sample of hospitalized patients with first-episode psychosis. J Am Acad Psychiatry Law. 2011;39(1):57–64.
63. Risperidone [package insert]. Titusville, NJ: Ortho-McNeil-Janssen Pharmaceuticals, Inc.; 2009.
64. Rogers E, Kash- MacDonald M, Olschewski A. Systematic Review of Supported Housing Literature, 1993–2008. Boston: Boston University, Sargent College, Center for Psychiatric Rehabilitation; 2009.
65. Rosenheck R, Leslie D, Keefe R, McEvoy J, Swartz M, Perkins D, Stroup S, Hsiao JK, Lieberman J. CATIE Study Investigators Group. Barriers to employment for people with schizophrenia. Am J Psychiatry. 2006;163(3):411–7. https://doi.org/10.1176/appi.ajp.163.3.411. PMID: 16513861.
66. Samara MT, Leucht C, Leeflang MM, Anghelescu IG, Chung YC, Crespo-Facorro B, Elkis H, Hatta K, Giegling I, Kane JM, Kayo M, Lambert M, Lin CH, Möller HJ, Pelayo-Terán JM, Riedel M, Rujescu D, Schimmelmann BG, Serretti A, Correll CU, Leucht S. Early improvement as a predictor of later response to antipsychotics in schizophrenia: a diagnostic test review. Am J Psychiatry. 2015;172(7):617–29. https://doi.org/10.1176/appi.ajp.2015.14101329. Epub 2015 Jun 5. PMID: 26046338.
67. Schneider M, Regente J, Greiner T, Lensky S, Bleich S, Toto S, Grohmann R, Stübner S, Heinze M. Neuroleptic malignant syndrome: evaluation of drug safety data from the AMSP program during 1993–2015. Eur Arch Psychiatry Clin Neurosci. 2020;270(1):23–33. https://doi.org/10.1007/s00406-018-0959-2. Epub 2018 Nov 30. PMID: 30506147.
68. Siskind D, Hahn M, Correll CU, Fink-Jensen A, Russell AW, Bak N, Broberg BV, Larsen J, Ishøy PL, Vilsbøll T, Knop FK, Kisely S, Ebdrup BH. Glucagon-like peptide-1 receptor agonists for antipsychotic-associated cardio-metabolic risk factors: a systematic review and individual participant data meta-analysis. Diabetes Obes Metab. 2019;21(2):293–302. https://doi.org/10.1111/dom.13522. Epub 2018 Oct 7. PMID: 30187620.
69. Stein LI, Test MA. Alternative to mental hospital treatment. I. Conceptual model, treatment program, and clinical evaluation. Arch Gen Psychiatry. 1980;37(4):392–7. https://doi.org/10.1001/archpsyc.1980.01780170034003. PMID: 7362425.
70. Stubbs B, Williams J, Gaughran F, Craig T. How sedentary are people with psychosis? A systematic review and meta-analysis. Schizophr Res. 2016;171(1–3):103–9. https://doi.org/10.1016/j.schres.2016.01.034. Epub 2016 Jan 21. PMID: 26805414.
71. Substance Abuse and Mental Health Services Administration. National consensus on mental health recovery and systems transformation. Rockville: Department of Health and Human Services; 2005.
72. Takeuchi H, Siu C, Remington G, Fervaha G, Zipursky RB, Foussias G, Agid O. Does relapse contribute to treatment resistance? Antipsychotic response in first- vs. second-episode schizophrenia. Neuropsychopharmacology. 2019;44(6):1036–1042. doi: https://doi.org/10.1038/s41386-018-0278-3. Epub 2018 Nov 22. PMID: 30514883; PMCID: PMC6462044.
73. Tandon R, Nasrallah HA, Keshavan MS. Schizophrenia, "just the facts" 4. Clinical features and conceptualization. Schizophr Res. 2009;110(1–3):1–23. https://doi.org/10.1016/j.schres.2009.03.005. Epub 2009 Mar 27. PMID: 19328655.
74. Thorazine [package insert]. Greenville, SC: PAI Pharmaceutical Associates; 1998.

75. Tsoi DT, Porwal M, Webster AC. Interventions for smoking cessation and reduction in individuals with schizophrenia. Cochrane Database Syst Rev. 2013, Issue 2. Art. No.: CD007253. https://doi.org/10.1002/14651858.CD007253.pub3. Accessed 20 February 2021.
76. Varshney M, Mahapatra A, Krishnan V, Gupta R, Deb KS. Violence and mental illness: what is the true story? J Epidemiol Community Health. 2016;70(3):223–5. https://doi.org/10.1136/jech-2015-205546. Epub 2015 Aug 28. PMID: 26320232; PMCID: PMC4789812.
77. Wildgust HJ, Hodgson R, Beary M. The paradox of premature mortality in schizophrenia: new research questions. J Psychopharmacol. 2010;24(4 Suppl):9–15. https://doi.org/10.1177/1359786810382149. PMID: 20923916; PMCID: PMC2951588.
78. Wykes T, Huddy V, Cellard C, McGurk SR, Czobor P. A meta-analysis of cognitive remediation for schizophrenia: methodology and effect sizes. Am J Psychiatry. 2011;168(5):472–85. https://doi.org/10.1176/appi.ajp.2010.10060855. Epub 2011 Mar 15. PMID: 21406461.
79. Ziaaddini H, Kheradmand A, Vahabi M. Prevalence of cigarette smoking in schizophrenic patients compared to other hospital admitted psychiatric patients. Addict Health. 2009 Summer;1(1):38–42. PMID: 24494081; PMCID: PMC3905500.
80. Ziprasidone [package insert]. New York, NY: Pfizer; 2014.

Chapter 5
Obsessive Compulsive Disorder

5.1 Introduction and Epidemiology

Case Example 5.1
Mr. B., a 32-year-old male, presents to his PCP after being referred by the local emergency room. He had presented 3 days ago with complaints of acute chest pain and shortness of breath. His cardiac work-up, including EKG and enzymes, was negative. As he was low risk for coronary artery disease and he admitted to being under a great deal of stress, he was given a diagnosis of a panic attack. He tells his PCP that while this was the most severe panic attack he has had, he has been having them for many months and has had an increase in anxiety over the last year. In order to help make a definitive diagnosis of panic disorder, his PCP asked him if his attacks were spontaneous or triggered by specific circumstances or thoughts. Mr. B. was initially cagey with his answer, seeming to imply that certain thoughts were triggering his panic attacks. He eventually admitted that he was hoping only to get treatment for the attacks and not discuss his thoughts. When asked why, he replied that the thoughts were embarrassing, and he was ashamed of them—afraid to say them out loud. He finally admitted that he was having thoughts that he was harming people by thinking about them. When the image or thought of someone he knew popped into his head, he had the feeling that this meant that he had accidently hurt them or sexually molested them in some way. When these thoughts got too strong, he would have a panic attack. He is adamant that he would never do this, and whats more he knows he hasn't. He is afraid that he has anyway, however, and spends a great deal of time reviewing his actions to

R. Hudak, J. M. Gannon, *Handbook of Psychiatric Disorders in Adults in the Primary Care Setting*, Current Clinical Practice,
https://doi.org/10.1007/978-3-030-98709-1_5

reassure himself that no abuse took place. Due to the intrusive, nonsensical nature of these thoughts, the PCP diagnosed him as having OCD and that the panic attacks were simply secondary to the primary disorder. It was decided not to start him on medications due to the length of time it takes medications to work, and instead he was referred to a psychiatrist and therapist specializing in OCD treatment.

Obsessive-compulsive disorder (OCD) is one of the most common and disabling of all psychiatric disorders. It is estimated to affect between 2% and 3% of all individuals [16] which would make it the fourth most common psychiatric disorder behind simple phobias, substance use disorders, and major depressive disorder [37]. OCD causes significant morbidity and disability in its sufferers. The World Health Organization has listed it as one of the top 10 causes of all disability, both medical and psychiatric, worldwide, which highlights its significant psychosocial burden [31]. It has been estimated that the average person with OCD will lose 3 years of wages during their lifetime, and at least a third of patients will report occupational difficulty. People with OCD are also less likely to marry than the general population, and when they do, they are more likely to experience marital difficulties [16].

The age of onset of OCD is somewhat difficult to state definitively due to the various definitions of age of onset in various studies. Some studies determined the age of onset to be around the age of 10 years [43], while others have stated that the average age of onset is 21 years [37]. However, since many OCD patients will tell you they first developed lesser, subclinical obsessions at much younger ages and it is not unusual for patients to state that their first memories are of OCD thoughts, a childhood age of onset is likely in many cases. Interestingly, OCD is unusual among psychiatric illnesses in that the symptoms present the same in childhood as in adulthood (with the possible exception that children may have less insight into their symptoms). Therefore, it should be expected that patients presenting with OCD can be found in virtually every age group.

The course of OCD is that of a chronic, lifelong illness. Patients rarely achieve remission of their disorder and the likelihood of complete remission in adults is very low [7]. Instead, most patients are advised that with proper treatment, the goal is that they will learn to manage their OCD symptoms, rather than their symptoms managing them. Typically, OCD symptoms will fluctuate over the lifespan of a sufferer, with the symptoms waxing and waning at different points in their life. With a good history, patients like Mr. B. will admit to some degree of intrusive thoughts starting at a very young age.

The course of OCD in patients has historically been divided into three categories [17]:

1. Episodic course with periods of incomplete remission
2. Phasic course with periods of complete remission between exacerbations

3. Continuous and unremitting course with most patients experiencing some fluctuations in the levels of symptoms and a minority of patients experiencing a chronic and deteriorative course

Studies show that while most patients have the episodic course of OCD, the advent of modern treatments increases the possibility of remission; despite this, relapses are still common after remission [26]. Many patients who report significant improvement after treatment will still meet criteria for OCD; however, symptom reduction can still lead to significant clinical improvement and greater functionality even if the primary symptoms remain. Patients should be educated at the outset of treatment that symptom resolution is not necessarily the goal, but that improvement should be great enough that the patient feels that they can control their OCD symptoms, rather than the symptoms control them.

Treatment resistance is a significant issue with OCD, as it is a chronic illness that is typically present for the life of the individual. It has been estimated that between 40% and 60% of people with OCD are considered to be treatment resistant [35]. However, it must be emphasized that while a formal definition of treatment-resistant OCD does not exist, treatment response is often defined as a 25–30% reduction in symptoms [35] which means that even patients defined as clinical responders can be left with symptoms that are clinically marked and disabling. People with a mild level of OCD (which is defined as a score of less than 16 on the Yale-Brown Obsessive Compulsive Scale) may still have significant levels of OCD requiring intervention [21]. While most clinicians ideally would refer someone with a treatment-resistant psychiatric illness to a psychiatric specialist, that is not always possible, especially in more rural areas where specialty psychiatric care can be difficult to come by. Therefore, a familiarity with standard OCD protocols is vital so that the appropriate clinical decisions and treatments are made. However, even when patients are being seen by psychiatrists, it is important for primary care to be aware of proper treatment protocols for OCD, as the medications used in OCD are prescribed in doses outside of the protocols used for other psychiatric disorders.

5.2 OCD in the Medical Setting

The role of the primary care physician is vital in the proper diagnosis and treatment of OCD. According to the International OCD Foundation, it can be 14–17 years after the onset of symptoms until the OCD sufferer obtains appropriate, evidence-based treatment. Most patients with OCD do not initially present to a psychiatrist; the majority of the time they will present to their PCP with complaints related to the OCD symptoms but will not complain of their OCD symptoms directly. Mr. B. above is a typical example. This can occur for many reasons. Certainly, most people are not familiar with the concept of intrusive thoughts, and therefore the general public just is not aware of this phenomenon, much less that it is abnormal. However, perhaps the greatest reason is simply the nature of OCD itself: by definition, obsessions are embarrassing and cause shame. Their inherent nature is itself responsible for patients not wanting to discuss them. Therefore, it is vital that physician and other primary care providers understand what OCD is, how it may present, and to have appropriate clinical suspicion that OCD may be an underlying reason for a patient's visit in a wide variety of circumstances. The primary care office can be directly responsible for reducing the lengthy amount of time from illness onset until OCD patients receive appropriate, evidence-based treatment.

There are numerous complaints that people with OCD may present to the primary care physician with other than obsessions or compulsions. See Table 5.1 for a list of typical chief complaints. People with excessive anxiety may also have similar chief complaints (see Chap. 2). Other psychiatric complaints will be commonly given, while the patient does their best to hide or downplay symptoms of OCD. Panic attacks and anxiety are two of the common chief complaints. Depression is another common complaint, due to both the high comorbidity of major depressive disorder and OCD, but also since dealing with OCD is very difficult and dysphoric. Complaints of sleep disturbances and other vague, somatic complaints are typical, and patients who seem somatically preoccupied (i.e., hypochondriasis) should be screened for OCD. Patient may complain of "racing thoughts" or "increased energy" due to the anxiety that OCD can create. Nonspecific physical complaints that occur secondary to anxiety are often seen, such as tics or muscle twitches, chest pain, GI disturbances, shortness of breath, or dizziness. Dermatologic findings secondary to compulsive behavior are common and can include dry and chapped hands and lips, gum lesions, and eczema or nonspecific dermatitis from overwashing or use of harsh chemicals on the skin. Screening for anxiety or obsessive-compulsive disorders is critical in patients with unexplained physical complaints. If there is suspicion that the patient may have OCD as an underlying cause, the use of appropriate screening questions should be performed. Screening questions are listed in Table 5.2. Please keep in mind that OCD can present as virtually any intrusive thought that one can imagine—OCD is not just an illness of cleaning or checking. However, those two symptoms are among the most common OCD symptoms, and so question about them will pick up many people with OCD.

Table 5.1 Possible presentations for people with obsessive-compulsive disorders or anxiety disorders

Panic attacks
Anxiety or depression
Sleep disturbances
Complaints of "racing thoughts" or "increased energy"
Tics or muscle twitches
Chest pain or shortness of breath
GI distress or vague GI complaints
Dizziness
Skin lesions, chapped hands, eczema
Chapped or dry lips or gum/cheek lesions from overcleaning

Table 5.2 Screening questions for OCD

Do you have to wash your hands excessively?
Do you have to check things over and over?
Do you have thoughts that bother you or make you anxious?
Do you have thoughts that do not make sense, that seem silly or weird, or that you cannot get rid of?
Are there certain behaviors that you feel compelled to do repeatedly that may seem silly or weird?

5.3 Diagnosis and Presentation of OCD

The diagnosis of OCD is a relatively straightforward diagnosis, especially compared to many of the other diagnostic criteria found in the DSM 5. To meet the criteria for OCD, a person simply has to have either obsessions or compulsions or both, the obsessions or compulsions must be time-consuming (e.g., take more than 1 hour a day) or cause clinically significant distress, and the symptoms are not attributable to the physiological effects of a substance or another medical condition and are not better explained by another psychiatric disorder (e.g., an individual who hears voices telling them to wash their hands repeatedly would not meet criteria for OCD). The key is the proper recognition and diagnosis of obsessions and compulsions. Obsessions are defined by DSM 5 as:

1. Recurrent and persistent thoughts, urges, or images that are experienced, at some time during the disturbance, as intrusive and unwanted, and that in most individuals cause marked anxiety or distress
2. The individual attempts to ignore or suppress such thoughts, urges, or images or to neutralize them with some other thought or action (i.e., by performing a compulsion)

Compulsions are defined by DSM 5 as:

1. Repetitive behaviors (e.g., handwashing, ordering, checking) or mental acts (e.g., praying, counting, repeating words silently) that the individual feels driven to perform in response to an obsession or according to rules that must be applied rigidly.
2. The behaviors or mental acts are aimed at reducing anxiety or distress or preventing some dreaded event or situation; however, these behaviors or mental acts are not connected in a realistic way with what they are designed to neutralize or prevent or are clearly excessive.

The lay concept that OCD is the act of keeping things neat and clean is nothing at all like actual nature of OCD. Likewise, the lay concepts of obsessions and compulsions are qualitatively different than the psychiatric definition.

Obsessions are intrusive thoughts, urges, or images. In other words, they are thoughts that the person does not desire to have and does not wish to have. The very presence of the thought makes the person who has it uncomfortable. The OCD sufferer (at least early in the course of the illness) will be aware that the thought they are experiencing is silly and untrue. However, the thought causes significant distress, and they try to push it out of their mind, which leads to the thought returning even stronger at another time. The content of the obsession can literally be about any topic. While the content of some obsessions is common among OCD sufferers and is generally recognized even by clinicians who are not OCD specialists (e.g., the fear that unknown and unseen germs can cause death), some obsessional content can strike professionals as very unusual (e.g., the thought that a man could trap his adult daughter in an ordinary envelop while paying bills and causing her to suffocate and die; or the intrusive image of a woman with postpartum obsessions holding her newborn's bloody cornea in her hands after she imagines that she might rip it out of his eye). It is vital to note that these thoughts, images, or urges are unwanted by the person and are against their value system. In the example provided, the woman with the intrusive image of harm toward her newborn is at no risk of real harm.

It is common for patients like Mr. B. to minimize or attempt to hide their OCD symptoms due to the extreme embarrassment and shame associated with them.

As with obsessions, compulsions are defined differently by psychiatry than the common usage. Compulsive acts are not addictive behaviors, nor are they behaviors that provide pleasure on some level. Compulsions are acts that the person does not wish to perform but feel that they must in order to prevent a bad outcome. For example, in the instance of the woman with postpartum harm urges, she would repeatedly check her baby's eye to ensure that it was still intact and that she had not actually damaged it. The more she checked to ensure that the eye was OK, the more anxious she became because she could never be certain that she had not actually done harm. Note that this is very different from an addictive behavior which results in the pleasure of a euphoric high. Even later in addiction when using drugs is as much about preventing withdrawal symptoms as it is about getting high, it is still not compulsive; it is a purposeful, intentional, and wanted behavior. The most common obsessions and compulsions provide a useful marker as to the symptoms most likely to be seen in the primary care office. See Tables 5.3 and 5.4 [11].

Table 5.3 The rate of obsessions in OCD patients

Primary obsession	Percentage of OCD patients
Contamination	38
Fear of harming self or others	24
Symmetry concerns	10
Religious (scrupulosity)	6
Sexual	6
Hoarding obsessions	5
Unacceptable urges	4
Miscellaneous	1

Table 5.4 The rate of compulsions in OCD patients

Primary compulsion	Percentage of OCD patients
Checking	28
Cleaning/washing	27
Miscellaneous	12
Repeating	11
Mental rituals	11
Ordering	6
Hoarding	4
Counting	2

5.4 Treatment

5.4.1 Exposure with Response Prevention

The treatment of OCD involves an integrated approach—patients should be offered a combination of cognitive behavioral therapy (CBT)—particularly a specific CBT known as Exposure with Response Prevention (E/RP) and, if necessary, medication management, specifically the use of selective serotonin reuptake inhibitors (SSRIs). Many patients with a mild-to-moderate level of OCD can be offered E/RP as first-line therapy without the addition of medication management. Medication management may be useful in patients with moderate-to-severe levels of OCD, although a trial of E/RP alone is not unwarranted if the patient desires [24].

Clinical Tip
Behavioral therapy, specifically E/RP, is a first-line therapy for OCD, with the addition of SSRIs usually reserved for moderate-to-severe cases or per patient request.

The use of appropriate E/RP in patients with OCD cannot be overstated. Some studies have found that E/RP is superior to medication use for OCD [12], and one study suggested that while medication and E/RP are both superior to placebo, E/RP plus medication is in fact no better than E/RP alone [13]. The bottom line is clear: E/RP is the primary choice of treatment for all patients. Medication management can be a useful adjunct, but medication management alone cannot equal the effects of E/RP. However, there can be significant difficulty in finding a qualified E/RP therapist to refer your patients to. E/RP is usually not taught at most graduate schools. In order to get trained in E/RP, most therapists have to seek out proper instruction on their own after graduation. To further confuse matters, many therapists are trained in therapeutic techniques that are often colloquially called "exposure therapy." These therapies are *not* the same thing as E/RP, and they are not interchangeable. Most of the so-called exposure therapies can and have been used as placebo in research trials. Obviously, no primary care physician wants to refer one of their patients to someone who is going to practice a treatment that is considered placebo. So how does the person who is not a trained psychiatrist figure out the right person in your community to refer your patients to who need E/RP? Fortunately, there are some helpful hints that we can give you.

First, look at the therapists list from the International OCD Foundation, at www.IOCDF.org. They maintain a list of therapists who express an interest in OCD or have declared themselves to be OCD specialists. While just listing yourself as an OCD professional is no guarantee, of course, that the therapist has been trained in E/RP, it certainly greatly increases your likelihood. A therapist on that website who states that they have completed BTTI (Behavior Therapy Training Institute) has indeed completed formal training in E/RP. Another option is to inquire if any potential therapists have trained in an OCD specialty clinic. Such a therapist can be assumed to have appropriate experience as well. There are some useful questions that you can ask prospective therapists, or *questions that you can give to your patients when they are making inquiries,* to help ensure that they are getting a qualified therapist:

- "What techniques do you use to treat OCD?" If the therapist gives a vague answer or simply says CBT without mentioned E/RP, there is a good chance they do not have OCD training.
- "Do you use Exposure with Response Prevention to treat OCD?" Again, therapists who give vague answers or who only state that they do exposures may not be using evidence-based therapy.
- "Where did you get your training in OCD?" Therapists who state that they are a member of the IOCDF or who state that they have attended specialized training through the IOCDF or other specialty treatment centers are more likely to have received the appropriate training.
- "Do you leave your office to do OCD therapy?" It is a good sign if they say yes, as it is typical to go out in the community while practicing E/RP.
- "What are your feelings about OCD medications?" While E/RP is indeed a first-line treatment for OCD, most OCD specialists recognize the utility of medications and will have a positive attitude about them. Be wary of therapists who have negative attitudes toward medications—they are more likely to practice forms of therapy other than CBT and E/RP.

5.5 Treatment

5.5.1 Pharmacotherapy

Medication treatment of OCD involves relatively straightforward protocols; however, the protocols for SSRI pharmacotherapy for OCD differ than the protocols for other psychiatric conditions, particularly compared to mood disorders. Thus, practitioners need to familiarize themselves not only with the medications that are OCD specific, but with the unique dosing and responses for OCD. See Fig. 5.1 for a basic OCD algorithm that can be followed in the primary care office. The medications

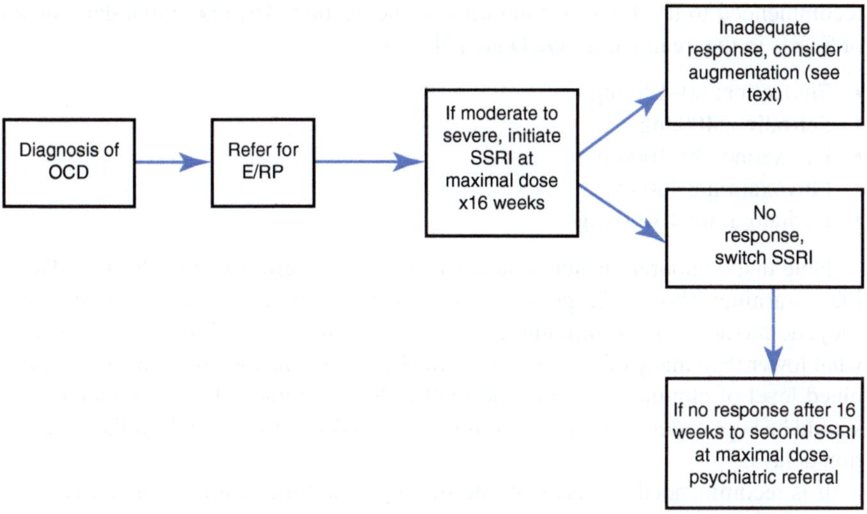

Fig. 5.1 OCD treatment algorithm in primary care

that are the treatment of choice for OCD are the selective serotonin reuptake inhibitors (SSRIs) as well as a single tricyclic antidepressant (TCA) that acts as an SSRI: clomipramine [2]. There are currently five medications that are approved for OCD treatment in adults: fluoxetine, sertraline, paroxetine, fluvoxamine, and clomipramine. There are two additional SSRIs that are not approved for OCD treatment in the USA but work equally well for OCD: citalopram and escitalopram [2]. There are four medications approved in the USA for children with OCD: fluoxetine, sertraline, fluvoxamine, and clomipramine [15]. All of the SSRIs are equally efficacious for OCD. There have been suggestions that clomipramine may be numerically advantageous over the SSRIs in OCD, but this has never been demonstrated definitively [2]. Because clomipramine is a TCA and has the typical associated side effects which can be problematic in some people, it is recommended that two SSRIs be tried and failed before using clomipramine.

SSRIs are prescribed according to different protocols for OCD than when used for major depressive disorder. Patients with OCD often require higher dosing of the SSRI and may also require a greater length of trial (12–16 weeks) for full efficacy. While some patients with OCD will respond at low-to-mid-range doses of SSRIs, most will need high doses in order to get adequate treatment. Generally, if patients are treatment naïve or if they have previously responded well to low SSRI doses, they can be offered the option of trying a low-to-mid-range dose first before trying a maximal dose. The disadvantage with this strategy is that if they do not respond initially, they will have to be titrated up to the full anti-obsessional dose and wait for another 12–16 weeks to gauge response. Many patients do not wish to prolong a possible therapeutic response and will opt for an initial titration to the maximum dose. If a patient is not treatment naïve or if they have failed other SSRI trials in the past, there is no reason to offer them an intermediate dose; they should be recommended to try the maximum dose of medication. The maximum daily doses of SSRIs in the treatment of OCD are [21, 24]:

- Fluoxetine: 80–120 mg
- Sertraline: 400 mg
- Paroxetine: 80–100 mg
- Fluvoxamine: 450 mg
- Escitalopram: 40–60 mg

Note that citalopram is not included as it is not a useful OCD medication due to FDA warnings about QTc prolongation above 40 mg daily. The anti-obsessional tricyclic medication, clomipramine, has a maximum dose of 250 mg a day, somewhat lower than many of the other TCA medications. The total tricyclic level (combined level of clomipramine plus desmethylclomipramine—the active metabolite) should be kept under 500 ng/ml to minimize the risk of seizures and cardiac conduction delays.

It is recommended to start with the starting dose for a minimum of 1 week and increase by the same starting or titration dose on a weekly basis (or as tolerated) until the patient has reached the target or maximum dose. Starting doses are typically within FDA parameters and in most patients would be:

- Fluoxetine 10–20 mg
- Sertraline 25–50 mg
- Paroxetine 10–20 mg
- Fluvoxamine 25–50 mg
- Escitalopram 5–10 mg

The starting and titration dose may need to be half in elderly or sensitive patients, but the end target dose is usually the same. It is important to note that the therapeutic dose for anti-obsessional response is, in many cases, above the maximum daily amount approved by the FDA. For example, the target OCD dose of sertraline is 400 mg/day, while the FDA has approved sertraline at a maximum of 200 mg/day. It is vital to note that these supramaximal doses are either scientifically validated [33] or recommended by expert consensus certified by the American Psychiatric Association [24]. Therefore, prescribing SSRIs in a manner consistent with these guidelines is not the liability that some physicians may fear, but is indeed backed up by research, experience, and consensus. Prescribing SSRIs at these doses sometimes will result in pushback from pharmacists, insurance companies, or even psychiatrists who are not familiar with OCD guidelines. Be prepared to stand your ground with these appropriate and recommended clinical practices. Pharmacists can be told that these doses are correct as prescribed if you are questioned. If insurance companies refuse to pay, prior authorization or appeal may not work, but these medications are generally inexpensive, and many people can afford to pay out of pocket at retail price or with help from online coupons.

As mentioned above, the definition of a therapeutic SSRI trial for OCD differs from antidepressant protocol. In order to determine if a patient has responded or will respond to medication treatment, the initial medication must be used at the maximum dose for a 12–16-week trial. For example, this means that if sertraline is titrated up to an anti-obsessional dose of 400 mg daily over a 1-month period, the patient must be on the full 400 mg dose for 12–16 weeks before it can be determined if they have had an appropriate response or not. If they start to notice a decrease in symptoms only at the end of this 12–16-week period, the trail can be extended further in order to achieve maximal benefit. If the patient is a treatment-naïve patient who elects to try an intermediate dose first (e.g., 200 mg daily), a response can only be determined after 12–16 weeks. If there is not enough of a benefit after that time, the dose can be titrated to 400 mg, but another 12–16-week trial period at that dose is indicated.

To sum up, a therapeutic trial of an SSRI or clomipramine for OCD is defined as the use of the medication at the maximum dose for a period of 12–16 weeks. At the end of this trial, a medication can be assessed for response. If the patient has responded adequately, the medication should be maintained. If the patient has had minimal improvement, further action may be warranted. How is response evaluated? The easiest way to do this in the primary care setting is based on his and the patient's psychosocial functioning. In other words, are they satisfied with their level of response? Are they able to engage in their preferred activities? Are they functioning at school and work appropriately? Is the OCD not interfering in their family or romantic relationships? If the answers to these questions are yes, it can be assumed that the person has achieved a reasonable response. Further increases or medication augmentation would be at the request of the patient if they desired a greater response. However, if a more formal assessment of the severity of symptoms is required, a self-report scale can be given to the patient that they can fill out pre- and posttreatment. The Y-BOCS is a 10-question OCD rating scale scored from 0 to 40 points that measures the severity of OCD [42]. The patient can fill it out in the waiting room and the scores placed in the chart. An improvement in their score of >25% is considered by many authors to be a significant response [35]. A copy of the Y-BOCS can be found on the website for the International OCD Foundation here:

- https://iocdf.org/wp-content/uploads/2014/08/Assessment-Tools.pdf

5.6 Maintenance Versus Discontinuation of Medications

OCD is a chronic illness that is generally present throughout the lives of most sufferers; therefore, ongoing treatment possibly including the chronic use of medications will be the case for many individuals. It is not unusual to be asked by the patient how long they will need to be on medications, and patients should be counseled that they will likely need ongoing treatment which may include medications, therapy, or both. Symptom relapse is typically lower in patients who continue medications [10], and therefore our recommendation is that patients who experience minimal side effect issues consider taking medications indefinitely. The dose of medication prescribed during maintenance treatment is typically the same dose as during the acute phase. If the patient opts for lowering the dose or stopping medications, the patient should be maintained at the acute phase dose for a minimum of 1–2 years after adequate response is achieved. Any medication taper after that point should be performed very slowly—over 4–6 months or more. Patients should be made aware that if they opt for a taper, reinstatement of the medication back to the prior dose in the case of exacerbation may not result in the same clinical benefits as the original trial [9].

5.7 SSRI Prescribing Practice

When prescribing SSRIs, the starting dose (listed in Table 5.5) is given for 1–2 weeks minimum or until the patient is comfortably tolerating the medication. Titration, when needed, is the same dosage as the starting dosage until the target dose is achieved or target clinical symptoms have sufficiently improved. In elderly patients, the starting and titration dose should be halved, and the time between dose increases should be lengthened; however, target doses should remain the same in most cases. In patients who have recently stopped medications suddenly for any reason, they usually can be started back on the full dose of their medication if it has been 2 weeks or less since their last dose. Longer periods than that, and medication should be started back at the starting dose.

The SSRIs are usually given in the morning. Occasionally, paroxetine causes sedation in some patients and can be switched to bedtime dosing if that occurs. Medications can be given with or without food although it is generally recommended that they be taken after breakfast to minimize GI side effects. One exception is sertraline, which must be given after a meal to improve absorption.

Patients should be encouraged to always take sertraline after a meal, to increase efficacy and decrease side effects. Other SSRIs may be given with or without food.

Table 5.5 CYP450 inhibitory potential of SSRIs and SNRIs

CYP isoenzyme	Citalopram	Fluoxetine	Fluvoxamine	Paroxetine	Sertraline
CYP1A2	+/–	+	+++	+	+/–
CYP2C19	?	++	+++		+
CYP2D6	+	+++	+	+++	+
CYP3A4	?	++	++	+/–	+/–

Table adapted from Page and Hudak [34]
Key: +/– unlikely, ? unknown, + mild, ++ moderate, +++ substantial

5.8 SSRI Side Effects

Typical side effects of SSRIs include excessive yawning, headache, GI distress (nausea, dyspepsia, constipation, diarrhea), vivid dreams or nightmares, and tremors [2]. These side effects often are transient and are usually managed conservatively, using over-the-counter analgesics for headache, stool softeners for constipation, and H2 antagonists for dyspepsia. Starting at a lower dose and maintaining that dose for a few weeks prior to titration are often sufficient for side effect management:

- *Sexual side effects* are among the most troubling side effects that can occur with chronic, ongoing use of SSRI therapy and are reported in approximately a third of patients on SSRI therapy [5]. The most common reported problems are loss of libido, delayed orgasm or anorgasmia, erectile dysfunction (males), and lack of lubrication (females). Often, a careful history will determine that the complaints of erectile dysfunction or lack of lubrication are not primary issues per se, but are the result of severe anorgasmia. There are numerous strategies that can be used in patients suffering from sexual side effects, such as a careful history regarding the nature of the actual side effects, their usual sexual habits, and their partner's (if there is one) knowledge of the situation. It should be noted that many patients state that the sexual side effects can remit over time, often taking many months or more; as a result, further intervention other than patience may not always be necessary. The addition of bupropion at a dose of 300 mg daily has been shown to reduce sexual side effects from SSRIs [2]. Buspirone can be used safely at doses between 20 and 60 mg daily and can help reverse sexual side effects [38]. If the patient does not wish to take a medication chronically in order to reverse sexual side effects, the use of cyproheptadine 4 mg orally 1–2 hours prior to sexual activity can reduce sexual side effects [40]. We recommend this be used no more than 3 times per week. Another method that can be used is the drug holiday method. We recommend that the patient's medication be stopped the day before planned sexual activity. On the day that sexual activity occurs, the person can delay their dose until afterward. The medication can then be resumed on a normal basis the following day; this results in only one total missed dose. Patients should not do this more than one time per week in order to minimize missed dosages. The drug holiday method is not recommended with fluoxetine (due to its long half-life), and caution should be used with paroxetine due to its potent discontinuation syndrome (see below).
- *Movement disorders such as myoclonus* are defined as sudden, abrupt, shock-like involuntary movements caused by muscle contractions. Nocturnal jaw clenching may also occur. Usually, lowering the dose or switching meds can help, but these side effects may spontaneously remit as well [45].
- A *frontal lobe amotivational syndrome* can occur, characterized by apathy, affective blunting, and memory issues. Complaints of sedation may accompany this. (Note: excessive yawning is also a side effect of SSRIs and is not associated with fatigue.) This side effect may be more common in OCD patients as it may occur

at higher doses and may not improve with time as opposed to some other SSRI side effects [30]. The most common strategies to manage this include lowering the dose or switching agents. In our practice, we have had success using modafinil at usual therapeutic doses to counteract this side effect.

- Any of the SSRIs may lead to *weight gain* with long-term usage. This side effect may be more noticeable in chronic conditions such as OCD as this may be associated with long-term use [8]. Management of this side effect is usually conservative, with recommendations given around lifestyle changes such as appropriate diet and exercise.
- *Excessive sweating* is a common complaint. Conservative management works in most cases, which simply involves recommending the patient have a change of bed clothes available to change into in the middle of the night. While there is little data on pharmacological management of this side effect, benztropine at 0.5 mg nightly can be tried [2].
- *Hyponatremia* is a rare (0.5% per year incidence) problem that can occur with SSRIs; elderly, female, and patients using concomitant diuretics are in the highest-risk category. This typically occurs within a few weeks of medication initiation or dose increase [29]. Symptoms typically include muscle cramps, fatigue, delirium, and seizures.
- *SSRI discontinuation syndrome* can occur with the abrupt discontinuation of many antidepressants, including the SSRIs (with the possible exception of fluoxetine due to its extended half-life). While it does not demand medical intervention, the symptoms can be quite distressing and even disabling; dizziness, light-headedness, insomnia, fatigue, anxiety, headache, nausea, and sensory disturbances described as electric sensations in the head or limbs (colloquially known as "brain zaps") are reported most commonly [47]. While symptoms are acute, resolution can be achieved rapidly by reinstating the full dose of the medication. Very slow and extended tapers can ameliorate this problem in most patients. In the case of someone on a maximum dose of an SSRI, the taper period may last 6 months or longer to reduce the risk of discontinuation syndrome. This also has the side benefit of decreasing the risk of relapse, as slower tapers of medications can reduce the possibility of OCD reoccurring after medications are stopped.
- *Serotonin syndrome* is a rare but serious medical condition that includes symptoms such as mental status changes, gastrointestinal symptoms, autonomic instability (tachycardia, hypertension, and hyperthermia), and neuromuscular abnormalities including myoclonus, hyperreflexia, hypertonicity, and rigidity; clinically, it presents very much like neuroleptic malignant syndrome [3, 4]. It has been most commonly associated with combinations of serotonergic agents but has been reported to occur with single agents. Treatment is usually supportive and includes discontinuation of the serotonergic agent; the addition of the 5-HT 2a antagonist cyproheptadine may also be of benefit [4].
- *Gastrointestinal bleeding* is a potential side effect of SSRI use and may be exacerbated with the concomitant use of nonsteroidal anti-inflammatory agents [29]. The use of medications to reduce the risk of GI bleeding may be warranted in high-risk patients [1].

5.9 Drug Interactions and Medication Choice

In the absence of data that would guide the choice of medication, usually the choice of SSRI is based on a few factors. First, patient preference cannot be discounted: if a patient has decided that they want to try a particular SSRI and communicate that they are hopeful about it, it is certainly reasonable to start that medication. If there is a family history with positive response to a particular SSRI, that medication should be considered. Past history is also a vital component in choice of medication: if someone has failed a particular SSRI, it is obviously best practice to try a different SSRI. If a patient has not met the criteria for a therapeutic trial for a certain SSRI (see above for definition of a therapeutic trial), that medication can still be initiated. However, often patients will have a negative attitude toward that medication, and if there is a different SSRI that has not been tried before, the best strategy may be to use the medication they are naïve to. The side effect profile of the various medications may be considered: for example, paroxetine may be avoided in patients who are especially concerned about weight gain and sedation or if discontinuation syndrome is a concern [41]. Women of childbearing years are a special case, and while there is no definitive information in this area, sertraline is the medication that is most recommended for women who are pregnant [46] and likely is the best choice in this population. Sertraline is associated with a higher rate of gastrointestinal side effects, especially diarrhea; fluoxetine is associated with greater rates of agitation and insomnia [28].

Patients who are somatically preoccupied and concerned about side effects from SSRIs are often more willing to accept clomipramine, which is a TCA and acts as a serotonin reuptake inhibitor. Because its side effects are predictable—sedation, orthostatic hypotension, and anticholinergic symptoms—these patients are often willing to accept this medication knowing that they can plan on these side effects without worrying about the additional side effects that SSRIs may cause and that they often hear about from others or read about online.

Drug-drug interactions are also important considerations when choosing specific SSRI pharmacotherapy. The action of the SSRI on the cytochrome P450 system is the most relevant piece of information when evaluating drug interactions with SSRIs, as many of the medications are potent inhibitors of various isoenzymes. Fluvoxamine is a significant inhibitor of the CYP1A2 isoenzyme, while paroxetine and fluoxetine are inhibitors of the CYP2D6 isoenzyme. Sertraline, citalopram, and escitalopram are not potent inhibitors of the CYP450 enzyme system and may be considered preferred medications in patients on multiple medications where drug-drug interactions are a concern [18]. See Table 5.5. Medications that are metabolized through the CYP450 system may have plasma levels increased if that specific isoenzyme is inhibited by an SSRI (or other CYP inhibitor). A list of common medications that are metabolized by specific isoenzymes are listed in Table 5.6. This is not meant to be a comprehensive list but to provide a guide to clinicians; consulting appropriate references on specific medications when prescribing is recommended when looking at potential drug-drug interactions. Other common isoenzyme

Table 5.6 Important substrates of CYP isoenzymes

1A2	2C19	2D6	3A4
Caffeine, theophylline, clozapine, clomipramine	Proton pump inhibitors, diazepam	Many tricyclic antidepressants (TCAs), beta-blockers, antiarrhythmic agents, atomoxetine, duloxetine, risperidone, codeine, hydrocodone, oxycodone, dextromethorphan	Calcium channel blockers, erythromycin, alprazolam, midazolam, triazolam, statins (HMG-CoA reductase inhibitors), HIV protease inhibitors, venlafaxine, mirtazapine, trazodone, ziprasidone

Table adapted from [22, 44]

Table 5.7 Other important CYP isoenzyme inhibitors

1A2	2D6	3A4
Ciprofloxacin, cimetidine	Cimetidine	Erythromycin, ketoconazole, ritonavir, amiodarone, grapefruit

Table adapted from [44]

inhibitors that can influence the plasma levels of OCD medications, as well as other medications, are listed in Table 5.7. Please see Table 1.13 in Chap. 1 which contains a comprehensive list of CYP inhibitors and inducers in order to facilitate better recognitions of potential drug-drug interactions.

5.10 Treatment-Resistant OCD

As stated above, treatment-resistant OCD is a common phenomenon, occurring in approximately half of people with OCD [35]. Ideally, medication management for treatment-resistant OCD would not be imitated in the primary care setting, but rather by a psychiatrist specializing in OCD. However, it is important to have familiarity with the protocols that may be used in these instances.

Since the mid-2000s, there has been an increasing interest in the use of glutamatergic medications in OCD, primarily as SSRI augmentation, but also primary treatment as well [36]. Prior to the use of these medications, second-generation antipsychotics (SGA) were the primary augmenters of choice. While the evidence for SGAs for OCD augmentation is stronger than the evidence for glutamatergic medications, the risk/benefit ratio clearly favors the use of glutamatergic medications over antipsychotics, and our recommendation for psychiatrists is to give patients a trial of glutamatergic meds prior to trying SGAs [2]. One of the commonly used medications for OCD augmentation is memantine, a medication that is approved in the USA for the treatment of moderate-to-severe dementia of the Alzheimer's type [23]. It is used to augment the SSRI after a full trial has only yielded a modest benefit. It is prescribed in OCD at the same dosage as it is for

Alzheimer's dementia. Another medication that has received much attention is riluzole, which is approved by the FDA for the treatment of amyotrophic lateral sclerosis [27]. While the evidence for this compound is preliminary, it may eventually provide a reasonable alternative for OCD augmentation [19]. While it is a well-tolerated compound, it can cause increases in liver transaminases and requires regular monitoring [36].

Second-generation antipsychotics (SGAs) also have utility for OCD augmentation and are commonly prescribed when SSRI response is inadequate. We recommend that they be tried when glutamatergic augmentation has failed. The doses of these medications that are used are typically lower than when used for psychosis. The SGAs are not all created equal: this is a large, heterogenous group of medications and only some have been adequately studied as OCD augmentation. Ideally, a patient who is far enough along in OCD protocol treatment to be considered for antipsychotic augmentation will be with a psychiatrist knowledgeable in the treatment of OCD, but a brief overview is warranted. Risperidone has the most evidence for OCD augmentation of the second-generation antipsychotics and has demonstrated efficacy in a double-blind placebo-controlled trial [20], but it is worth pointing out that it is not as efficacious as E/RP as augmentation in treatment-resistant patients [14]. It is typically used at doses lower than used for psychosis, and 0.5–2 mg daily is recommended. Aripiprazole has evidence from small DB-RCT trials showing that it is effective as augmentation [32, 39] and is usually used at 2–15 mg daily. Olanzapine has some data from a small DB-RCT [25] and is usually used in doses of 2.5–15 mg daily. Quetiapine has some mixed data [6] and is generally used at doses of 50–200 mg daily. Please see Chap. 4 for a full discussion on the appropriate prescribing practices for antipsychotic medication. One salient feature with all of the second-generation antipsychotics is that the possibility exists of exacerbating OCD symptoms, rather than improvement. In particular, risperidone, olanzapine, quetiapine, and clozapine (not recommended for OCD augmentation) have all been reported to induce or worsen OCD symptoms. Most of the other second-generation antipsychotics have little evidence for use in OCD and are not recommended.

In severe cases of treatment-resistant OCD, neurosurgical interventions may be utilized. Deep brain stimulation (DBS) involves the implantation of electrodes, with the nucleus accumbens being the most common target. Various ablative procedures can be performed as well, usually a capsulotomy or cingulotomy, the disadvantage over DBS being that ablative procedures are not reversible. These interventions are not performed in general psychiatric settings but should only be considered in settings that specialize in OCD treatment. Newer biological interventions are also being studied, with deep transcranial magnetic stimulation (dTMS) having been recently cleared by the FDA. Note that dTMS used for OCD is a different procedure using a different machine and magnetic coil than TMS when it is used for major depressive disorder.

5.11 When to Refer

When a primary care physician decides to refer a patient out for specialty care is always dependent upon the training and the comfort level of the practitioner; much will depend on the resources available in the community. Because the first line of treatment in OCD is E/RP, referral to a therapist well versed in E/RP is always the first referral that must be made, of course. While the timing of when a referral to a psychiatrist occurs is up to the comfort level of the primary care physician in most respects, certain general rules apply. If there is an OCD specialty treatment center located in an academic setting, an initial referral immediately upon suspicion of the diagnosis is appropriate. Not only would appropriate E/RP be available in such a setting, but the possibility of research or academic study of OCD patients who are naïve to treatment or not on medications is always a possibility in such a setting. Therefore, the PCP would be encouraged not to initiate medication treatment but to refer instead. A list of OCD specialty clinics can be found here: https://iocdf.org/. Because of the length of time it takes to titrate an OCD medication, plus the 3-month or more waiting period as a trial for medication response, there often is not a need to immediately start medication in the primary care setting if specialty care is fairly readily available. This is why, in the case of Mr. B. above, referral without starting meds is perfectly appropriate.

In the absence of an OCD specialty center, immediate referral for therapy to an E/RP specialist is indicated. The above link can also be used to find appropriate therapy referrals. A separate search for psychiatric (medication) treatment may also be utilized at the above website.

It is certainly reasonable to start anti-obsessional medication in the primary care setting prior to referring to a psychiatrist, especially if there is no OCD specialty center available locally. As a rule of thumb, we would recommend referral to a psychiatrist if a patient has failed one full, appropriate trial of an SSRI. Some PCPs may feel comfortable switching to a second SSRI at maximum dose and awaiting another full trial, but if psychiatric care is available locally, most patients who are treatment resistant in that fashion would likely benefit from referral.

In general, referral to mental health specialists should occur:

- When the patient requests E/RP or other specialized behavioral therapy.
- In the case of diagnostic uncertainty, when treatment protocols are dependent upon an exact and correct diagnosis.
- Failure of one to two SSRIs at maximum dose each for 12–16 weeks.
- Patient becomes a high utilizer of primary care office or resources.
- The PCP's own comfort level and experience.

5.12 Conclusion

OCD is a serious psychiatric condition and is one of the most common psychiatric disorders. Patients typically present to providers in the medical setting prior to any psychiatric care, and proper psychiatric care can be delayed for years after symptom onset. Therefore, proper recognition of this disorder in the primary care setting is paramount. Proper treatment includes Exposure with Response Prevention Therapy and possibly the use of medications as well. SSRIs, as well as clomipramine, are the preferred medications of choice, and medications are used in higher doses and for longer periods of time than when used for mood disorders.

References

1. Andrade C, Sharma E. Serotonin reuptake inhibitors and risk of abnormal bleeding. Psychiatr Clin North Am. 2016;39(3):413–26. https://doi.org/10.1016/j.psc.2016.04.010. Epub 2016 Jun 28. PMID: 27514297.
2. Borue X, Sharma M, Hudak R. Biological treatments for obsessive-compulsive and related disorders. J Obsessive Compuls Relat Disord. 2015;6:7–26.
3. Boyer EW, Shannon M. The serotonin syndrome. N Engl J Med. 2005;352(11):1112–20. https://doi.org/10.1056/NEJMra041867. Erratum in: N Engl J Med. 2007 Jun 7;356(23):2437. Erratum in: N Engl J Med. 2009 Oct 22;361(17):1714. PMID: 15784664.
4. Caroff SN, Watson CB, Rosenberg H. Drug-induced hyperthermic syndromes in psychiatry. Clin Psychopharmacol Neurosci. 2021;19(1):1–11. https://doi.org/10.9758/cpn.2021.19.1.1. PMID: 33508784; PMCID: PMC7851465.
5. Clayton AH, Pradko JF, Croft HA, Montano CB, Leadbetter RA, Bolden-Watson C, Bass KI, Donahue RM, Jamerson BD, Metz A. Prevalence of sexual dysfunction among newer antidepressants. J Clin Psychiatry. 2002;63(4):357–66. https://doi.org/10.4088/jcp.v63n0414. PMID: 12000211.
6. Dold M, Aigner M, Lanzenberger R, Kasper S. Antipsychotic augmentation of serotonin reuptake inhibitors in treatment resistant obsessive-compulsive disorder: a meta-analysis of double-blind, randomized, placebocontrolled trials. Int J Neuropsychopharmacol. 2013;16(3):557–74. https://doi.org/10.1017/S1461145712000740. Epub 2012 Aug 29. PMID: 22932229.
7. Eisen JL, Goodman WK, Keller MB, Warshaw MG, DeMarco LM, Luce DD, Rasmussen SA. Patterns of remission and relapse in obsessive-compulsive disorder: a 2-year prospective study. J Clin Psychiatry. 1999;60(5):346–51; quiz 352. https://doi.org/10.4088/jcp.v60n0514. PMID: 10362449.
8. Ferguson JM. SSRI antidepressant medications: adverse effects and tolerability. Prim Care Companion J Clin Psychiatry. 2001;3(1):22–7. https://doi.org/10.4088/pcc.v03n0105. PMID: 15014625; PMCID: PMC181155.
9. Figee M, Denys D. New pharmacotherapeutic approaches to obsessive-compulsive disorder. CNS Spectr. 2009;14(2 Suppl 3):13–23. https://doi.org/10.1017/s1092852900027255. PMID: 19238126.
10. Fineberg NA, Pampaloni I, Pallanti S, Ipser J, Stein DJ. Sustained response versus relapse: the pharmacotherapeutic goal for obsessive-compulsive disorder. Int Clin Psychopharmacol. 2007;22(6):313–22. https://doi.org/10.1097/YIC.0b013e32825ea312. PMID: 17917549.
11. Foa EB, Kozak MJ, Goodman WK, Hollander E, Jenike MA, Rasmussen SA. DSM-IV field trial: obsessive-compulsive disorder. Am J Psychiatry. 1995;152(1):90–6. https://doi.org/10.1176/ajp.152.1.90. Erratum in: Am J Psychiatry 1995 Apr;152(4):654. PMID: 7802127.
12. Foa EB, Franklin M, Kozak M. Psychosocial treatment for obsessive compulsive disorder: literature review. In: Swinson RP, Antony MM, Rachman S, Richter RA, editors. Obsessive compulsive disorder: theory, research and treatment. USA: American Psychological Association: Guilford Press; 1998. p. 258–76.

13. Foa EB, Liebowitz MR, Kozak MJ, Davies S, Campeas R, Franklin ME, Huppert JD, Kjernisted K, Rowan V, Schmidt AB, Simpson HB, Tu X. Randomized, placebo-controlled trial of exposure and ritual prevention, clomipramine, and their combination in the treatment of obsessive-compulsive disorder. Am J Psychiatry. 2005;162(1):151–61. https://doi.org/10.1176/appi.ajp.162.1.151. PMID: 15625214.
14. Foa EB, Simpson HB, Rosenfield D, Liebowitz MR, Cahill SP, Huppert JD, Bender J Jr, McLean CP, Maher MJ, Campeas R, Hahn CG, Imms P, Pinto A, Powers MB, Rodriguez CI, Van Meter PE, Vermes D, Williams MT. Six-month outcomes from a randomized trial augmenting serotonin reuptake inhibitors with exposure and response prevention or risperidone in adults with obsessive-compulsive disorder. J Clin Psychiatry. 2015;76(4):440–6. https://doi.org/10.4088/JCP.14m09044. PMID: 25375780; PMCID: PMC4524354.
15. Gilbert AR. Medication management of obsessive compulsive disorders in children and adolescents. In: Hudak R, Dougherty DD, editors. Clinical obsessive compulsive disorders in adults and children. United Kingdom: Cambridge University Press; 2011.
16. Goodman WK. Obsessive-compulsive disorder: diagnosis and treatment. J Clin Psychiatry. 1999;60 Suppl 18:27–32. PMID: 10487253.
17. Goodwin DW, Guze SB, Robins E. Follow-up studies in obsessional neurosis. Arch Gen Psychiatry. 1969;20(2):182–7. https://doi.org/10.1001/archpsyc.1969.01740140054006. PMID: 5763526.
18. Hemeryck A, Belpaire FM. Selective serotonin reuptake inhibitors and cytochrome P-450 mediated drug-drug interactions: an update. Curr Drug Metab. 2002;3(1):13–37. https://doi.org/10.2174/1389200023338017. PMID: 11876575.
19. Hirschtritt ME, Bloch MH, Mathews CA. Obsessive-compulsive disorder: advances in diagnosis and treatment. JAMA. 2017;317(13):1358–67. https://doi.org/10.1001/jama.2017.2200. PMID: 28384832.
20. Hollander E, Baldini Rossi N, Sood E, Pallanti S. Risperidone augmentation in treatment-resistant obsessive-compulsive disorder: a double-blind, placebo-controlled study. Int J Neuropsychopharmacol. 2003;6(4):397–401. https://doi.org/10.1017/S1461145703003730. PMID: 14604454.
21. Hudak R, Gopalan P, Dougherty DD. Treatment resistant obsessive compulsive disorder. In: Nemeroff CB, editor. Management of treatment resistant major psychiatric disorders. USA: Oxford University Press; 2012.
22. Kennedy SH, Lam RW, McIntyre RS, Tourjman SV, Bhat V, Blier P, Hasnain M, Jollant F, Levitt AJ, MacQueen GM, McInerney SJ, McIntosh D, Milev RV, Müller DJ, Parikh SV, Pearson NL, Ravindran AV, Uher R, CANMAT Depression Work Group. Canadian Network for Mood and Anxiety Treatments (CANMAT) 2016 clinical guidelines for the management of adults with major depressive disorder: Section 3. Pharmacological treatments. Can J Psychiatry. 2016;61(9):540–60. https://doi.org/10.1177/0706743716659417. Epub 2016 Aug 2. Erratum in: Can J Psychiatry. 2017;62(5):356. PMID: 27486148; PMCID: PMC4994790.
23. Koran LM, Aboujaoude E. Promising treatments for obsessive-compulsive disorder: a call for additional research. Curr Med Chem. 2018;25(41):5690–7. https://doi.org/10.2174/0929867324666170526120916. PMID: 28552055.
24. Koran LM, Hanna GL, Hollander E, Nestadt G, Simpson HB. Practice guideline for the treatment of patients with obsessive-compulsive disorder. USA: American Psychiatric Association; 2007.
25. Maina G, Pessina E, Albert U, Bogetto F. 8-week, single-blind, randomized trial comparing risperidone versus olanzapine augmentation of serotonin reuptake inhibitors in treatment-resistant obsessive-compulsive disorder. Eur Neuropsychopharmacol. 2008;18(5):364–72. https://doi.org/10.1016/j.euroneuro.2008.01.001. Epub 2008 Feb 15. PMID: 18280710.
26. Marcks BA, Weisberg RB, Dyck I, Keller MB. Longitudinal course of obsessive-compulsive disorder in patients with anxiety disorders: a 15-year prospective follow-up study. Compr Psychiatry. 2011;52(6):670–7. https://doi.org/10.1016/j.comppsych.2011.01.001. Epub 2011 Feb 23. PMID: 21349511; PMCID: PMC3683832.

27. Marinova Z, Chuang DM, Fineberg N. Glutamate-modulating drugs as a potential therapeutic strategy in obsessive-compulsive disorder. Curr Neuropharmacol. 2017;15(7):977–95. https://doi.org/10.2174/1570159X15666170320104237. PMID: 28322166; PMCID: PMC5652017.
28. Math SB, Janardhan Reddy YC. Issues in the pharmacological treatment of obsessive-compulsive disorder. Int J Clin Pract. 2007;61(7):1188–97. https://doi.org/10.1111/j.1742-1241.2007.01356.x. Epub 2007 May 18. PMID: 17511795.
29. Moret C, Isaac M, Briley M. Problems associated with long-term treatment with selective serotonin reuptake inhibitors. J Psychopharmacol. 2009;23(8):967–74. https://doi.org/10.1177/0269881108093582. Epub 2008 Jul 17. PMID: 18635702.
30. Murphy TK, Segarra A, Storch EA, Goodman WK. SSRI adverse events: how to monitor and manage. Int Rev Psychiatry. 2008;20(2):203–8. https://doi.org/10.1080/09540260801889211. PMID: 18386213.
31. Murray CJ, Lopez AD. The global burden of disease. USA: Harvard University Press; 1996.
32. Muscatello MR, Bruno A, Pandolfo G, Micò U, Scimeca G, Romeo VM, Santoro V, Settineri S, Spina E, Zoccali RA. Effect of aripiprazole augmentation of serotonin reuptake inhibitors or clomipramine in treatment-resistant obsessive-compulsive disorder: a double-blind, placebo-controlled study. J Clin Psychopharmacol. 2011;31(2):174–9. https://doi.org/10.1097/JCP.0b013e31820e3db6. PMID: 21346614.
33. Ninan PT, Koran LM, Kiev A, Davidson JR, Rasmussen SA, Zajecka JM, Robinson DG, Crits-Christoph P, Mandel FS, Austin C. High-dose sertraline strategy for nonresponders to acute treatment for obsessive-compulsive disorder: a multicenter double-blind trial. J Clin Psychiatry. 2006;67(1):15–22. https://doi.org/10.4088/jcp.v67n0103. PMID: 16426083.
34. Page SA, Hudak R. Selective serotonin reuptake inhibitors in the treatment of obsessive-compulsive disorder. In: Hudak R, Dougherty DD, editors. Clinical obsessive compulsive disorders in adults and children. United Kingdom: Cambridge University Press; 2011.
35. Pallanti S, Quercioli L. Treatment-refractory obsessive-compulsive disorder: methodological issues, operational definitions and therapeutic lines. Prog Neuro-Psychopharmacol Biol Psychiatry. 2006;30(3):400–12. https://doi.org/10.1016/j.pnpbp.2005.11.028. Epub 2006 Feb 28. PMID: 16503369.
36. Pittenger C, Krystal JH, Coric V. Glutamate-modulating drugs as novel pharmacotherapeutic agents in the treatment of obsessive-compulsive disorder. NeuroRx. 2006;3(1):69–81. https://doi.org/10.1016/j.nurx.2005.12.006. PMID: 16490414; PMCID: PMC3593363.
37. Rasmussen SA, Eisen JL. The epidemiology and differential diagnosis of obsessive compulsive disorder. J Clin Psychiatry. 1994;55 Suppl:5–10; discussion 11–4. PMID: 7961532.
38. Rosen RC, Lane RM, Menza M. Effects of SSRIs on sexual function: a critical review. J Clin Psychopharmacol. 1999;19(1):67–85. https://doi.org/10.1097/00004714-199902000-00013. PMID: 9934946.
39. Sayyah M, Sayyah M, Boostani H, Ghaffari SM, Hoseini A. Effects of aripiprazole augmentation in treatment-resistant obsessive-compulsive disorder (a double blind clinical trial). Depress Anxiety. 2012;29(10):850–4. https://doi.org/10.1002/da.21996. Epub 2012 Aug 29. PMID: 22933237.
40. Schweitzer I, Maguire K, Ng C. Sexual side-effects of contemporary antidepressants: review. Aust N Z J Psychiatry. 2009;43(9):795–808. https://doi.org/10.1080/00048670903107575. PMID: 19670052.
41. Shrestha P, Fariba K, Abdijadid S. Paroxetine. 2020 Oct 6. In: StatPearls [Internet]. Treasure Island (FL): StatPearls Publishing; 2021. PMID: 30252278.
42. Storch EA, Rasmussen SA, Price LH, Larson MJ, Murphy TK, Goodman WK. Development and psychometric evaluation of the Yale-Brown Obsessive-Compulsive Scale – Second Edition. Psychol Assess. 2010;22(2):223–32. https://doi.org/10.1037/a0018492. PMID: 20528050.
43. Swedo SE, Rapoport JL, Leonard H, Lenane M, Cheslow D. Obsessive-compulsive disorder in children and adolescents. Clinical phenomenology of 70 consecutive cases. Arch Gen Psychiatry. 1989;46(4):335–41. https://doi.org/10.1001/archpsyc.1989.01810040041007. PMID: 2930330.

44. The Medical Letter on Drugs and Therapeutics, September 21. 2020;62(1607):e152– e153.
45. Vandel P, Bonin B, Leveque E, Sechter D, Bizouard P. Tricyclic antidepressant-induced extrapyramidal side effects. Eur Neuropsychopharmacol. 1997;7(3):207–12. https://doi.org/10.1016/s0924-977x(97)00405-7. PMID: 9213080.
46. Womersley K, Ripullone K, Agius M. What are the risks associated with different Selective Serotonin Re-uptake Inhibitors (SSRIs) to treat depression and anxiety in pregnancy? An evaluation of current evidence. Psychiatr Danub. 2017;29(Suppl 3):629–44. PMID: 28953843.
47. Zajecka J, Tracy KA, Mitchell S. Discontinuation symptoms after treatment with serotonin reuptake inhibitors: a literature review. J Clin Psychiatry. 1997;58(7):291–7. https://doi.org/10.4088/jcp.v58n0702. PMID: 9269249.

Chapter 6
Obsessive-Compulsive and Related Disorders

6.1 Introduction

Case Example 6.1
Mr. S. was a 25-year-old male seen in a specialty OCD clinic. He had a comorbid diagnosis of OCD and body dysmorphic disorder. His OCD involved a fear of germs and contamination and consumed his thoughts all day long. As he participated in OCD treatment, his symptoms dramatically improved, and he experienced a marked decrease in his preoccupation with his OCD symptoms. However, as his OCD improved, he had more time to focus on his BDD symptoms (fear that his penis was deformed). As his OCD improved, he thought about his penis more and more, becoming more depressed until he became acutely suicidal and required psychiatric hospitalization.

At one time, obsessive-compulsive disorder (OCD) was categorized as one of the anxiety disorders. However, since the 1990s, psychiatrists started to recognize the fact that OCD did not properly fit into the category of anxiety disorders, as it was not a disorder of anxiety, but a disorder of intrusive thoughts (obsessions) and repetitive behaviors that someone feels compelled to perform (compulsions). These symptoms may indeed result in anxiety but were not caused by anxiety. At the same time, it was felt that there were other psychiatric disorders that had some similarities to OCD and perhaps belonged in an obsessive-compulsive spectrum of disorders. When the DSM 5 was released in 2013, this was codified when a new category of disorders was added—the obsessive-compulsive and related disorders. The disorders that were grouped in the obsessive-compulsive and related disorders (OCRD)

R. Hudak, J. M. Gannon, *Handbook of Psychiatric Disorders in Adults in the Primary Care Setting*, Current Clinical Practice,
https://doi.org/10.1007/978-3-030-98709-1_6

included disorders from other groupings in DSM as well as disorders that had not been formally recognized prior to that time. These OCRD include OCD, of course, as well as body dysmorphic disorder (BDD), hoarding disorder (HD), trichotillomania or hair-pulling disorder (HPD), and excoriation or skin-picking disorder (SPD). HPD and SPD are sometimes referred to as body-focused repetitive behaviors (BFRBs) as there are numerous other BFRBs of clinical significance, including nail biting, lip licking, lip biting, and cheek chewing. Because of the still relatively new diagnosis and classifications, terminology can seem confusing when doing literature searches, especially by non-psychiatric specialists; this should be a self-correcting problem over time.

It is vital for medical practitioners and primary care physicians to become familiar with the OCRD, because the majority of these patients do not initially present to mental health professionals. People with BDD usually present to physicians such as cosmetic surgeons in an attempt to fix their perceived defect. Patients with a BFRB often don't talk about their symptoms to medical professionals (including psychiatrists) as they believe they simply have a "bad habit" and don't even realize that the BFRB is considered a psychiatric disorder that has evidence-based treatment. The sequelae from HD can be significant, and there are numerous documented cases of people who have died as a result of their hoarding behaviors from such reasons as structural collapse of the dwelling or being unable to exit in the case of fire. Untreated OCRD can have vast and significant psychosocial consequences for both the patient and the community at large. Eighty percent of cosmetic surgeons have unknowingly operated on patients who have had BDD [49], and 40% of surgeons have been threatened by a patient with BDD who was unhappy with their outcome [62]. There are numerous articles written in the cosmetic surgery literature [58], dermatological literature [25], and dental literature [27] among others, demonstrating the significant impact that OCRD have upon other specialties. The non-psychiatric medical practitioner must learn how to recognize these disorders, properly engage and manage them in their practices, and make appropriate referrals to mental health professionals specializing in these disorders.

Any patient with any one of the obsessive-compulsive and related disorders is at an increased risk for having another OCRD. Therefore, proper evaluation of an OCRD patient includes screening for the other OCRD.

6.2 Body Dysmorphic Disorder

6.2.1 Introduction and Epidemiology

BDD is a relatively common disorder, and its rate in the general population has been estimated at between 0.7% and 2.4%, making it somewhat more common than other psychiatric disorders such as schizophrenia or anorexia nervosa [4]. Approximately

10% of patients in a dermatology setting and as many as 50% of patients in cosmetic surgery settings have BDD [4]. The disorder typically begins in early adolescence [39], and similar to OCD, its clinical features in adults and children are similar [44]. The gender ratio is fairly even, with studies showing a female-to-male ratio of 3:2 [39] with clinical features in men and women being generally similar. There do not appear to be major differences across cultures in the features of BDD, although this has not received sufficient study [39]. BDD is considered a chronic condition and does not typically remit without treatment [43]. Another important feature of BDD is that patients tend to have poor or absent insight and do not realize that they are suffering from a disorder [37]. Patients generally do not perceive that they have a psychiatric disorder and are unaware that their perceived defects are slight or non-existent. They often will describe symptoms of what they will label as "paranoia": the belief that they are being scrutinized by others in a negative way because of their offensive appearance. As a result, many patients with BDD are reluctant to talk about their symptoms or share them with their doctor.

Quality of life is generally poor in patients with BDD. Forty-three percent of patients have had psychiatric hospitalizations, 36% are unable to work, and 31% of patients are completely housebound due to their BDD [39]. Patients with BDD tend to have a poorer quality of life than people with major depressive disorder or post-traumatic stress disorder. Patients with BDD are much less likely to marry than even patients with OCD [39].

Suicidality is one of the most important considerations when seeing patients with BDD. Eighty percent of patients with BDD reported suicidal ideations within the past year [4]. When comparing the rate of suicidality of BDD patients with other psychiatric disorders, BDD patients have a higher likelihood of suicide than virtually every other psychiatric disorder [23]. As the case example of Mr. S. illustrates, the emergence of suicidal ideation can occur in an almost paradoxical manner (in his case, while he was experiencing significant improvement in his comorbid psychiatric disorder). This only emphasizes the need for appropriate recognition of this serious disorder.

6.2.2 BDD in the Medical Setting

Due to the poor insight associated with BDD, most patients do not complain that they are preoccupied with concerns about their appearance, but instead have complaints about their appearance itself. Patients will ask for referrals to cosmetic surgeons, cosmetic dentists, and dermatologists. They may have scars from attempts to self-correct their appearance. Approximately one third of BDD patients have problems with skin picking in an attempt to remove perceived blemishes or lesions [41]. While they may use their fingers, implements such as pins, needles, razor blades, or knives can be used causing considerable dermatological damage [39]. The self-surgery that BDD patients can engage in can cause significant scarring and possibly be life-threatening [35] and may be an exception to the fact that most BDD patients are normal in appearance. Skin picking in an attempt to improve appearance is not considered to be skin-picking disorder: careful screening to distinguish both disorders from each other is critical due to the differences in morbidity and mortality.

The need to properly screen for and manage BDD is not just vital for the patients' welfare: patients with BDD who are properly diagnosed can be incredibly disruptive in the medical setting, causing disproportionate staff resource utilization and turmoil in the office.

Case Example 6.2
Mrs. D was a 51-year-old female, who made appointments with her dermatologist on a monthly basis. On the day of this appointment, the staff had realized that they had accidently scheduled her for a typical appointment slot, which was generally two patients every 15 minutes in this private practice. Due to her numerous complaints, she often used up an hour or more of the doctor's time. They also belatedly realized that they had scheduled another very similar patient in the same time slot. The staff was anxious and on edge, knowing that they would get in trouble for making such a mistake. When they gave the doctor a printout of his schedule for the day, they whited out the afternoon, stating that the printer was broken. Then, while he was in with patients that morning, they called patients to cancel and reschedule to make the afternoon more doable. When they finally revealed what happened, most of the lunch hour in the clinic was lost due to the staff and doctor's anxiety. When the patient did come, she had a list of more than 14 places on her skin that she wanted examined and had numerous questions, concerns, and anxiety about each one. Virtually everything she was concerned about were normal skin features such as pores or hair follicle that she would examine with magnifying mirrors. Even with a scheduled hour to examine her, the dermatologist was still running behind on his other patients the rest of the afternoon due to the length of the appointment.

Case Example 6.2 was observed while the author was on a medical student rotation during the fourth year of medical school. The disruption to the normal routine of the office was significant obviously, but it was only after psychiatric training that the author in hindsight realized this was almost certainly a case of BDD. While this private office had handled other difficult and unusual cases during the rotation (such as delusional parasitosis), there was no patient who caused the disruptions this patient did. Obviously, the rearranging of the schedule the staff had to do not only disrupted other patients of that day but would have significantly reduced the revenue of the clinic that day due to the decreased volume of patients. In retrospect, had the doctor been able to recognize, diagnose, and properly engage and refer this BDD patient, the positive outcome would have been significant—not just for the patient but for the office practice as well. As BDD is a common disorder—and found in higher percentages in medical settings [25, 27, 58]—it behooves all physicians to be aware of this disorder.

6.2.3 Diagnosis and Presentation of BDD

Patients with body dysmorphic disorder have intense preoccupations with one or more perceived flaws in their appearance. They believe that they are ugly, unattractive, or hideous for others to look at. Any body part can be the focus of their preoccupations, but the most common areas of concern are the face, skin, and hair [43]. Other common areas of concern include the eyes, teeth, overall weight, breasts, legs, lips, chin, nose, eyebrows, or genitals [14]. Patients with BDD will often spend hours a day performing rituals or repetitive behaviors in response to the concerns about their appearances. These rituals will usually involve checking their appearance, comparing themselves to others, camouflaging or hiding their perceived defects, or seeking reassurance from others about their appearance. Excessive tanning, excessive grooming (shaving, combing, hair plucking, or skin picking), covering areas of concern with clothing, excessive body building, checking in mirrors, and touching the area of concern are possible compulsive behaviors that BDD patients engage in. Seeking cosmetic surgery or other cosmetic procedures is very common among BDD patients, and they commonly present to cosmetic surgeons, dermatologists, or cosmetic dentistry. See Table 6.1 for the diagnostic criteria for BDD. The criteria for BDD include three insight specifiers: with good or fair insight, with poor insight, or with absent/delusional insight. Insight tends to be low in patients with BDD, with BDD patients more likely to fall into the absent/delusional belief category than other OC-related disorders [54]. Their belief about their perceived deformity may be so strong that it can appear to be delusional or psychotic

Table 6.1 DSM 5 diagnostic criteria for body dysmorphic disorder

A. Preoccupation with one or more perceived defects or flaws in physical appearance that are not observable or appear slight to others
B. At some point during the disorder, the individual performs repetitive behaviors (e.g., mirror checking, excessive grooming, skin picking, reassurance seeking) or mental acts (e.g., comparing their appearance with others) in response to the appearance concerns
C. The preoccupation causes clinically significant distress or impairment in social, occupational, or other areas of functioning
D. If the preoccupation is with weight or body fat, the symptoms are not better explained by an eating disorder
Specifier: *With muscle dysmorphia* this applies when the individual is preoccupied with concerns that their body is too small or not muscular enough
Specifier: *Degree of insight*: with good or fair insight; with poor insight; with absent insight/delusional beliefs

in nature: however, despite this presentation it is not considered a psychotic disorder, and antipsychotics have minimal benefit in the treatment of these patients [42].

BDD is distinct from eating disorders. If the concerns are about weight or body size, the diagnosis may be an eating disorder such as anorexia nervosa and not BDD. Immediate psychiatric referral is imperative in such an instance.

Patients with BDD have obsessions concerning the way that they look, believing that they are hideous, unattractive, deformed, or abnormal in some way. They will look normal and appropriate, or even attractive, to others, but are unable to be reassured that they are not a freak or monster. While the face (especially the nose), head, and skin are the most common focuses of obsessive preoccupations, it can occur on any part of the body. It does not just have to be one part of the body, and in many instances, they will focus on multiple parts of the body. The person engages in compulsive behaviors that are designed to diminish the anxiety caused by their intense preoccupations. The purpose of those behaviors is generally to check, hide, or fix the perceived appearance defects, which is time-consuming and difficult to control [39]. The behaviors that the person engages in will include examining themselves in mirrors, excessive grooming, clothing that masks areas of their bodies, excessive tanning, and skin picking. Patients who engage in compulsive skin picking may use surgical implements to do so, leading to scarring or even life-threatening complications such as rupturing major blood vessels [39]. The scarring from such self-surgery may cause deformity and would be an exception to the rule that BDD patients look normal. The compulsions will take 3–8 hours per day in about 40% of patients, and in one quarter of patients, they will spend over 8 hours a day on rituals [4]. As is the case with OCD, these compulsive behaviors are not pleasurable and do not give enjoyment or satisfaction but instead are an attempt (usually unsuccessful) to give relief to severe distress and anxiety.

Seeking cosmetic surgery is a common practice among BDD patients. It is a vital point for clinicians to realize that cosmetic procedures do not help with BDD symptoms. Patients are rarely satisfied with their outcomes postsurgery, and their preoccupations will continue either on the prior area of focus or to a new area. As noted above, 40% of cosmetic surgeons have been threatened by BDD patients unhappy with their treatments. There are numerous articles written in the cosmetic surgery literature [58], dermatological literature [25], and dental literature [27] among others, demonstrating the significant impact that OCRD have upon those specialties. The proper recognition of BDD by any doctor providing cosmetic treatment is not only important to proper patient management but also for the safety of physicians and medical staff. Therefore, cosmetic procedures are not recommended for patients with BDD, and instead psychiatric referral is strongly encouraged at that point. It is of course possible that patients with BDD may have actual flaws that could benefit from surgical or other medical intervention. However, it is our recommendation that cosmetic procedures do not take place in these patients. Instead, referral to specialists in BDD is the proper course of action, and surgical procedure should only take place in patients who are in appropriate treatment and only with coordination of the psychiatric treatment team.

Clinical Tip
Even BDD patients with actual physical flaws should not be offered cosmetic procedures until appropriate psychiatric treatment is in place and psychiatrist, surgeon, and patient all agree the patient is stable.

Engaging BDD patients properly is critical in order to properly treat and refer these people. See Table 6.2 for tips in engaging and evaluating these patients. If BDD is suspected, appropriate screening questions should be administered. Asking them a question such as "Are you worried about an imagined defect in your appearance?" is not a screening question that is going to lead to a meaningful exchange. Instead, a better screening question would be "Are you unhappy with how you look?" Follow it up by asking how much this concern preoccupies them and how much time they spend worrying about it. Do not attempt to reassure them or tell them that they look normal. Ask about the other areas of the body that patients with BDD may focus on. Screen for the various compulsions and rituals that BDD patients may engage in, such as tanning, weightlifting, concealing, touching, and checking. Take their concerns seriously and don't dismiss them. Emphasize that this is a common and treatable disorder and that it is possible to decrease their level of concern. The focus of treatment initially is to decrease their excessive preoccupation, thus reducing their distress. The goal is not to "convince" them that they look normal. If cosmetic surgery is brought up, tell patients that you recommend against it at this time, as it does not resolve the intense preoccupations. Instead, ask them to delay until after psychiatric treatment, and emphasize that effective psychiatric treatment exists for this disorder. Finally, reading recommendations and self-education can help, and giving patients the recommendation to read *The Broken Mirror* by K Phillips [38] can be an important initial intervention.

Table 6.2 Screening questions and engaging BDD patients

Ask: "Are you unhappy with your appearance?"
Ask: "Does this concern preoccupy you?" "How much time do you spend thinking about this?"
Screen: Ask about other areas of the body that are commonly seen as areas of concern in BDD
Screen: Determine that no eating disorder is present. If patient screens positive for eating disorder, immediate psychiatric referral is indicated
Screen: Determine if OCD, social anxiety, or substance use disorders are present
Establish a therapeutic alliance, and provide education on BDD. Recommend *The Broken Mirror* by K Phillips
Discourage surgery, asking them to delay until after psychiatric treatment is established and psychiatrist feels it is appropriate
Inform them that the initial focus of treatment is to reduce their distress and excessive preoccupation

6.2.4 Treatment of BDD

As with OCD, the first-line and primary form of treatment for BDD is psychotherapy, specifically cognitive behavioral therapy (CBT), as CBT has the greatest evidence base for BDD treatment [59]. Usually an integrated approach is used—patients are offered CBT—particularly a specific form of CBT known as Exposure with Response Prevention (E/RP) and, if necessary, medication management, specifically the use of selective serotonin reuptake inhibitors (SSRIs). Many patients with a mild-to-moderate level of BDD can be offered E/RP as first-line therapy without the addition of medication management. Medication management may be useful in patients with moderate-to-severe levels of BDD, although a trial of E/RP alone is not unwarranted if the patient desires. While medication management can be a useful adjunct, medication management alone cannot equal the effects of CBT. See Fig. 6.1 for an algorithmic approach to BDD in the primary care setting.

The type of therapy used in BDD is the same as used in OCD: Exposure with Response Prevention is the core of the treatment, with some additional techniques added to improve efficacy, such as cognitive restructuring, which helps the patient identify inaccurate beliefs and develop new and more accurate thoughts. However, there are numerous barriers to patients getting appropriate CBT for BDD; only 17.4% of patients with BDD receive appropriate CBT for their disorder [30]. Similar to OCD, there is a marked lack of therapists who are appropriately trained to deliver CBT in patients with BDD. In addition, the intense shame and stigma that BDD patients feel make it difficult to seek mental health services. However, supportive and nonjudgmental encouragement from the referents in the primary care setting can help to overcome that barrier.

When searching for a therapist to refer your patients to for BDD, it is vital that the therapist has formal training in the treatment of BDD which unfortunately is not always easy to find in many locations. The best first step is to check the therapists list from the International OCD Foundation, at www.IOCDF.org. They maintain a list of therapists

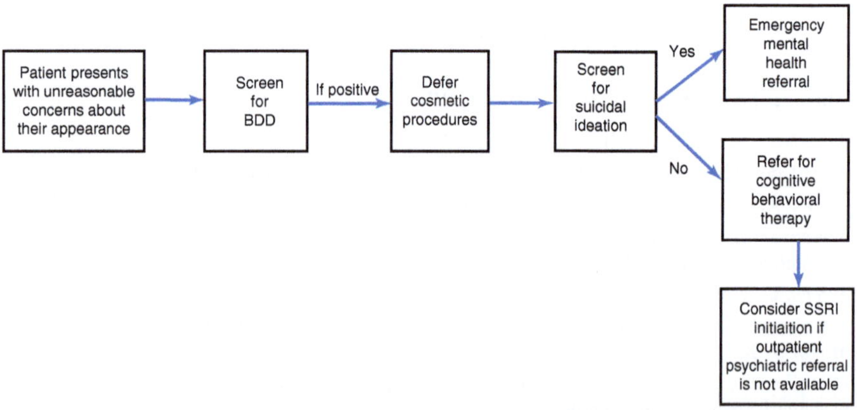

Fig. 6.1 Approach to BDD in the primary care setting

who express an interest in obsessive-compulsive and related disorders (OCRD) or have declared themselves to be OCRD specialists. While just listing yourself as an OCRD professional is no guarantee, of course, that the therapist has been trained in E/RP, it certainly greatly increases your likelihood. A therapist on that website who states that they have completed BTTI (Behavioral Therapy and Training Institute) has indeed completed formal training in E/RP. Another option is to inquire of potential therapists if they have trained in an OCD or BDD specialty clinic. Such a therapist can be assumed to have the appropriate experience as well. There are some useful questions that you can ask prospective therapists, or *questions that you can give to your patients when they are making inquiries*, to help ensure that they are getting a qualified therapist:

- "What techniques do you use to treat BDD?" If the therapist gives a vague answer or simply says CBT without mentioned E/RP, there is a good chance they do not have OCD training.
- "Do you use Exposure with Response Prevention to treat BDD?" Again, therapists who give vague answers or who only state that they do "exposures" may not be using appropriate therapy.
- "Where did you get your training in BDD?" Therapists who state that they are a member of the IOCDF, or who state that they have attended specialized training through the IOCDF, are more likely to have received the appropriate training.
- "What are your feelings about anti-obsessional medications?" While CBT is indeed first-line treatment for BDD, most specialists recognize the utility of medications and will have a positive attitude about them. Be wary of therapists who have negative attitudes toward medications—they are more likely to practice forms of therapy other than CBT and E/RP.

6.2.5 *Treatment of BDD*

6.2.5.1 Pharmacotherapy

Despite the significant potential for suicidality in BDD, there have been relatively few studies examining the overall pharmacotherapy for BDD. Based on what is known at this time, the use of SSRIs at the same protocols for OCD in regard to dosing and length of clinical trial is recommended for BDD [26]. The use of the tricyclic antidepressant, clomipramine, which acts as an SRI, can also be prescribed. While patients can consider a trial of the SSRI at lower dosages, generally titration up to the target maximum dose for BDD is warranted in most instances. Please see below in Hoarding section for dosing of SSRIs and clomipramine for BFRBs, as it is the same for all of the OCRD. It is recommended to start with the starting dose for a minimum of 1 week and increase by the same starting or titration dose on a weekly basis (or as tolerated) until the patients have reached the target or maximum dose. The starting and titration dose may need to be half the dose listed in elderly or sensitive patients, but the end target dose is usually the same. Of note, we currently do not recommend the initiation of citalopram for OCRD, as its potential to induce cardiac induction delays limits its ability to be used at full, anti-obsessional doses. It is important to note that the maximum dose is, in many cases, above the maximum daily amount as recommended by the FDA. For example, the maximum OCD dose of sertraline is 400 mg/day, while the FDA has approved sertraline at a maximum of 200 mg/day. In the column labeled "Occasional dose," the recommended doses used are generally above FDA maximum approved dosing. It is vital to note that these supramaximal doses are scientifically validated [34]. Therefore, prescribing SSRIs in a manner consistent with these guidelines is not the liability that some physicians may fear, but is indeed backed up by research, experience, and consensus. Prescribing SSRIs at these doses sometimes will result in pushback from pharmacists, insurance companies, or even psychiatrists who are not familiar with OCRD guidelines. Be prepared to stand your ground with these appropriate and recommended clinical practices. Pharmacists can be told that these doses are correct as prescribed if you are questioned. If insurance companies refuse to pay, prior authorization or appeal may not work, but these medications are generally inexpensive, and many people can afford to pay out of pocket at retail price or with help from online coupons.

The definition of a therapeutic SSRI trial for BDD differs from antidepressant SSRI protocol. In order to determine if a patient has responded or will respond to medication treatment, the initial medication must be used at the maximum dose for 12–16 weeks. For example, this means that if sertraline is titrated up to an anti-obsessional dose of 400 mg daily over a 1-month period, the patient must be on the full 400 mg dose for 12–16 weeks before it can be determined if they have had a response or not. If they start to notice a decrease in symptoms only at the end of this 12–16-week period, the trial can be extended further in order to achieve maximal benefit. If the patient is a treatment-naïve patient who elects to try an intermediate dose first (e.g., 200 mg daily), any response can only be determined after 12–16 weeks. If there is not enough of a benefit after that time, the dose can be titrated to 400 mg, but another 12–16-week trial period at that dose is warranted. See Table 6.5 for dosage recommendations for BDD.

Starting and titration doses for elderly or sensitive patients are often 50% of the usual dose. The adage "start low and go slow" applies here. However, elderly patients quite often require the same high-end dosages that other adults need for adequate response. Therefore, don't stay low—continue to titrate the SSRI as necessary.

See below for a discussion on the side effects of SSRI therapy.

While the initial steps for pharmacotherapy for all of the OCRD are going to be the same for all of the OCRD (use of SSRIs or clomipramine titrated to the maximum dose for a 12–16-week trial), there are some specific differences for the individual OCRD that are worth considering. In the case of BDD, the modifier for "absent insight/delusional beliefs" will apply to a great number of the patients seen. However, even patients who appear to have delusional beliefs can respond well to SSRI therapy alone [40]. Numerous studies have shown no benefits with antipsychotic augmentation for treatment-resistant BDD [10], and therefore the use of antipsychotics in BDD would rarely, if ever, be initiated in the medical setting by non-psychiatric physicians.

6.2.6 *When to Refer for BDD*

The threshold for when a primary care physician decides to refer a patient out for specialty care is always dependent upon the training and the comfort level of the practitioner; much will depend on the resources available in the community. Because the first line of treatment in BDD is CBT, referral to a therapist well versed in the treatment of BDD is always the first referral that must be made, of course. While the timing of when a referral to a psychiatrist occurs is up to the comfort level of the primary care physician in most respects, certain general rules apply.

BDD patients should always be referred for CBT. Referral to a psychiatrist specializing in BDD is appropriate for most cases as well.

Due to the fact that BDD patients have a high risk of suicidal behavior and due to the complex nature of BDD phenomenology, referral to a psychiatrist should be made for virtually all patients at the time of referral for CBT. If there is an OCD or BDD specialty treatment center located in an academic setting, an initial referral immediately upon suspicion of the diagnosis is appropriate. Not only would appropriate E/RP be available in such a setting, but the possibility of research or academic study of OCD patients who are naïve to treatment or not on medications is always a possibility. Therefore, the PCP would be encouraged not to initiate medication treatment but instead to refer their patient for specialty psychotherapy and pharmacotherapy. Only in areas where psychiatric care is difficult to obtain will most primary care physicians initiate pharmacotherapy in BDD patients.

Cases like Mr. S. illustrate the potentially difficult nature in treating this disorder. There can be a paradoxical response: the patient can become increasingly suicidal as their overall mental status seemingly is improving. Assess document symptoms, and communicate them to the psychiatric referral is often the ideal course of action.

6.3 Hair-Pulling Disorder (Trichotillomania) and Skin-Picking Disorder (Excoriation Disorder) and the Other Body-Focused Repetitive Behavior Disorders

6.3.1 *Introduction and Epidemiology*

Trichotillomania, now often referred to as hair-pulling disorder (HPD) due to the fact that it has no correlation with bipolar disorder, was classified as an impulse control disorder in DSM-IV. Skin-picking disorder (SPD) was not officially recognized as a psychiatric disorder in DSM-IV at all despite the serious and potentially fatal nature of the illness. HPD and SPD are now rightfully recognized as obsessive-compulsive and related disorders (OCRD) and are often referred to as body-focused repetitive behaviors (BFRBs) as there are numerous other body-focused behaviors that patients can suffer from, such as nail biting, lip licking or biting, and cheek chewing. The illnesses all share similar symptom presentation, course of illness, and genetic vulnerabilities [56]. The BFRBs can be discussed together because of similarities in etiological factors as well as in phenomenology [52]; additionally, their treatment can be discussed together as well.

The diagnosis of trichotillomania (and hence the other BFRBs as well) has changed over time. DSM-IV had listed trichotillomania as an impulse control disorder, and part of the criteria stated that the person must have an increasing sense of tension prior to the act of pulling and feel pleasure, gratification, or relief when pulling out their hair. DSM 5 abandoned this part of the criteria, as it is known that any BFRB can occur with a variety of emotional states, including anxiety, boredom, pleasure, and with varying degrees of conscious awareness. This change in criteria increased the estimated lifetime prevalence of trichotillomania to 3% [11] as the more inclusive criteria more accurately reflect the features of the disorder. While skin picking has been noted in the literature for decades, its recent recognition as a nosologically separate disorder means that numbers (and other research findings) may not be as well delineated. Its prevalence is estimated to be as high as 5.4% [24]. Females are markedly more affected than males with BFRBs, and it is estimated that there is a 10:1 female-to-male ratio for trichotillomania [14]. The average age of onset is 13 years [29]. It is a chronic condition, tending to wax and wane over the lifespan. The site of the BFRB can remain stable, or it can shift over time as well. Trichotillomania and skin picking in particular can lead to severe disfigurement or even death resulting from secondary medical complications.

6.3.2 BFRBs in the Medical Setting

The vast majority of people with any type of BFRB initially present to non-psychiatric physicians. They will rarely complain of the symptoms of the disorder itself, but instead are there for treatment of the consequences. In other words, they do not ask for help with the actual BFRB but will ask for treatment for resulting hair or skin sequelae. Most people aren't aware that BFRBs represent a psychiatric disorder, much less one with evidence-based treatment: they simply believe that they have a "bad habit." The BFRB symptoms are usually accompanied by a significant amount of shame or guilt (making patients reluctant to disclose their symptoms), and there may be associated anxiety or depressive symptoms as well.

Hair pulling can occur on any site in the body. The most common site is the scalp (73%). However, other areas of the body are also affected, including eyebrows (56%), eyelashes (53%), pubic hair (46%), and legs (15%) [60]. Upon physical examination, irritation and follicle damage may be noted. Typically, atypical regrowth of hair is observed—specifically hair regrowth at different lengths which can be considered pathognomonic [5]. Patients will often examine the hair after it is pulled and may rub it on their lips, mouth it, or eat the hair.

Some people with skin picking will report that acne, bumps, or other skin blemishes can trigger the picking, but the excoriation will occur even after the initial condition clears [21]. The site of skin picking may be concentrated in one area: however, patients have an average of 4.5 locations on the body where picking may occur. The person may use fingernails to pick or may choose a variety of implements, such as knives, tweezers, pins, etc. [21] as well as topical analgesics. Medical complications from skin picking can be severe and can include infections and severe blood loss, and death is a possible outcome. Patients may need skin grafts, transfusions, or reconstructive surgery as well as antibiotic therapy.

A thorough physical examination should occur in all BFRB patients to ensure that the physical damage has not resulted in a systemic illness such as bacteremia, cellulitis, or osteomyelitis [21]. In the experience of the authors, BFRBs occur commonly in patients with intellectual and developmental disabilities, and these patients should be screened closely. Medical conditions that can result in skin picking and other BFRBs, such as amphetamine abuse, scabies, etc., should also be ruled out appropriately.

6.3.3 *Diagnosis and Presentation of BFRBs*

As noted above, the criteria for trichotillomania and excoriation or skin-picking disorder have changed over the years. No longer are emotional states a required part of the diagnosis. To make the diagnosis, a patient simply has to have the body-focused behavior, make repeated attempt to stop the behavior, have clinically significant distress, and symptoms are not attributable to another medical or psychiatric condition. If the behavior is hair pulling, a diagnosis of trichotillomania (hair-pulling disorder) is made. If it is skin picking, a diagnosis of excoriation (skin-picking) disorder is given. If the behavior is any other body-focused repetitive behavior, the correct diagnosis is Other Specified Obsessive-Compulsive and Related Disorder. See Table 6.3 for the full diagnostic criteria.

Table 6.3 DSM 5 diagnostic criteria for body-focused repetitive behaviors

A. Recurrent behavior (hair pulling, skin picking, nail biting, lip or cheek chewing, etc.) that causes clinically significant symptoms
B. Repeated attempts to stop the behaviors
C. The behavior causes clinically significant distress or impairment in social, occupational, or other important areas of functioning
D. The behavior is not attributable to another medical condition
E. The behavior is not better explained by the symptoms of another mental disorder (e.g., attempts to correct a flaw in body dysmorphic disorder)

Note: If the BFRB is hair pulling, the official diagnosis is trichotillomania (hair-pulling disorder). If skin picking, excoriation (skin-picking) disorder. Any other BFRB is Other Specified Obsessive-Compulsive and Related Disorder

Patients with BFRBs will usually present to the primary care office, dermatologist, or occasionally dentists or podiatrists. They rarely will complain about the primary behavior; instead, they will ask for help regarding the result of the BFRB such as hair loss, skin or lip lesions, injuries to the nail bed, etc. The reason that patients don't mention the behavior is usually twofold: (1) the behavior is a source of a great deal of shame and embarrassment and (2) the person considers it to be a "habit" and feel they are to blame. They are typically not aware of its nature as a psychiatric disorder with a biological basis and evidence-based treatment.

Patients with trichotillomania generally present with bald patches in the area(s) affected. Atypical hair regrowth is typically noted: hairs will be growing back at different lengths, and this can be considered pathognomonic for trichotillomania. Patients will often mouth the hair after pulling, rub the hair on the lips, and occasionally bite or ingest the hair. Trichobezoars are a potential complication, and sequelae associated with them (e.g., weight loss, iron deficiency anemia, malabsorption, and obstruction) should be considered [5]. Mouthing and eating behavior can also occur with skin picking and other BFRBs as well. Other skin conditions that can present as picking include scabies, atopic dermatitis, psoriasis, and blistering skin disorders among others [21]. Examples of other medical conditions that can present with hair loss include alopecia areata and telogen effluvium [1].

When examining a patient with alopecia, hair regrowth of different lengths at the site can be considered pathognomonic for hair-pulling disorder.

Medical work-up should be done as clinically necessary and will focus on other possible causes of the hair or skin condition, as well as potential sequelae. A general history and physical is typically enough to diagnose a BFRB; however, if necessary, tests like a punch biopsy can help confirm a diagnosis of trichotillomania [36]. Exams including microscopic examination of lesions for scabies, a Wood's lamp examination for fungal infections, patch testing for allergies, skin biopsies, and laboratory investigations of thyroid, parathyroid, liver, and kidney function can be performed to rule out other causes of skin lesions [21].

6.3.4 *Treatment of Body-Focused Repetitive Behaviors*

Generally, medication treatment for BFRBs will not commonly be initiated for patients in the medical setting for adult patients with appropriate intellectual development. This, of course, depends on the availability of psychiatric care in the community. First-line treatment for BFRBs is a psychotherapy called habit reversal training (HRT). In most cases, once a BFRB is identified in the medical setting, a referral to a trained therapist should be the first step. As is the case with E/RP for OCD and BDD, trained therapists are not always easy to find, as most graduate schools do not routinely teach HRT. Finding a trained and skilled therapist is important for these disorders, as many of the traditional techniques that are taught routinely to psychotherapists do not work for BFRBs and in fact can be considered placebo. Please see above for suggestions in the BDD section on finding qualified practitioners of HRT. In addition to the referral list from the IOCDF mentioned above, as well as the screening questions that you or the patient can ask a prospective therapist, there is an additional organization that trains therapists in HRT. The organization formerly known as the Trichotillomania Learning Center is now known as The TLC Foundation for BFRBs. They maintain a website at www.bfrb.org. They conduct trainings in HRT for professional therapists and maintain a list of qualified therapists. This is an excellent reference that you can pass on to your patients as well.

6.3.5 Pharmacotherapy of BFRBs

In areas where psychiatric care is not available, the primary care physician may need to initiate pharmacotherapy. This should be reserved for patients who have failed HRT or cannot participate in HRT for various reasons. Interestingly, there has been significant research within the last decade opening up new potential avenues of treatment. Historically, SSRIs have been the first line of treatment for BFRBs [5]. Clomipramine, a tricyclic antidepressant that acts as a serotonin reuptake inhibitor, has been studied as a treatment for various BFRBs. The evidence for clomipramine is stronger than that of SSRIs [3] and can therefore be considered a first-line treatment ahead of SSRIs. However, side effects to clomipramine may make it difficult to be used routinely first line in clinical use [34]. As a result, in most cases it may make sense to try one to two SSRIs at standard OCRD doses prior to trying clomipramine. See Table 6.5 for dosage recommendations. Of note, starting and titration doses for elderly or sensitive patients are often 50% of the usual dose. The adage "start low and go slow" applies here. However, elderly patients quite often require the same high-end dosages that other adults need for adequate response. Therefore, don't stay low—continue to titrate the SSRI as necessary.

The definition of a therapeutic SSRI trial for OCD differs from antidepressant protocol. In order to determine if a patient has responded or will respond to medication treatment, the initial medication must be used at the steady-state dosing for 12–16 weeks. For example, this means that if sertraline is titrated up to an anti-obsessional dose of 400 mg daily over a 1-month period, the patient must be on the full 400 mg dose for 12–16 weeks before it can be determined if they have had a response or not. If they start to notice a decrease in symptoms only at the end of this 12–16-week period, the trial can be extended further in order to achieve maximal benefit. If the patient is a treatment-naïve patient who elects to try an intermediate dose first (e.g., 200 mg daily), a response can only be determined after 12–16 weeks. If there is not enough of a benefit after that time, the dose can be titrated to 400 mg, but another 12–16-week trial period at that dose is warranted.

Medications that act on the glutamatergic system have been receiving increased interest in the treatment of OCRD. In the case of BFRBs, there has been a study showing n-acetylcysteine (NAC) as having a positive effect for trichotillomania in adults at doses ranging from 1200 to 2400 mg/day [20] and another one at dosages of 1200–3000 mg/day for excoriation disorder [22]. NAC appears to be well tolerated by patients, and it was studied as both a stand-alone medication and an add-on to more traditional SSRI medication. Due to the fact that SSRIs and CMI have a longer track record of use, it is our current recommendation that CMI be used first line if tolerated and SSRIs as a second line if CMI does not work or is intolerable due to side effects. NAC can be used second line after SSRIs and is appropriate as an augmenting medication as well.

Of note, there has been some work with second-generation antipsychotics and BFRBs. Olanzapine at 2–10 mg/day was found to be helpful in patients with trichotillomania [53] and may be a potential augmenting agent in patients with severe, nonresponsive symptoms. However, due to usual antipsychotic side effects, this medication should not be routinely used and would rarely be prescribed in a primary care setting. If it is prescribed, please see Chap. 4 for more complete information on the prescribing of antipsychotic medications. There are numerous other medications that have received varying degrees of interest in the past, such as naltrexone, but have not demonstrated good efficacy and are not recommended. See Fig. 6.2 for an algorithmic approach to BFRBs in the primary care setting.

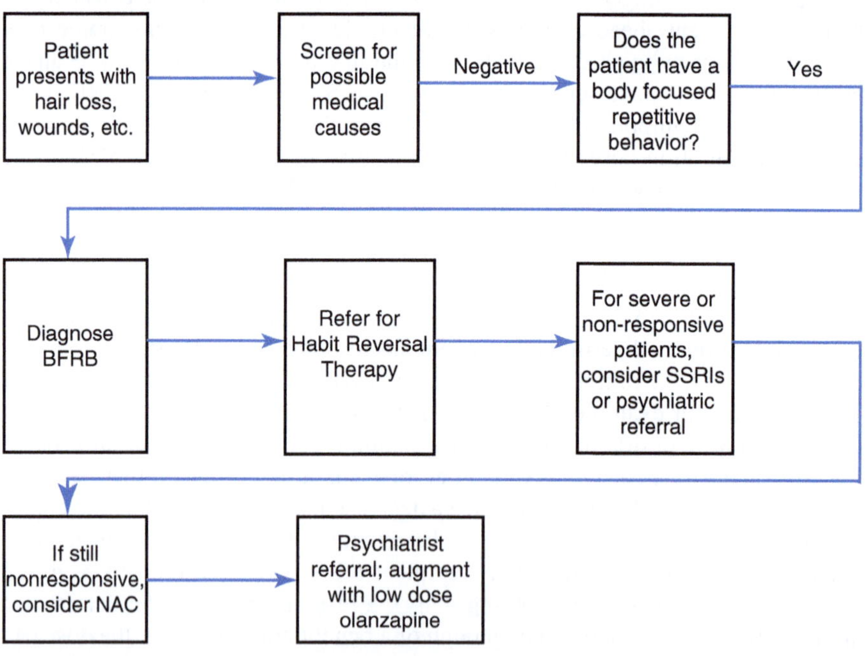

Fig. 6.2 Approach to BFRBs in the primary care setting

6.3.6 When to Refer for BFRBs

When to refer a patient out for specialty care from the general medical setting is always dependent upon the training and the comfort level of the practitioner; much will depend on the resources available in the community. Because the first line of treatment in BFRBs is CBT—specifically habit reversal training (HRT)—referral to a therapist well versed in the treatment of BFRBs is always the first referral that must be made. While the timing of when a referral to a psychiatrist occurs is up to the comfort level of the primary care physician in most respects, certain general rules apply. If the patient does not respond appropriately to properly applied HRT, medications should be initiated at that time. Failure of a first-line medication (e.g., failure of an SSRI at appropriate dosage) is a valid reason to refer the patient to a psychiatrist comfortable in the treatment of BFRBs. If the patient has significant medical complications from the BFRB (i.e., infections, anemia, cosmetically significant scarring), psychiatric intervention is recommended. Any comorbid psychiatric symptoms, especially mood, psychotic, or suicidal symptoms, should be evaluated by a psychiatrist as well. Lastly, the level of comfort in treating BFRBs for the primary care physician will determine when a referral to a psychiatrist is made.

6.4 Hoarding Disorder

6.4.1 Introduction and Epidemiology

Hoarding disorder has received a lot of public attention in recent years, in no small part to high-profile cases shown in the news and numerous television reality shows. Despite this, it was not formally recognized as a psychiatric disorder prior to DSM 5 in 2013. It used to be considered to be a subtype of OCD; research has helped demonstrate that it is indeed a separate diagnosis due to differences in onset, course of illness, degree of insight, and treatment response [33]; this has helped facilitate research as well [13]. Hoarding disorder (HD) is an important illness for the primary care physician to be able to recognize and begin appropriate interventions due to its chronic and debilitating nature and due to the marked public health concerns that accompany it. HD is a very common disorder, affecting as much as 5% of the population [48] with the problem increasing with age and an even higher prevalence among patients over 70 [13]. While the age of onset typically occurs during childhood [15], it rarely comes to medical attention at that age due to parents forcing their children to clean. Public health concerns are numerous. Patients have significant impairments in the activities of daily living, such as cleaning and cooking, due to clutter, and significant difficulties in occupational functioning are often present [19]. The clutter can present serious safety risks not only to the occupants of the home but for the community in general, due to risk of fire, poor sanitation, food contamination, malnutrition, medical problems, and falls [13, 19]. Hoarders have a 5-year mortality rate of 50% [46]. Legal issues are common as well; 64% of public health departments reported receiving a complaint regarding hoarding or clutter within the past 5 years [18], and risk of eviction is high [55]. Numerous deaths as a result of hoarding have been reported with some cases becoming famous (i.e., the Collyer brothers of New York City). Animal hoarding can be particularly severe—these patients tend to have limited insight and the public health implications are enormous [45].

Comorbidities are common in HD, and therefore proper screening of patients for related medical and psychiatric conditions is paramount. Over 90% of patients with HD have another psychiatric disorder: ADHD, schizophrenia, eating disorders, traumatic brain injury, and dementia are commonly present, as well as anxiety, mood, and personality disorders. Substance use disorders are also commonly found [19]. Medical problems other than dementias are common as well, and HD are 78% more likely to have obesity and 64% more likely to suffer from chronic medical conditions [55]. Therefore, if hoarding is noted in a patient in the primary care setting, the medical screening and diagnostic process is not over and in fact is only beginning.

6.4.2 *Hoarding Disorder in the Medical Setting*

As with the other obsessive-compulsive and related disorders, patients will rarely present with a complaint of clutter. Typically, the physician will only hear about it from family members or from legal authorities (e.g., county health departments). Since these cases may garner media attention, the primary care practitioner may initially hear about the behavior in local newscasts or from legal authorities. Once a complaint about clutter is brought to your attention, certain steps should be taken. First, a determination should be made if the clutter is clinically significant. In other words, does it meet the diagnostic criteria (see below): living spaces rendered not usable for their original purpose. If the patient does appear to have HD, an examination for both psychiatric and medical comorbidities should occur next. Special attention should be paid to dementia/cognitive screening as this is a significant comorbidity.

> The primary care provider may be asked to interact with the local health department in cases of severe hoarding or even have hoarding patients brought to them by local authorities.

6.4.3 Diagnosis and Presentation of Hoarding Disorder

The main feature in patients with HD is the inability to throw away items that appear to others to have little intrinsic value. The accumulation of these items causes clutter to a degree that living spaces in the house can no longer be used for their intended purpose. For example, counters may be piled with so much clutter that food preparation is impossible. Beds, sofas, chairs, and tables may be unusable due to clutter, and entire rooms may become impassible. Patients may have problems with excessive acquiring or items that are not needed, while others simply cannot discard what they already have. There is typically an emotional attachment to the hoarded objects. They tend to have poor psychosocial functioning (i.e., not allowing visitors in the house). Insight can range from good to absent but is typically lower than OCD [8]. Patients with comorbid neurocognitive dysfunctions are especially likely to have poorer insight. See Table 6.4 for diagnostic criteria for hoarding disorder.

Animal hoarding is a serious potential presentation of HD. DSM 5 defines it as "the accumulation of a large number of animals and a failure to provide the minimal standards of nutrition, sanitation, and veterinary care and to act on the deteriorating condition of the animals including disease, starvation, and death) and the environment (e.g., severe overcrowding, extremely unsanitary conditions)." Some authors believe that this represents a distinct nosological category [45] and insight is particularly poor in this group of patients [17].

Table 6.4 DSM 5 diagnostic criteria for hoarding disorder

A: Persistent difficulty discarding or parting with possessions, regardless of their actual value
B: This difficulty is due to a perceived need to save the items and to distress associated with discarding them
C: The difficulty discarding possessions results in the accumulation of possessions that congest and clutter active living areas and substantially compromise their intended use. If living areas are uncluttered, it is only because of the interventions of third parties
D: The hoarding causes clinically significant distress or impairment in social, occupational, or other important areas of functioning (including maintaining a safe environment for self and others)
E: The hoarding is not attributable to another medical condition (e.g., brain injury, cerebrovascular disease, Prader-Willi syndrome)
F: The hoarding is not better explained by the symptoms of another mental disorder (e.g., obsessions in OCD, decreased energy in MDD, delusions in schizophrenia or another psychotic disorder, cognitive deficits in neurocognitive disorders, restricted interests in autism)

6.4.4 Treatment of Hoarding Disorder

There is still not enough known about the treatment for hoarding disorder [13], and this may be due in part to the fact that it was not recognized as a separate, stand-alone disorder until DSM 5 was released in 2013. The use of cognitive behavioral therapy is considered the primary treatment for hoarding disorder at this time. Community-based support groups for hoarding have been used in many parts of the USA—these groups are often led by a professional therapist and may be free to attend. Like other OCRD, the CBT techniques used for treating hoarding disorder are not typically taught in graduate schools, and most therapists are likely not familiar with this disorder unless they have sought out specialized training. Therapists who have experience in hoarding disorder or special training from the International OCD Foundation are preferred (www.iocdf.org). The organization has a list of such therapists on its website and is a useful resource to both providers and patients. See Fig. 6.3 for an algorithmic approach to hoarding in the primary care setting.

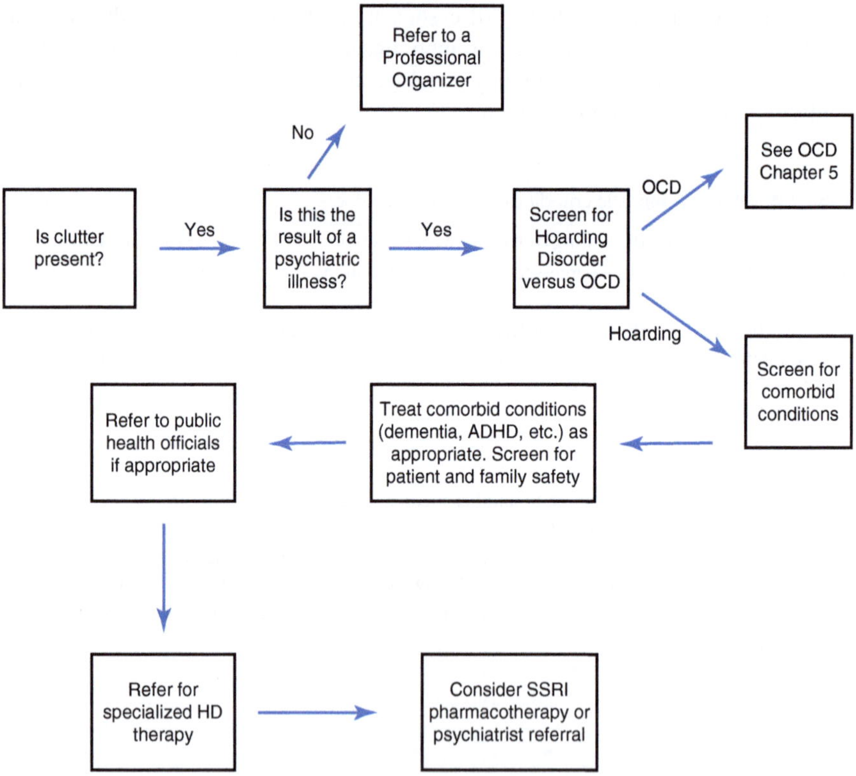

Fig. 6.3 Approach to hoarding in the primary care setting

Professional organizers can be helpful in the treatment of HD. Sometimes, patients will present to professional organizers believing that their hoarding is a result of disorganization and not a mental disorder. As they go into their clients' homes, they can contribute a useful allied support for HD patients in conjunction with their psychotherapist. Referrals for professional organizers who are familiar with hoarding disorder can be found through the National Association of Professional Organizers (www.napo.net).

6.5 Pharmacotherapy of Hoarding Disorder (and Other OCRD)

As of this writing, there are no treatment guidelines for the pharmacotherapy of HD [45]. Medication treatment should be considered an adjunct to cognitive behavioral therapy. Traditionally, SSRIs have been used in the treatment of HD, and studies indicate that they are indeed the most effective medications and should be considered first-line pharmacotherapy [45]. When patients present with comorbid ADHD, the use of stimulant medications may also be of benefit [13]. The recommended clinical practice is to use SSRIs for HD and other OCRD in a similar manner as for OCD—medications will typically be titrated up to the maximum dosages, particularly in patients who do not respond to lower doses. See Table 6.5 for dosage recommendations.

A recommended therapeutic trial of any one medication involves the medication being used at the maximum dose for a period of 12–16 weeks. Unlike antidepressant therapy, when patients are given SSRIs as anti-obsessionals, no clinical

Table 6.5 Dosing of serotonin reuptake inhibitors in obsessive-compulsive and related disorders

Anti-obsessional	Starting and titration dose (mg/day)[a]	Maximum dose (mg/day)	Occasional dose (mg/day)
Fluoxetine	20	80	120
Sertraline	50	400	400
Paroxetine	20	80	100
Fluvoxamine	50	400	450
Escitalopram	10	40	60
Clomipramine	25	250	250[b]

Adapted from Hudak et al. [26]

[a]Medications may be started at this dose and titrated by the same amount until maximum dose is reached. In elderly or sensitive patients, consider using half this dose, but the maximum dose remains the same. Titration of dose is typically done on a weekly basis but can be done more or less often depending on patient's tolerability

[b]Doses of 250 mg clomipramine are not recommended, and total tricyclic level (combined level of clomipramine plus desmethylclomipramine—the active metabolite) should be kept under 500 ng/ml to minimize the risk of seizures and cardiac conduction delays

Note: Citalopram is no longer recommended to be prescribed in doses over 40 mg due to possible QTc prolongation which limits its utility in OCRD

response may be seen early on in the treatment course, with initial responses only occurring during the end of the 12–16-week trial. Since this is a disorder that affects the elderly so often, it is important to note that the adage of medication usage in geriatric patients—"start low, go slow"—applies here as well, but it is vital not to necessarily stay low. That patient population still may need maximal doses for full clinical benefit.

As is the case with BDD, the lack of insight that is common in HD does not imply that antipsychotic medications are useful in this disorder. Due to their limited benefit [28], the use of antipsychotic medications in HD is not recommended.

6.5.1 When to Refer Patients for Hoarding Disorder

Typically, all patients that present with hoarding disorder will require referral rather than treatment in the primary care office as was noted above. Psychotherapy is considered not just first-line treatment for HD, but in fact is the primary treatment. Cognitive behavioral therapy is the primary treatment used in HD, and community-based CBT group therapy is a successful and common referral [13]. As with the other OCRD, we recommend checking the referral list from the International OCD Foundation to find lists of qualified therapists (www.iocdf.org).

As patients with hoarding disorder are at markedly elevated risk for comorbid psychiatric disorders, a general psychiatric screening is probably advisable for most patients. Certainly, if this is not practical in the medical setting, referral to a psychiatrist is warranted. Pharmacotherapy is generally assumed to not be successful in HD; however, this is not always the case [50]. When pharmacotherapy for HD is necessary, SSRIs are typically used and at usual OCD protocols. Failure of even one medication trial should trigger a referral to a psychiatrist due to the possibility of uncovered comorbidities contributing to treatment resistance. In cases of severe hoarding where public health officials are involved or need to be notified due to a public health risk, in cases where patient or family is at risk, or if animal hoarding is present, psychiatric referral is strongly recommended.

6.5.2 SSRI Side Effects

Note: As the first-line pharmacotherapy of all of the OCRD is SSRIs, side effects can be discussed just once.

Typical side effects of SSRIs include excessive yawning, headache, GI distress (nausea, dyspepsia, constipation, diarrhea), vivid dreams or nightmares, and tremors [6]. These side effects often are transient and are usually managed conservatively, using over-the-counter analgesics for headache, stool softeners for constipation, and H2 antagonists for dyspepsia. Starting at a lower dose and maintaining that dose for a few weeks prior to titration are often sufficient for side effect management:

- *Sexual side effects* are among the most troubling side effects that can occur with chronic, ongoing use of SSRI therapy and are reported in approximately a third of patients on SSRI therapy [12]. The most common reported problems are loss of libido, delayed orgasm or anorgasmia, erectile dysfunction (males), and lack of lubrication (females). Often, a careful history will determine that the complaints of erectile dysfunction or lack of lubrication are not primary issues per se but are the result of severe anorgasmia. There are numerous strategies that can be used in patients suffering from sexual side effects, such as a careful history regarding the nature of the actual side effects, their usual sexual habits, and their partner's (if there is one) knowledge of the situation. It should be noted that many patients state that the sexual side effects can remit over time, often taking many months or more; as a result, further intervention other than patience may not always be necessary. The addition of bupropion at a dose of 300 mg daily has been shown to reduce sexual side effects from SSRIs [6]. Buspirone can be used safely at doses between 20 and 60 mg daily and can help reverse sexual side effects [47]. If the patient does not wish to take a medication chronically in order to reverse sexual side effects, the use of cyproheptadine 4 mg orally 1–2 hours prior to sexual activity can reduce sexual side effects [51]. Another method that can be used is the drug holiday method. We recommend that the patient's medication be stopped the day before planned sexual activity. On the day that sexual activity occurs, the person can delay their dose until afterward. The medication can then be resumed on a normal basis the following day; this results in only one total missed dose. Patients should not do this more than one time per week in order to minimize missed dosages. The drug holiday method is not recommended with fluoxetine (due to its long half-life), and caution should be used with paroxetine due to its potent discontinuation syndrome (see below).
- *Movement disorders such as myoclonus* are defined as sudden, abrupt, shock-like involuntary movements caused by muscle contractions. Nocturnal jaw clenching may also occur. Usually, lowering the dose or switching meds can help, but these side effects may spontaneously remit as well [57].
- A *frontal lobe amotivational syndrome* can occur, characterized by apathy, affective blunting, and memory issues. Complaints of sedation may accompany this. (Note: excessive yawning is also a side effect of SSRIs and is not associated with fatigue.) This side effect may be more common in OCRD patients as it may occur at higher doses and may not improve with time as opposed to some other SSRI side effects [32]. The most common strategies to manage this include lowering the dose or switching agents. In our practice, we have had success using modafinil at usual therapeutic doses to counteract this side effect.

- Any of the SSRIs may lead to *weight gain* with long-term usage. This side effect may be more noticeable in chronic conditions such as OCRD as this may be associated with long-term use [16]. Management of this side effect is usually conservative, with recommendations given around lifestyle changes such as appropriate diet and exercise.
- *Excessive sweating* is a common complaint. Conservative management works in most cases, which simply involves recommending the patient have a change of bed clothes available to change into in the middle of the night. While there is little data on pharmacological management of this side effect, benztropine at 0.5 mg nightly can be tried [6].
- *Hyponatremia* is a rare (0.5% per year incidence) problem that can occur with SSRIs; elderly, female, and patients using concomitant diuretics are in the highest-risk category. This typically occurs within a few weeks of medication initiation or dose increase [31]. Symptoms typically include muscle cramps, fatigue, delirium, and seizures.
- *SSRI discontinuation syndrome* can occur with the abrupt discontinuation of many antidepressants, including the SSRIs (with the possible exception of fluoxetine due to its extended half-life). While it does not demand medical intervention, the symptoms can be quite distressing and even disabling; dizziness, light-headedness, insomnia, fatigue, anxiety, headache, nausea, and sensory disturbances described as electric sensations in the head or limbs (colloquially known as "brain zaps") are reported most commonly [61]. While symptoms are acute, resolution can be achieved rapidly by reinstating the full dose of the medication. Very slow and extended tapers can ameliorate this problem in most patients. In the case of someone on a maximum dose of an SSRI, the taper period may last 6 months or longer to reduce the risk of discontinuation syndrome. This also has the side benefit of decreasing the risk of relapse, as slower tapers of medications can reduce the possibility of OCD reoccurring after medications are stopped.
- *Serotonin syndrome* is a rare but serious medical condition that includes symptoms such as mental status changes, gastrointestinal symptoms, autonomic instability (tachycardia, hypertension, and hyperthermia), and neuromuscular abnormalities including myoclonus, hyperreflexia, hypertonicity, and rigidity; clinically, it presents very much like neuroleptic malignant syndrome [7, 9]. It has been most commonly associated with combinations of serotonergic agents but has been reported to occur with single agents. Treatment is usually supportive and includes discontinuation of the serotonergic agent; the addition of the 5-HT 2a antagonist cyproheptadine may also be of benefit [9].
- *Gastrointestinal bleeding* is a potential side effect of SSRI use and may be exacerbated with the concomitant use of nonsteroidal anti-inflammatory agents [31]. The use of medications to reduce the risk of GI bleeding may be warranted in high-risk patients [2].

References

1. Alessandrini A, Bruni F, Piraccini BM, Starace M. Common causes of hair loss - clinical manifestations, trichoscopy and therapy. J Eur Acad Dermatol Venereol. 2021;35(3):629–40. https://doi.org/10.1111/jdv.17079. Epub 2021 Jan 8. PMID: 33290611.
2. Andrade C, Sharma E. Serotonin reuptake inhibitors and risk of abnormal bleeding. Psychiatr Clin North Am. 2016;39(3):413–26. https://doi.org/10.1016/j.psc.2016.04.010. Epub 2016 Jun 28. PMID: 27514297.
3. Baczynski C, Sharma V. Pharmacotherapy for trichotillomania in adults. Expert Opin Pharmacother. 2020;21(12):1455–66. https://doi.org/10.1080/14656566.2020.1761324. Epub 2020 Jul 7. PMID: 32633577.
4. Bjornsson AS, Didie ER, Phillips KA. Body dysmorphic disorder. Dialogues Clin Neurosci. 2010;12(2):221–32. https://doi.org/10.31887/DCNS.2010.12.2/abjornsson. PMID: 20623926; PMCID: PMC3181960.
5. Bloch M. Trichotillomania and other impulse control disorders. In: Hudak R, Dougherty D, editors. Clinical obsessive compulsive disorders in adults and children. Cambridge University Press, UK; 2011.
6. Borue X, Sharma M, Hudak R. Biological treatments for obsessive-compulsive and related disorders. J Obses Compul Relat Disorder. 2015;6:7–26.
7. Boyer EW, Shannon M. The serotonin syndrome. N Engl J Med. 2005;352(11):1112–20. https://doi.org/10.1056/NEJMra041867. Erratum in: N Engl J Med. 2007;356(23):2437. Erratum in: N Engl J Med. 2009;361(17):1714. PMID: 15784664
8. Brakoulias V, Milicevic D. Assessment and treatment of hoarding disorder. Australas Psychiatry. 2015;23(4):358–60. https://doi.org/10.1177/1039856215587235. Epub 2015 May 27. PMID: 26019288.
9. Caroff SN, Watson CB, Rosenberg H. Drug-induced hyperthermic syndromes in psychiatry. Clin Psychopharmacol Neurosci. 2021;19(1):1–11. https://doi.org/10.9758/cpn.2021.19.1.1. PMID: 33508784; PMCID: PMC7851465.
10. Castle D, Beilharz F, Phillips KA, Brakoulias V, Drummond LM, Hollander E, Ioannidis K, Pallanti S, Chamberlain SR, Rossell SL, Veale D, Wilhelm S, Van Ameringen M, Dell'Osso B, Menchon JM, Fineberg NA. Body dysmorphic disorder: a treatment synthesis and consensus on behalf of the International College of Obsessive-Compulsive Spectrum Disorders and the Obsessive Compulsive and Related Disorders Network of the European College of Neuropsychopharmacology. Int Clin Psychopharmacol. 2021;36(2):61–75. https://doi.org/10.1097/YIC.0000000000000342. PMID: 33230025; PMCID: PMC7846290.
11. Christenson GA, Pyle RL, Mitchell JE. Estimated lifetime prevalence of trichotillomania in college students. J Clin Psychiatry. 1991;52(10):415–7. PMID: 1938977.
12. Clayton AH, Pradko JF, Croft HA, Montano CB, Leadbetter RA, Bolden-Watson C, Bass KI, Donahue RM, Jamerson BD, Metz A. Prevalence of sexual dysfunction among newer antidepressants. J Clin Psychiatry. 2002;63(4):357–66. https://doi.org/10.4088/jcp.v63n0414. PMID: 12000211.
13. Davidson EJ, Dozier ME, Pittman JOE, Mayes TL, Blanco BH, Gault JD, Schwarz LJ, Ayers CR. Recent advances in research on hoarding. Curr Psychiatry Rep. 2019;21(9):91. https://doi.org/10.1007/s11920-019-1078-0. PMID: 31410591; PMCID: PMC7294597.
14. Diagnostic and statistical manual of mental disorders 5. American Psychiatric Association; USA: 2013.
15. Dozier ME, Ayers CR. The etiology of hoarding disorder: a review. Psychopathology. 2017;50(5):291–6. https://doi.org/10.1159/000479235. Epub 2017 Aug 16. PMID: 28810245; PMCID: PMC7294599.
16. Ferguson JM. SSRI antidepressant medications: adverse effects and tolerability. Prim Care Companion J Clin Psychiatry. 2001;3(1):22–7. https://doi.org/10.4088/pcc.v03n0105. PMID: 15014625; PMCID: PMC181155.

17. Ferreira EA, Paloski LH, Costa DB, Fiametti VS, De Oliveira CR, de Lima Argimon II, Gonzatti V, Irigaray TQ. Animal hoarding disorder: a new psychopathology? Psychiatry Res. 2017;258:221–5. https://doi.org/10.1016/j.psychres.2017.08.030. Epub 2017 Aug 18. PMID: 28843626.
18. Frost RO, Steketee G, Williams L. Hoarding: a community health problem. Health Soc Care Community. 2000;8(4):229–34. https://doi.org/10.1046/j.1365-2524.2000.00245.x. PMID: 11560692.
19. Gilliam CM, Tolin DF. Compulsive hoarding. In: Hudak R, Dougherty DD, editors. Clinical obsessive compulsive disorders in adults in children. Cambridge University Press, UK; 2011.
20. Grant JE, Odlaug BL, Kim SW. N-acetylcysteine, a glutamate modulator, in the treatment of trichotillomania: a double-blind, placebo-controlled study. Arch Gen Psychiatry. 2009;66(7):756–63. https://doi.org/10.1001/archgenpsychiatry.2009.60. PMID: 19581567.
21. Grant JE, Odlaug BL, Chamberlain SR, Keuthen NJ, Lochner C, Stein DJ. Skin picking disorder. Am J Psychiatry. 2012;169(11):1143–9. https://doi.org/10.1176/appi.ajp.2012.12040508. PMID: 23128921.
22. Grant JE, Chamberlain SR, Redden SA, Leppink EW, Odlaug BL, Kim SW. N-acetylcysteine in the treatment of excoriation disorder: a randomized clinical trial. JAMA Psychiat. 2016;73(5):490–6. https://doi.org/10.1001/jamapsychiatry.2016.0060. PMID: 27007062.
23. Harris EC, Barraclough B. Suicide as an outcome for mental disorders. A meta-analysis. Br J Psychiatry. 1997;170:205–28. https://doi.org/10.1192/bjp.170.3.205. PMID: 9229027.
24. Hayes SL, Storch EA, Berlanga L. Skin picking behaviors: an examination of the prevalence and severity in a community sample. J Anxiety Disord. 2009;23(3):314–9. https://doi.org/10.1016/j.janxdis.2009.01.008. Epub 2009 Jan 23. PMID: 19223150.
25. Herbst I, Jemec GBE. Body dysmorphic disorder in dermatology: a systematic review. Psychiatry Q. 2020;91(4):1003–10. https://doi.org/10.1007/s11126-020-09757-y. PMID: 32472234.
26. Hudak R, Borue X, Sharma M. Biological models and treatments for obsessive - compulsive related disorders for adults. In: Abramowitz JS, McKay D, Storch EA, editors. Wiley handbook of obsessive compulsive disorder. Wiley-Blackwell, USA; 2017.
27. James M, Clarke P, Darcey R. Body dysmorphic disorder and facial aesthetic treatments in dental practice. Br Dent J. 2019;227(10):929–33. https://doi.org/10.1038/s41415-019-0901-7. PMID: 31758136.
28. Kim D, Ryba NL, Kalabalik J, Westrich L. Critical review of the use of second-generation antipsychotics in obsessive-compulsive and related disorders. Drugs R D. 2018;18(3):167–89. https://doi.org/10.1007/s40268-018-0246-8. PMID: 30171515; PMCID: PMC6131117.
29. Mansueto CS, Stemberger RM, Thomas AM, Golomb RG. Trichotillomania: a comprehensive behavioral model. Clin Psychol Rev. 1997;17(5):567–77. https://doi.org/10.1016/s0272-7358(97)00028-7. PMID: 9260041.
30. Marques L, Weingarden HM, Leblanc NJ, Wilhelm S. Treatment utilization and barriers to treatment engagement among people with body dysmorphic symptoms. J Psychosom Res. 2011;70(3):286–93. https://doi.org/10.1016/j.jpsychores.2010.10.002. Epub 2010 Dec 16. PMID: 21334500.
31. Moret C, Isaac M, Briley M. Problems associated with long-term treatment with selective serotonin reuptake inhibitors. J Psychopharmacol. 2009;23(8):967–74. https://doi.org/10.1177/0269881108093582. Epub 2008 Jul 17. PMID: 18635702.
32. Murphy TK, Segarra A, Storch EA, Goodman WK. SSRI adverse events: how to monitor and manage. Int Rev Psychiatry. 2008;20(2):203–8. https://doi.org/10.1080/09540260801889211. PMID: 18386213.
33. Nakao T, Kanba S. Pathophysiology and treatment of hoarding disorder. Psychiatry Clin Neurosci. 2019;73(7):370–5. https://doi.org/10.1111/pcn.12853. Epub 2019 May 20. PMID: 31021515.
34. Ninan PT, Koran LM, Kiev A, Davidson JR, Rasmussen SA, Zajecka JM, Robinson DG, Crits-Christoph P, Mandel FS, Austin C. High-dose sertraline strategy for non-responders to acute treatment for obsessive-compulsive disorder: a multicenter double-blind trial. J Clin Psychiatry. 2006;67(1):15–22. https://doi.org/10.4088/jcp.v67n0103. PMID: 16426083.

35. O'Sullivan RL, Phillips KA, Keuthen NJ, Wilhelm S. Near-fatal skin picking from delusional body dysmorphic disorder responsive to fluvoxamine. Psychosomatics. 1999;40(1):79–81. https://doi.org/10.1016/S0033-3182(99)71276-4. PMID: 9989126.
36. Pereyra AD, Saadabadi A. Trichotillomania. 2020 Jul 3. In: StatPearls [Internet]. Treasure Island (FL): StatPearls Publishing; 2021. PMID: 29630238.
37. Phillips KA. Psychosis in body dysmorphic disorder. J Psychiatr Res. 2004;38(1):63–72. https://doi.org/10.1016/s0022-3956(03)00098-0. PMID: 14690771.
38. Phillips KA. The broken mirror. Oxford University Press; 2005.
39. Phillips KA. Body dysmorphic disorder. In: Hudak R, Dougherty DD, editors. Clinical obsessive-compulsive disorders in adults and children. Cambridge University Press, UK; 2011.
40. Phillips KA. Pharmacotherapy and other somatic treatments for body dysmorphic disorder. In: Phillips KA, editor. Body dysmorphic disorder: advances in research and clinical practice. New York: Oxford University Press, USA; 2017.
41. Phillips KA, Diaz SF. Gender differences in body dysmorphic disorder. J Nerv Ment Dis. 1997;185(9):570–7. https://doi.org/10.1097/00005053-199709000-00006. PMID: 9307619.
42. Phillips KA, Hollander E. Treating body dysmorphic disorder with medication: evidence, misconceptions, and a suggested approach. Body Image. 2008;5(1):13–27. https://doi.org/10.1016/j.bodyim.2007.12.003. Epub 2008 Mar 5. PMID: 18325859; PMCID: PMC2705931.
43. Phillips KA, Menard W, Fay C, Weisberg R. Demographic characteristics, phenomenology, comorbidity, and family history in 200 individuals with body dysmorphic disorder. Psychosomatics. 2005;46(4):317–25. https://doi.org/10.1176/appi.psy.46.4.317. PMID: 16000674; PMCID: PMC1351257.
44. Phillips KA, Didie ER, Menard W, Pagano ME, Fay C, Weisberg RB. Clinical features of body dysmorphic disorder in adolescents and adults. Psychiatry Res. 2006;141(3):305–14. https://doi.org/10.1016/j.psychres.2005.09.014. Epub 2006 Feb 23. PMID: 16499973; PMCID: PMC1592052.
45. Piacentino D, Pasquini M, Cappelletti S, Chetoni C, Sani G, Kotzalidis GD. Pharmacotherapy for hoarding disorder: how did the picture change since its excision from OCD? Curr Neuropharmacol. 2019;17(8):808–15. https://doi.org/10.2174/1570159X17666190124153048. PMID: 30678629; PMCID: PMC7059160.
46. Roane DM, Landers A, Sherratt J, Wilson GS. Hoarding in the elderly: a critical review of the recent literature. Int Psychogeriatr. 2017;29(7):1077–84. https://doi.org/10.1017/S1041610216002465. Epub 2017 Feb 6. PMID: 28162112.
47. Rosen RC, Lane RM, Menza M. Effects of SSRIs on sexual function: a critical review. J Clin Psychopharmacol. 1999;19(1):67–85. https://doi.org/10.1097/00004714-199902000-00013. PMID: 9934946.
48. Samuels JF, Bienvenu OJ, Grados MA, Cullen B, Riddle MA, Liang KY, Eaton WW, Nestadt G. Prevalence and correlates of hoarding behavior in a community-based sample. Behav Res Ther. 2008;46(7):836–44. https://doi.org/10.1016/j.brat.2008.04.004. Epub 2008 Apr 13. PMID: 18495084; PMCID: PMC2483957.
49. Sarwer DB, Spitzer JC. Body image dysmorphic disorder in persons who undergo aesthetic medical treatments. Aesthet Surg J. 2012;32(8):999–1009. https://doi.org/10.1177/1090820X12462715. Epub 2012 Sep 26. PMID: 23015692.
50. Saxena S. Pharmacotherapy of compulsive hoarding. J Clin Psychol. 2011;67(5):477–84. https://doi.org/10.1002/jclp.20792. Epub 2011 Mar 14. PMID: 21404273.
51. Schweitzer I, Maguire K, Ng C. Sexual side-effects of contemporary antidepressants: review. Aust N Z J Psychiatry. 2009;43(9):795–808. https://doi.org/10.1080/00048670903107575. PMID: 19670052.
52. Snorrason I, Belleau EL, Woods DW. How related are hair pulling disorder (trichotillomania) and skin picking disorder? A review of evidence for comorbidity, similarities and shared etiology. Clin Psychol Rev. 2012;32(7):618–29. https://doi.org/10.1016/j.cpr.2012.05.008. Epub 2012 Jul 20. PMID: 22917741.

53. Stewart RS, Nejtek VA. An open-label, flexible-dose study of olanzapine in the treatment of trichotillomania. J Clin Psychiatry. 2003;64(1):49–52. https://doi.org/10.4088/jcp.v64n0110. PMID: 12590623.
54. Toh WL, Castle DJ, Mountjoy RL, Buchanan B, Farhall J, Rossell SL. Insight in body dysmorphic disorder (BDD) relative to obsessive-compulsive disorder (OCD) and psychotic disorders: revisiting this issue in light of DSM-5. Compr Psychiatry. 2017;77:100–8. https://doi.org/10.1016/j.comppsych.2017.06.004. Epub 2017 Jun 8. PMID: 28651226.
55. Tolin DF, Frost RO, Steketee G, Gray KD, Fitch KE. The economic and social burden of compulsive hoarding. Psychiatry Res. 2008;160(2):200–11. https://doi.org/10.1016/j.psychres.2007.08.008. Epub 2008 Jul 1. PMID: 18597855; PMCID: PMC3018686.
56. Van Ameringen M, Simpson W, Patterson B, Dell'Osso B, Fineberg N, Hollander E, Hranov L, Hranov G, Lochner C, Karamustafalioglu O, Marazziti D, Menchon JM, Nicolini H, Pallanti S, Stein DJ, Zohar J. Pharmacological treatment strategies in obsessive compulsive disorder: a cross-sectional view in nine international OCD centers. J Psychopharmacol. 2014;28(6):596–602. https://doi.org/10.1177/0269881113517955. Epub 2014 Jan 15. PMID: 24429223.
57. Vandel P, Bonin B, Leveque E, Sechter D, Bizouard P. Tricyclic antidepressant-induced extrapyramidal side effects. Eur Neuropsychopharmacol. 1997;7(3):207–12. https://doi.org/10.1016/s0924-977x(97)00405-7. PMID: 9213080.
58. Wever CCC, Wever AMEA, Constantian M. Psychiatric disorders in facial plastic surgery. Facial Plast Surg Clin North Am. 2020;28(4):451–60. https://doi.org/10.1016/j.fsc.2020.06.003. Epub 2020 Sep 9. PMID: 33010863.
59. Wilhelm S, Weingarden H, Greenberg JL, McCoy TH, Ladis I, Summers BJ, Matic A, Harrison O. Development and pilot testing of a cognitive-behavioral therapy digital service for body dysmorphic disorder. Behav Ther. 2020;51(1):15–26. https://doi.org/10.1016/j.beth.2019.03.007. Epub 2019 Aug 7. PMID: 32005333.
60. Woods DW, Flessner C, Franklin ME, Wetterneck CT, Walther MR, Anderson ER, Cardona D. Understanding and treating trichotillomania: what we know and what we don't know. Psychiatr Clin North Am. 2006;29(2):487–501, ix. https://doi.org/10.1016/j.psc.2006.02.009. PMID: 16650719.
61. Zajecka J, Tracy KA, Mitchell S. Discontinuation symptoms after treatment with serotonin reuptake inhibitors: a literature review. J Clin Psychiatry. 1997;58(7):291–7. https://doi.org/10.4088/jcp.v58n0702. PMID: 9269249.
62. Ziglinas P, Menger DJ, Georgalas C. The body dysmorphic disorder patient: to perform rhinoplasty or not? Eur Arch Otorhinolaryngol. 2014;271(9):2355–8. https://doi.org/10.1007/s00405-013-2792-6. Epub 2013 Nov 5. PMID: 24190759.

Chapter 7
Post-traumatic Stress Disorder

E.F. is a 40-year-old divorced female who presents to your primary care clinic to establish care. She reports a history of fibromyalgia, tension headaches, and irritable bowel syndrome. Her chief complaint today is "I feel exhausted." on questioning, she notes chronic sleep difficulties that she describes as worsening. She further elaborates that she has difficulty falling asleep and staying asleep and gets as little as 3 hours of sleep a night. She then discloses that she tends to avoid sleep as she has trouble relaxing due to anxious anticipation of nightmares that often wake her up. The patient mumbles that these nightmares are about past "bad things" that happened to her years ago but quickly adds, "I really don't want to talk about it." She then notes that she sometimes thinks about these things during the day, even when she is actively trying not to, and certain places and objects can unexpectedly precipitate these memories. During the conversation, the patient suddenly becomes agitated and shouts, "you know what? I don't even know why I am telling you these things. No one can help me. I am a lost cause." Before the patient leaves the room, you manage to reassure her that you do, in fact, want to help her. She apologizes and becomes tearful, admitting that it is hard for her to "control [her] emotions" and "trust people."

7.1 Introduction and Epidemiology

Trauma is a normal, emotional response to a terrible event or events. Trauma-inducing events commonly include sexual and physical assault, child abuse, interpersonal violence, serious accidents, and natural disasters. Trauma can impact people in a myriad of different ways, influenced by the severity of the traumatic event(s), availability of

R. Hudak, J. M. Gannon, *Handbook of Psychiatric Disorders in Adults in the Primary Care Setting*, Current Clinical Practice,
https://doi.org/10.1007/978-3-030-98709-1_7

supports post traumatic event(s), accessibility of coping skills, and cultural considerations. After experiencing a traumatic event, an individual may experience a range of emotions, from fear and sadness to anger and denial. They may also feel disconnected from reality. Somatic experiences, including fatigue, feeling easily startled or restless, or having an upset stomach, are also common, as are cognitive concerns, such as having difficulty concentrating. Most of the time, these feelings and physical experiences will largely resolve within a few hours or days after the traumatic event and ultimately cause minimal disruption in day-to-day functioning. When these experiences persist and impact daily life, a trauma-related disorder should be suspected.

Post-traumatic stress disorder (PTSD) is the most diagnosed trauma-related disorder. It is unfortunately common, with lifetime prevalence rates, estimated from population surveys, of between 6% and 7% [13, 22]. Rates of PTSD stemming from a single traumatic event are estimated to be as high as 15% [2]. However, population prevalence rates at any given time are between 3% and 5% [7, 10]. This seeming discrepancy in prevalence rates can in part be explained by a reassuring clinical reality—most cases of PTSD are highly treatable [20] and resolve within a year of the incident trauma [12]. Most patients will, in fact, experience the most severe symptoms proximal to the traumatic event, with distress gradually decreasing in the first year after symptom onset [25]. Others will experience PTSD symptoms for several years before ultimately reaching remission. Overall, it is estimated that about 2/3 of patients diagnosed with PTSD go into complete symptom remission; the remaining 1/3 have a more chronic course [19], though even some of these patients may achieve periods of remission [4].

While PTSD is most frequently linked with traumatic events that can happen to anyone, it is also commonly associated with military combat. Active-duty military and recently returned veterans who served in Operation Enduring Freedom (OEF) and/or Operation Iraqi Freedom (OIF) demonstrated PTSD rates as high as 14% [26]. Separated OEF/OIF veterans' PTSD rates were closer to 8–9% [14, 16, 28]. While veterans overall may not have significantly higher rates of PTSD compared to those of the general population [13, 22], some reports suggest higher lifetime, war zone related (17.0% in men, 15.2% in women) prevalence of PTSD, and current, all cause prevalence (12.2% in men, 8.5% in women) of PTSD, among Vietnam War veterans [17].

Strong risk factors for PTSD development include the nature and severity of the traumatic event [31]; lack of pre-event social support and lack of expansion of support post-event have predictive effects [3]. Education, history of previous trauma, family psychiatric history, and adverse childhood experiences have also been associated with development of PTSD after trauma [3]. Gender, age at trauma, and race are predictive of PTSD in some, but not all, populations. Neither age nor race/ethnicity is associated with statistically different PTSD population prevalence rates [13]. Gender differences, however, are observed. Women have higher lifetime PTSD prevalence rates (8.6–9.7%) than do men (4.1–5.2%) [13, 22].

Personal psychiatric history has also been associated with the development of PTSD with trauma [3]. Over 80% of patients with PTSD have at least one other major psychiatric disorder [12]. PTSD is frequently comorbid to other psychiatric conditions, particularly mood, anxiety, dissociative, personality, somatization, and substance use disorders [1]. It is also thought to be underrecognized in serious mental illness, like bipolar disorder and schizophrenia, and as sequelae of major medical illness.

E.F.'s presentation is suggestive of PTSD (see diagnostic criteria below). She also presents with a history of medical disorders that have been specifically associated with PTSD, namely, fibromyalgia [11] *and irritable bowel syndrome* [21]. *Given her increased risk of serious medical conditions as explained below, routine health screenings should not be neglected.*

Primary care physicians and associated health professionals commonly encounter PTSD in routine practice. PCPs are often the first to diagnose and treat the disorder [6], and patients with PTSD might be overrepresented in a typical primary care patient panel. In a study of one primary care clinic, 11.8% of patients met criteria for PTSD [30]. Somatization is often seen in more severe PTSD cases, and patients with PTSD self-report poorer physical health, chronic pain, and lower overall functioning than those without PTSD [23]. PTSD patients do have objectively higher rates of medical comorbidities, with statistically elevated rates of diabetes mellitus, noncirrhotic liver disease, heart disease, hypercholesterolemia, stomach ulcer, HIV, and arthritis, even when adjusting for the presence of comorbid psychiatric disorders [23]. Given these findings, regular preventative and diagnostic care by PCPs is recommended.

7.2 Diagnosis and Presentation

PTSD is classified as a trauma- and stressor-related disorder. All the diagnoses in this category are tied to a core traumatic or stressful experience or experiences. PTSD and acute stress disorder are trauma-related disorders that occur on a longitudinal continuum, with acute stress disorder presenting with symptoms similar to those of PTSD but constrained to a relatively brief period. It often precedes the onset of PTSD. As previously noted, responses to traumatic life events vary widely from person to person and across experiences; sometimes, the severity of trauma responses, their time course, and the degree of impairment associated with them are suggestive of a psychiatric disorder. While traumatic events can precipitate general anxiety, when the core trauma symptoms are not fear or anxiety but rather dysphoria and anhedonia, anger and aggression, or dissociation, this is suggestive of the presence of a trauma- and stressor-related disorder.

The following table (Table 7.1) is a summary of PTSD criteria as established in the Diagnostic and Statistical Manual of Mental Disorders: DSM 5 [5]. For simplicity, the criteria presented are specific to adults. Children can experience PTSD, though intrusion symptoms may be experienced as repetitive play with traumatic themes and frightening dreams without clear content. The symptoms are otherwise

Table 7.1 Criteria for PTSD

Exposure to a traumatic event(s) (can include actual or threatened death, sexual violence, and physical injury) through: 1. Direct experience(s). 2. In person witnessing of the trauma(s). 3. Learning about traumatic event(s) experienced by family members or close friends (note that if death occurred, it must have been violent or accidental). 4. Experiencing repeated exposure to details of traumatic events, usually in the context of work (e.g., police officers, first responders, etc.).
Recurrent intrusion symptoms (must experience one or more, associated with the traumatic event(s)): 1. Intrusive involuntary memories of the traumatic event(s). 2. Distressing dreams (the content and/or affect should be related to the traumatic event(s)). 3. Dissociative reactions in which the individual acts like the traumatic event is reoccurring, e.g., flashbacks. 4. Intense, prolonged psychological distress at exposure to "triggers," i.e., internal or external cues that symbolize or remind the patient of the traumatic event(s). 5. Intense, prolonged physiological reactions to "triggers".
Persistent avoidance symptoms (must experience one or more, associated with the traumatic event(s)): 1. Avoidance or efforts to avoid distressing trauma-associated thoughts, feelings, or memories. 2. Avoidance of or efforts to avoid external reminders that cause distressing trauma-associated thoughts, feelings, or memories. These reminders can include people, places, activities, conversations, etc.
Negative alterations in thoughts and feelings (must experience two or more, associated with the traumatic event(s)): 1. Inability to remember an important aspect of the traumatic event(s), usually due to dissociate amnesia. 2. Negative, persistent, exaggerated beliefs about oneself, others, and/or the broader world, e.g., "I am a bad person," "I am a complete wreck," "people are not to be trusted," "the world is not at all safe," etc. 3. Persistent, distorted thoughts or beliefs about the consequences or causes of the traumatic event(s) that lead the patient to misattribute blame, e.g., onto himself/herself or others. 4. Persistent negative emotional state, e.g., fear, shame, guilt, anger, etc. 5. Markedly diminished interest in or withdrawal from activities. 6. Feelings of detachment or estrangement from others. 7. Persistent inability to experience positive emotions, e.g., loving feelings, happiness, etc.
Marked alterations in arousal and reactivity (must experience two or more, associated with the traumatic event(s)): 1. Irritable behavior and angry outbursts with verbal or physical aggression toward people or objects, usually with little to no provocation. 2. Reckless or self-destructive behavior. 3. Hypervigilance. 4. Exaggerated startle response. 5. Problems with concentration. 6. Sleep disturbance, e.g., restless sleep or difficulty falling or staying asleep.

From DSM 5 [5]

similar for children over the age of 6 years and adults. Core symptoms of PTSD can be divided into experiencing or being a witness to traumatic event, experiencing intrusive symptoms of the traumatic event, avoiding stimuli associated with the traumatic event, having negative thoughts/feelings associated with the traumatic event, and having hyperarousal symptoms. Symptoms must last at least 1 month, cause significant distress and/or impairment in functioning, and not be attributable to another medical condition or medications/substances. Reoccurring episodes of depersonalization (feelings of being detached from one's body or mental processes) and/or derealization (feeling as though the external world is unreal) also commonly occur with PTSD. These dissociative symptoms can be added as qualifiers to a formal PTSD diagnosis and are considered separately from the core criteria dissociative reactions of the disorder.

Individuals with acute stress disorders are those who experienced an acute stress reaction to a traumatic event. Acute stress reactions (sometimes called combat and operational stress reactions in the military) are normal. While they can be quite profound, they usually respond to reassurance, rest, and a safe environment and occur over a limited time frame of a few hours to days. Acute stress disorders involve acute stress reactions that lead to functional impairment and/or profound distress and last for more than a few days. Trauma exposure criteria are identical to that of PTSD. Like with PTSD, symptoms cannot be attributable to another medical condition, medications, or substances. While not all PTSD patients will have experienced an acute stress disorder, patients with acute distress disorder whose symptoms last for more than a month will usually progress to PTSD. The acute stress disorder diagnosis is helpful in that it allows for early intervention to prevent PTSD development. Criteria of acute stress disorder are summarized in Table 7.2.

E.F. likely meets criteria for PTSD. She notes having had at least one traumatic experience years ago. She has nightmares, intrusive thoughts about the trauma event(s), and physiologic reactivity at trauma cues. Avoidance symptoms are hinted at by E.F.'s not wanting to discuss her trauma, and negative, persistent beliefs are manifest in her not being able to trust others and that she cannot be helped. Both sleep disturbance and her irritable behavior/outburst are likely arousal symptoms. Given that the patient hints at experiencing significant issues in interpersonal relationships and has multiple diagnoses that could point to somatic symptoms, she may have complex PTSD.

"Complex PTSD" is not an official DSM 5 diagnosis but is widely acknowledged in the field. Most guidelines do not recommend any specific treatment for complex PTSD diverging from that of PTSD. Generally, individuals who have this type of PTSD not only meet criteria for PTSD, but they also have fairly profound behavioral, emotional, and dissociative symptoms as well as somatization and significant disturbances in interpersonal relationships [4]. Complex PTSD is often associated with prolonged and/or repeated traumas, such as might occur with childhood sexual abuse, imprisonment, or torture [19].

In the DSM 5 [5], several other psychiatric disorders are grouped under the trauma- and stressor-related disorders category. These include reactive attachment

Table 7.2 Criteria for acute stress disorder

Exposure to trauma(s) (can include actual or threatened death, sexual violence, and physical injury) through: 1. Direct experience(s). 2. In person witnessing of the trauma(s). 3. Learning about traumatic event(s) experienced by family members or close friends (note that if death occurred, it must have been violent or accidental). 4. Experiencing repeated exposure to details of traumatic events, usually in the context of work (e.g., police officers, first responders, etc.).
Must experience nine (or more) of the following symptoms from any of the five categories, beginning or worsening after the trauma(s): Intrusion symptoms 1. Recurrent, involuntary, and intrusive distressing memories of the trauma(s) 2. Recurrent distressing dreams in which the content and/or affect of the dream are related to the trauma(s) 3. Dissociative reactions (e.g., flashbacks) in which the individual feels or acts as if the trauma(s) were reoccurring 4. Intense or prolonged psychological distress or marked physiological reactivity in response to "triggers" or cues that remind the patient of the trauma(s) Negative mood 5. Persistent inability to experience positive emotions (e.g., inability to experience happiness, satisfaction, loving feelings). Dissociative symptoms 6. An altered sense of reality or of one's self 7. Inability to remember an important aspect of the event(s), i.e., dissociative amnesia Avoidance symptoms 8. Efforts to avoid distressing memories, thoughts, or feelings about or closely associated with the trauma(s) 9. Efforts to avoid external reminders (e.g., people, places, conversations, activities, objects, situations) that arouse distressing memories, thoughts, or feelings about or closely associated with the trauma(s) Arousal symptoms 10. Sleep disturbance 11. Irritable behavior and angry outbursts (with little or no provocation) toward people or objects 12. Hypervigilance 13. Problems with concentration 14. Exaggerated startle response

From DSM 5 [5]

disorder and disinhibited social engagement disorder; as these are primarily disorders of childhood, they are out of the scope of this chapter. Adjustment disorder is the other condition included in this diagnostic grouping. Adjustment disorders are quite common in the general population, with up to 20% of individuals seeking mental health care meeting criteria for adjustment disorders [5]. Like with the other diagnoses in trauma- and stressor-related disorders, symptoms are associated with an identifiable stressor or set of stressors. The response to these stressors should include "marked distress" that is "out of proportion to the severity or intensity of the stressor." Relevant cultural and environmental factors that may be influencing the clinical presentation should also be taken into account. The distress experienced must lead to significant impairment in functioning. Some symptoms of depression and/or anxiety can be present, though full diagnostic criteria for mood or anxiety disorders should not be met. Examples of stressors that can precipitate adjustment disorders can include job loss, difficulties in school, natural disasters, and divorce. Stressors can have a sudden onset or be more insidious; they can be time limited or more chronic. In general, adjustment disorders do not include what would be considered normal grief or bereavement. Symptoms must begin within 3 months of the stressor and last no longer than 6 months after the stressor resolves. Patients with adjustment disorders often respond very well to psychotherapy and do not often require medication management with psychotropics, though judicious use of as needed medications for anxiety or difficulty sleeping may be appropriate.

7.3 PTSD in the Medical Setting

Screening for PTSD symptoms in patients who have survived traumatic events, have high occupational risks for PTSD, or have served in combat can be helpful, as can screening in patients who repeatedly present for nonspecific physical health complaints [19]. While screeners are not diagnostic, they can be quite helpful to PCPs in starting a conversation with patients to clarify symptoms and for assessing need for psychiatry referral [20]. PTSD screeners can be given to a patient starting 1 month after a traumatic event. Commonly used screeners in the USA include the Primary Care PTSD Screen (PC-PTSD) and the PTSD Checklist (PCL). The PC-PTSD is shown below. On this screener, more than three "yes" answers is suggestive of PTSD and would merit further follow-up.

The primary care PTSD screen for DSM-5 (PC-PTSD-5)
In the past month, have you… (YES/NO response)
1. Had nightmares about the event(s) or thought about the event(s) when you did not want to?
2. Tried hard not to think about the event(s) or went out of your way to avoid situations that reminded you of the event(s)?
3. Been constantly on guard, watchful, or easily startled?
4. Felt numb or detached from people, activities, or your surroundings?
5. Felt guilty or unable to stop blaming yourself or others for the event(s) or any problems the event(s) may have caused?

Referral to therapy and/or psychiatric services should be considered for all patients with suspected PTSD. Patients with a moderate-to-high risk of lethality and/or comorbid psychiatric (including substance use) diagnoses should always be referred. As with any psychiatric condition, referral to higher levels of care, including inpatient hospitalization, is indicated if the patient's symptoms are such that the patient presents with significant risk of harming themselves or others. For patients who do not require higher levels of care, collaborative care arrangements between primary care teams and PTSD competent behavioral health services are highly recommended [4]. Good collaborative models allow for stepped approaches to treatment while ensuring primary care continuity. If referral to a nonaffiliated behavioral health professional is necessary, selecting specialists competent in treating trauma and who can provide (or at least facilitate) both psychiatric and psychological treatment is indicated. Close PCP follow-up of patients with PTSD should continue, regardless of engagement in behavioral health treatment, given the high rates of serious medical comorbidity in this population.

Offering E.F. a referral to trauma-informed behavioral health services would be appropriate. Regardless of whether E.F. decides to engage, however, she will continue to require close medical follow-up. Partnering with her in engaging in routine healthcare screening, like for breast cancer, cervical cancer, hypertension, hyperlipidemia, and diabetes, cannot be overemphasized.

A patient presenting with acute distress disorder should have very close PCP follow-up. "Watchful waiting," including by PCPs, has been the long-standing treatment recommendation for acute stress disorder. More recent evidence supports referral for trauma-focused cognitive behavioral therapy (TFCBT) [20] or a therapy with both trauma exposure and cognitive restructuring components [4] if available. Of note, other psychological interventions have not been well studied in this population, but extreme caution in the use of therapies without an evidence base is merited given that psychological debriefing (a traditional approach to acute stress disorder) is now contraindicated as it is associated with worse outcomes [20]. Treating acute stress disorder with medication is generally not indicated. Some guidelines warn explicitly against prescribing benzodiazepines [20] given concerns for delayed recovery and risks associated with this class of medications.

Patients with PTSD, especially complex PTSD, can be challenging to engage and treat in a medical setting. These patients may, on the one hand, present frequently to PCPs for nonspecific somatic complaints while simultaneously engaging in high-risk behaviors and not following up with basic preventative care. Difficulty with forming and maintaining personal relationships may also make it difficult for some patients with PTSD to form healthy relationships with PCPs. In extreme cases, these patients, especially those with comorbid substance use disorder and/or personality disorder, can be disruptive in clinic and evoke a lot of frustration in office staff. Trauma-informed models of primary care delivery are thus highly recommended; training to attain trauma-informed status is sometimes available to PCP offices (e.g., as offered by the National Council) and should include all staff, including front desk staff. Clinics that provide trauma-informed care offer a safe, patient strength-based, nurturing, and empowering clinical environment for patients and staff; incorporate screenings for ongoing and past trauma, substance use disorders, and mood disorders; and ensure evidence-based treatment and referral for trauma-related disorders [18].

7.4 Treatment of PTSD

7.4.1 Psychotherapy

Quality psychotherapy is the cornerstone of PTSD treatment [4]. Patients with PTSD, not unlike most patients with mental illness, strongly benefit from forming a treating relationship with someone who skillfully and objectively listens while offering unconditional, positive support. At the same time, some types of psychotherapeutic treatments have a much stronger evidence base than others. Generally, effective treatments are "manualized" psychotherapies entailing specific protocols focused on exposure and/or cognitive restructuring [4]. These trauma-focused therapies not only have large effect sizes in clinical trials, but they significantly outperform evidence-based PTSD treatment with psychotropics [19]. That said, patient nonresponse rates and dropout rates are frequently high, even in the context of controlled clinical trials [27, 29]. Clinical considerations, including comorbid mental health and substance use disorders, are important to keep in mind when selecting treatment options with patients, as are retention and response to past treatment trials. Most importantly, understanding patient preference for specific treatment modalities is critical. Some patients, for example, may not feel "ready" for therapies incorporating trauma visualization or cue exposure but will engage with examining negative cognitions, behavioral activation, and psychoeducation. Referral to a therapist who will work with the patient in their preferred modality is paramount in ensuring participation. A good therapist will, over time, work with the patient to adapt the therapy to continue to meet their needs as their recovery progresses.

The manualized psychotherapeutic treatments with the strongest evidence base include trauma-focused cognitive behavioral therapy (TFCBT) and the closely related cognitive processing therapy and cognitive therapy as well as prolonged exposure therapy [1, 4]. Cognitive processing therapy and prolonged exposure therapy are the best studied psychotherapeutic interventions for PTSD [29]. Brief eclectic psychotherapy, eye movement desensitization and reprocessing (EMDR), and narrative exposure therapy are also frequently recommended [1, 4]. Each of these therapies can be provided in as little as 8–12 sessions, though more sessions may be required, especially if the patient has sustained multiple traumas.

TFCBT and related therapies (cognitive processing therapy and cognitive therapy) involve processing trauma memories and related emotions; help restructure trauma-related negative cognitions, including blaming oneself for the trauma and/or about viewing the world as unsafe; and include psychoeducation about managing reactions to trauma, including flashbacks [20]. These therapies also aim to reduce avoidant behavior, increase adaptive behaviors, and repair damaged relationships.

Prolonged exposure therapy incorporates exposure through the patient's repeatedly recounting the trauma narrative while being asked to simultaneously visualize it. Exposure to real-life trauma cues, e.g., new stories about traumatic events that cue physiologic reactivity, is also an important part of treatment. Emotional processing with trauma exposure is facilitated [4], while psychoeducation about physical and psychological reactions to trauma is also provided [19]. Narrative exposure therapy also relies on imagery and patient narrative, though it incorporates a whole life narrative and so is most frequently utilized when a patient has multiple traumas across their lifespan. Brief eclectic psychotherapy also involves trauma imagery and written narrative processing but incorporates cognitive restructuring and relaxation techniques. As it is based more in psychodynamic therapy, it also involves attention to greater meaning and, ultimately, entails metaphorical ritual closing of the traumatic event.

EMDR incorporates patient visualization and narration to process the most distressing mental image associated with the trauma alongside the emotions and negative cognitions associated with it. Bilateral eye movements, finger tapping, or auditory tones can all be used during visualization to help create an awareness of the external world, promote relaxation, and facilitate cognitive processing. EMDR is conducted in a phased manner with integrated psychoeducation and promotion of coping skills to manage distressing symptoms occurring both during the sessions and between visits.

7.4.2 Pharmacology

Psychopharmacologic agents are considered second-line treatment for PTSD. For patients who do not engage in therapy or for whom evidence-based therapies are not readily available, treatment with psychiatric medication often becomes the default option. Choosing medication with the strongest evidence base, with the least risk of serious side effects, and in review of the patient's personal medical history, family medical history, and past treatment response is critical. Moreover, informed patient preference is critically important. Given extremely high levels of psychiatric and substance use comorbidity in PTSD, however, it is not unusual for patients with PTSD to already be prescribed psychiatric medications at the time of PTSD diagnosis. Some of these medications may have beneficial effects on PTSD symptoms as well as on the primary psychiatric condition for which they are indicated. These medications can be continued and/or optimized to better target the PTSD symptoms.

There are several medications with good evidence for use in reducing the severity of PTSD symptoms, though clinical trials demonstrating efficacy also revealed only small-to-medium treatment effect sizes. The following table (see Table 7.3) summarizes several professional guidelines' pharmacologic treatment recommendations. Primary treatments and add-on treatments are included. Of note, while the use of add-on treatments is common in PTSD, there is less evidence supporting this practice.

Based on available trials and expert consensus, the primary psychopharmacologic treatment of PTSD consists of medications from the selective serotonin reuptake inhibitor (SSRI) antidepressant class. Of note, sertraline and paroxetine are the only FDA-approved treatments for PTSD. Effective dosing of antidepressants for

Table 7.3 Evidence-based pharmacologic treatments of PTSD

Primary treatments of PTSD	Add-on treatments for PTSD
Sertraline (VA, NICE, AUS, APA Psychol) Paroxetine (VA, NICE, AUS, APA Psychol) Fluoxetine (VA, NICE, AUS, APA Psychol) Venlafaxine (VA, NICE, AUS (if SSRI fails), APA Psychol) Other SSRIs (NICE) Prazosin (PTSD-associated nightmares; VA (neither recommend for or against))	Prazosin (VA – PTSD-associated nightmares, neither recommend for or against; AUS) Quetiapine (AUS (second line))

VA VA/DOD Clinical Practice Guideline for the Management of Posttraumatic Stress Disorders and Acute Stress Disorder [4], *APA Psychol* Clinical Practice Guideline for the Treatment of Posttraumatic Stress Disorder (PTSD) in Adults [1], *NICE* post-traumatic stress disorder [20], *AUS* Australian Guidelines for the Prevention and Treatment of Acute Stress Disorder, Posttraumatic Stress Disorder and Complex PTSD [19]

PTSD may require dosing in the upper end of the recommended range approved for major depressive disorder, for example, 200 mg of sertraline or 60 mg of fluoxetine. Common side effects of antidepressants include appetite and weight changes, headache, upper and lower GI complaints, and sexual side effects. More information on these side effects can be reviewed in other chapters of this book.

Use of the α_1-adrenergic antagonist prazosin for PTSD-associated nightmares also has relatively good support in the literature, although not all clinical trials have been positive [24]. Prazosin can be prescribed at doses as high as 10–16 mg at night, though therapeutic efficacy is often seen in doses between 2 and 6 mg [8]. Prazosin should generally be initiated at 1 mg nightly and increased quite slowly, over the course of several weeks, to reduce risks of orthostatic hypotension and its sequelae. Monitoring orthostatic vitals and symptoms should be done regularly during dose titration.

The use of antipsychotics in PTSD is not well supported. The VA guidelines strongly recommend against the use of risperidone and, to a lesser extent, other antipsychotics [4], though the NICE guidelines note that they can be used with careful monitoring [20]. Australian guidelines [19] recommend quetiapine as a second-line adjuvant and a third-line primary treatment, though they stipulate that doses should be much lower than those prescribed for schizophrenia, e.g., 300 mg versus 600 mg. Clinical indicators for antipsychotic prescription include the presence of severe, disabling behaviors and extreme hyperarousal and/or psychotic/psychotic-like symptoms that have not responded to other treatments [20]. It is important to note, however, that there is little evidence that these medications are efficacious for PTSD symptoms, and their use must be carefully monitored given associated risks of metabolic syndrome and movement disorders. Some experts would argue that the risks of antipsychotic prescribing exceed the potential benefits [4]. We would recommend that the decision to start an antipsychotic for PTSD be deferred to psychiatry.

Treatment with benzodiazepines, while formally a common practice, is no longer recommended [4, 20]. Some lower-quality evidence suggests that use of benzodiazepines in PTSD may be associated with overall worse outcomes, increased illness severity, and increased comorbidity [9]. Overall, the literature suggests that there is minimal to no benefit in using benzodiazepines in the treatment of PTSD, and the risks of prescribing this class of medications outweigh the benefits [4].

In recent years, exploration of the use of psychedelics for PTSD has yielded quite promising results, especially in the case of 3,4-methylenedioxymethamphetamine (MDMA). Thus, notwithstanding its classification as a Schedule 1 medication and despite its reputation as a "party drug," MDMA was designated by the US Food and Drug Administration (FDA) as a "breakthrough therapy" in 2017, enabling further research trials. Of note, in research trials so far, MDMA administration has been embedded in specific psychotherapy protocols. MDMA sessions last 5–8 hours, are proceeded and followed by preparatory and integration psychotherapy sessions, take place within comfortable clinic environments, and are facilitated by two therapists [15]. This is important to highlight in that MDMA has so far been considered a "psychotherapy enhancer" rather than a standalone treatment. Given this, it is likely that MDMA will ultimately require administration by trained behavioral health staff and as part of manualized psychotherapy. Much more research, however, is needed before MDMA can be safely recommended for clinical use.

7.5 Conclusions

Community rates of PTSD and other trauma-related disorders are high and greatly impact the quality of life of those who suffer from them. Close monitoring by PCPs is recommended given high rates of comorbid medical problems, common psychiatric comorbidities, and substance use disorders. While pharmacological treatment options are limited, evidence-based psychotherapies are quite effective. Access challenges, however, are often substantial, and retention rates are a common limitation. While new treatment avenues are on the horizon, it is important to highlight that most people with PTSD substantially improve over time, especially with treatment.

References

1. American Psychological Association Guideline Development Panel for the Treatment of PTSD in Adults. Clinical Practice Guideline for the Treatment of Posttraumatic Stress Disorder (PTSD) in Adults. 2017 February 24; 1–119.
2. Breslau N. The epidemiology of posttraumatic stress disorder: what is the extent of the problem? J Clin Psychiatry. 2001;62(Suppl17):16–22.
3. Brewin CR, Andrews B, Valentine JD. Meta-analysis of risk factors for posttraumatic stress disorder in trauma-exposed adults. J Consult Clin Psychol. 2000;68(5):748–66.
4. Department of Veteran's Affairs, Department of Defense. VA/DOD Clinical Practice Guideline For the Management of Posttraumatic Stress Disorders and Acute Stress Disorder, Version 3. 2017 June; 1–200.

5. Diagnostic and Statistical Manual of Mental Disorders: DSM 5. 5th ed., American Psychiatric Association, 2013.
6. Grinage BD. Diagnosis and management of post-traumatic stress disorder. Am Fam Physician. 2003;68(12):2401–8.1.
7. Goldstein RB, Smith SM, Chou SP, et al. The epidemiology of DSM-5 posttraumatic stress disorder in the United States: results from the National Epidemiologic Survey on Alcohol and Related Conditions-III. Soc Psychiatry Psychiatr Epidemiol. 2016;51(8):1137–48.
8. Green B. Prazosin in the treatment of PTSD. J Psychiatr Pract. 2014;20(4):253–9. https://doi.org/10.1097/01.pra.0000452561.98286.1e.
9. Guina J, Rossetter SR, De RB, Nahhas RW, Welton RS. Benzodiazepines for PTSD: A systematic review and meta-analysis. J Psychiatr Pract. 2015;21(4):281–303.
10. Harvard Medical School, 2007. National Comorbidity Survey (NCS). (2017, August 21). Retrieved from https://www.hcp.med.harvard.edu/ncs/index.php. Data Table 7.2: 12-month prevalence DSM-IV/WMH-CIDI disorders by sex and cohort.
11. Häuser W, Galek A, Erbslöh-Möller B, Köllner V, Kühn-Becker H, Langhorst J, Petermann F, Prothmann U, Winkelmann A, Schmutzer G, Brähler E, Glaesmer H. Posttraumatic stress disorder in fibromyalgia syndrome: prevalence, temporal relationship between posttraumatic stress and fibromyalgia symptoms, and impact on clinical outcome. Pain. 2013;154(8):1216–23. https://doi.org/10.1016/j.pain.2013.03.034. Epub 2013 Apr 2
12. Kessler RC, Sonnega A, Hughes M, Nelson CB. Posttraumatic stress disorder in the National Comorbidity Survey. Arch Gen Psychiatry. 1995;52(12):1048–60.
13. Kessler RC, Berglund P, Demler O, Jin R, Merikangas KR, Walters EE. Lifetime prevalence and age-of onset distributions of DSM-IV disorders in the national comorbidity survey replication. Arch Gen Psychiatry. 2005;62(6):593–602.
14. Kessler RC, Heeringa SG, Stein MB, et al. Thirty-day prevalence of DSM-IV mental disorders among nondeployed soldiers in the US Army: results from the Army study to assess risk and resilience in Service Members (Army STARRS). JAMA Psychiatry. 2014;71(5):504–13.
15. Krediet E, Bostoen T, Breeksema J, van Schagen A, Passie T, Vermetten E. Reviewing the potential of psychedelics for the treatment of PTSD. Int J Neuropsychopharmacol. 2020;23(6):385–400. https://doi.org/10.1093/ijnp/pyaa018. PMID: 32170326; PMCID: PMC7311646.
16. LeardMann CA, Smith TC, Smith B, Wells TS, Ryan MA. Baseline self reported functional health and vulnerability to post-traumatic stress disorder after combat deployment: prospective US military cohort study. BMJ. 2009;338:b1273.
17. Marmar CR, Schlenger W, Henn-Haase C, et al. Course of posttraumatic stress disorder 40 years after the Vietnam war: findings from the national Vietnam Veterans longitudinal study. JAMA Psychiatry. 2015;72(9):875–81.
18. Machtinger EL, Cuca YP, Khanna N, Rose CD, Kimberg LS. From treatment to healing: the promise of trauma-informed primary care. Womens Health Issues. 2015;25(3):193–7. https://doi.org/10.1016/j.whi.2015.03.008.
19. National Health and Medical Research Council. Australian Guidelines for the Prevention and Treatment of Acute Stress Disorder, Posttraumatic Stress Disorder and Complex PTSD. 2020 June 23.
20. National Institute for Health and Care Excellence (NICE). Post-traumatic stress disorder. London: NICE; 2018. p. 1–49. (NICE Guideline [NG116]).
21. Ng QX, Soh AYS, Loke W, Venkatanarayanan N, Lim DY, Yeo WS. Systematic review with meta-analysis: the association between post-traumatic stress disorder and irritable bowel syndrome. J Gastroenterol Hepatol. 2019;34(1):68–73. https://doi.org/10.1111/jgh.14446. Epub 2018 Sep 10
22. Pietrzak RH, Goldstein RB, Southwick SM, Grant BF. Prevalence and Axis I comorbidity of full and partial posttraumatic stress disorder in the United States: results from wave 2 of the National Epidemiologic Survey on Alcohol and Related Conditions. J Anxiety Disord. 2011a;25(3):456–65.

23. Pietrzak RH, Goldstein RB, Southwick SM, Grant BF. Medical comorbidity of full and partial posttraumatic stress disorder in US adults: results from Wave 2 of the National Epidemiologic Survey on Alcohol and Related Conditions. Psychosom Med. 2011b;73(8):697–707. https://doi.org/10.1097/PSY.0b013e3182303775. Epub 2011 Sep 23. PMID: 21949429; PMCID: PMC3188699.
24. Raskind MA, Peskind ER, Chow B, Harris C, Davis-Karim A, Holmes HA, Hart KL, McFall M, Mellman TA, Reist C, Romesser J, Rosenheck R, Shih MC, Stein MB, Swift R, Gleason T, Lu Y, Huang GD. Trial of Prazosin for Post-Traumatic Stress Disorder in Military Veterans. N Engl J Med. 2018;378(6):507–17. https://doi.org/10.1056/NEJMoa1507598.
25. Rothbaum B, Foa E. Subtypes of posttraumatic stress disorder and duration of symptoms. In: Davidson J, Foa E, editors. Posttraumatic stress disorder: DSM-IV and beyond. Washington, DC: American Psychiatric Press; 1994. p. 23–35. [F].
26. Schell TL, Marshall GN. Survey of individuals previously deployed for OEF/OIF. Invisible wounds of war: psychological and cognitive injuries, their consequences, and services to assist recovery. 2008. p. 87–115.
27. Schottenbauer MA, Glass CR, Arnkoff DB, Tendick V, Gray SH. Nonresponse and dropout rates in outcome studies on PTSD: review and methodological considerations. Psychiatry. 2008;71(2):134–68. https://doi.org/10.1521/psyc.2008.71.2.134.
28. Smith TC, Ryan MA, Wingard DL, Slymen DJ, Sallis JF, Kritz-Silverstein D. New onset and persistent symptoms of post-traumatic stress disorder self reported after deployment and combat exposures: prospective population based US military cohort study. BMJ. 2008;336(7640):366–71.
29. Steenkamp MM, Litz BT, Hoge CW, Marmar CR. Psychotherapy for military-related PTSD: a review of randomized clinical trials. JAMA. 2015;314(5):489–500. https://doi.org/10.1001/jama.2015.8370.
30. Stein MB, McQuaid JR, Pedrelli P, Lenox R, McCahill ME. Posttraumatic stress disorder in the primary care medical setting. Gen Hosp Psychiatry. 2000;22:261–9.
31. Van Ameringen M, Mancini C, Patterson B, Boyle MH. Post-traumatic stress disorder in Canada. CNS Neurosci Ther. 2008;14:171–81.

Chapter 8
ADHD in the Primary Care Setting

8.1 Introduction and Epidemiology

Case Example 8.1
Ms. G. is a 26-year-old woman who presented with a chief complaint of "I think I have ADHD and I need accommodations for test taking." She states that she has decided to go back to college but is having significant issues with focus and concentration. She has trouble in lectures but especially has difficulty with test taking. She states that these problems started at a very early age—she always had these issues growing up in school, but never complained about it, and was never evaluated or treated for it, as she was able to overcome it with coping skills. More details were requested about her inability to focus. She stated that it was particularly difficult to concentrate while looking at numbered lists as the steps would seem to "flip" or change places while looking at it. This also occurred with certain numbered pairs, leading to the especially problematic issues with test taking. No primary problems related to focus were identified. She was told that these symptoms most likely represented a learning disorder rather than ADHD which she readily accepted upon explanation. She was told accommodations for test taking were completely reasonable and that referral for therapy was indication which she accepted. No medication treatment was indicated.

Attention deficit hyperactivity disorder (ADHD) is a condition that is commonly diagnosed and treated in childhood. While it was at one time thought to be solely a childhood illness, we now know that it persists into adulthood and often goes undetected until that time. Because the majority of the initial diagnosis in children occurs in the primary care setting, adult patients are also likely to present to primary care settings for initial diagnosis and treatment [13]. Although complaints of lack of

R. Hudak, J. M. Gannon, *Handbook of Psychiatric Disorders in Adults in the Primary Care Setting*, Current Clinical Practice,
https://doi.org/10.1007/978-3-030-98709-1_8

focus or inattention can occur across many psychiatric symptoms and disorders (e.g., anxiety or mood disorders among others) and due to the fact that the first-line medications for this disorder include Schedule II medications, familiarity with the protocols for treating ADHD is essential knowledge for the primary care physician.

Research into adult ADHD is still lacking compared to children, but it is a disorder that is underrecognized and can lead to lifelong function impairments.

ADHD is relatively common: the prevalence in adults aged 20 to 64 is 4.4%, although the rate of ADHD in college students may be as high as 12% [3]. It is frequently underdiagnosed, with less than 20% of adults with ADHD having been given diagnosis or treatment [14]. While it is commonly believed that about 50% of children will grow out of their ADHD in adulthood, it is more likely that adult patients will experience fluctuating symptoms, with periods of remission in most cases, yet also experience periods of reoccurrence as well [17]. The fluctuation in symptoms that the person experiences throughout their life is due to circumstances: it is secondary to changes in external demands or supports and not because of improvement or worsening in the disorder itself. ADHD has a high comorbidity with other psychiatric illnesses that may mask its diagnosis [15]. ADHD is three times more common in individuals diagnosed with mood disorders and 1.7 more times common in people diagnosed with bipolar disorder [16]. Those with ADHD are more likely to have substance use disorders as well: 26% of individuals use cocaine and 10% meet criteria for a cocaine use disorder [11].

Because ADHD can cause significant socio-occupational dysfunction, such as lower education attainment, inability to maintain employment, and lesser occupational productivity [14], better identification and appropriate treatment and referral can result in better outcomes for an overlooked population.

8.2 ADHD in the Medical Setting

ADHD can present in numerous ways in the medical setting. Driving is an issue for ADHD patients that can obviously lead to problems or complaints in the primary care setting. Adults with ADHD are more likely to violate traffic laws including excessive speeding and to have higher rates of risk-taking behavior and resultant collisions [6]. They are more likely to engage in distracted driving due to their problems with attention, and issues with impulse control lead to greater rates of road rage [3]. Appropriate treatment of ADHD can lead to a significant reduction in the rate of traffic accidents including death [4].

Documentation of safe driving practices is recommended when seeing and treating patients with ADHD.

Patients with ADHD are noted to suffer from greater risks of certain medical problems. Some authors have found that ADHD patients have increased risks of obesity, diabetes, and asthma although the relationship between ADHD and these disorders is not always clear [8]. Ninety percent of patients with ADHD have psychiatric comorbidities, including mood disorders, anxiety disorders, OCD, intermittent explosive disorder, and substance use disorders [14]. Due to their propensity for impulsive behavior and driving, they are at a slightly higher risk of premature death due to accidents. Red flags for the possible presence of ADHD in adults include [3]:

- Organizational problems.
- Erratic occupational or academic performance.
- Anger control issues.
- Difficulty maintaining self-regulating activities, such as sleeping patterns.
- Difficulty managing finances.
- Addictive behavior.
- Frequent accidents or reckless driving.
- Family history of ADHD.
- Low self-esteem or chronic underachievement.

It is common for people to present to their primary care physician with complaints of deficits in attention. Some of the most common conditions that should be included in the differential diagnosis include hearing impairment, thyroid disease, lead toxicity, hepatic disease, sleep apnea, and drug interactions [13]. Many psychiatric disorders can have inattention as a prominent symptom; this should not be considered to be ADHD as the inattention symptoms in these instances would be expected to go away once the primary disorder is treated. Excessive anxiety and anxiety disorders commonly present with inattention as a primary complaint. OCD, major depressive disorder, bipolar disorder, personality disorders, and substance use disorders also will present with inattention or hyperactivity. As noted with Ms. G., a learning disability can have a very similar chief complaint. See Table 8.1 for a list of differential diagnoses.

Table 8.1 Differential diagnosis of ADHD

Psychiatric	Medical
Excessive anxiety or anxiety disorders	Sleep disorders
OCD	Thyroid disease
Major depressive disorder	Hepatic disease
Bipolar disorder	Drug interactions
Substance use disorder	Hearing impairment
Personality disorders	Lead toxicity
Malingering	Medication and substances including anticholinergics, antihistamines, steroids, anticonvulsants, opioids and other pain medications, benzodiazepines, caffeine, nicotine
Intellectual or developmental disability	Seizure disorder
Learning disorder	

Ms. G had none of the impulsive behavior that can be seen in ADHD; instead she mixed up lists and numbers, more indicative of a learning disability.

ADHD should present with symptoms prior to the age of 12 years (note: in prior editions of the DSM, the symptoms needed to be present prior to the age of 7). Therefore, when the complaints of inattention are not of this long-standing nature, a medical or psychiatric cause is most likely to blame. A complaint of ADHD-like symptoms therefore demands a careful screening, appropriate laboratory tests, and physical exam.

Rating scales and questionnaires have been developed to screen for ADHD; many of these are readily available on the Internet, and patients often take such tests and present to the office with them in hand. However, there are no screening tests that are considered sufficiently accurate enough to make a diagnosis on their own. Instead, making a diagnosis of ADHD depends upon obtaining a detailed patient history and assessing current symptoms and level of functioning. Screening tests can be useful, however, in helping to obtain information from both the patient and collateral sources as well as to help document changes that occur with time and/or treatment. One scale that has been validated as a screening tool to identify patients who require more comprehensive evaluation is the Adult Attention-deficit/hyperactivity disorder Self-Report Scale (ASRS) which was developed by the World Health Organization [2]. This screening tool, as well as other resources, is available for free on the website of the Canadian ADHD Resource Alliance at www.caddra.ca.

8.3 Diagnosis and Presentation of ADHD

Evaluation and management of ADHD can be appropriately done in the primary care setting, particularly if an appropriate stepwise approach is taken [13]. This includes:

- Screening and evaluation of symptoms present in the past 6 months.
- Establishing that a childhood history of symptoms prior to the age of 12 years is present by obtaining a developmental history (e.g., elementary school functioning, childhood behavior, etc.)
- Screening for functional impairments in social, occupational, and academic settings.
- Obtaining a psychiatric history and review of symptoms to rule out other disorders.
- Obtaining a family history for ADHD, drug use, and criminal behavior.
- Performing a physical exam with emphasis on neurologic examination and the thyroid, as well as contraindications to stimulant therapy (e.g., hypertension).

Impairment in ADHD must occur in at least two spheres: social functioning (friends, family), occupational functioning, and academic functioning.

The *inattention* of ADHD refers to wandering off task, lacking persistence, difficulty sustaining focus, and being disorganized. *Hyperactivity* manifests as extreme restlessness and wearing others out with high levels of activity. *Impulsivity* refers to hasty actions that occur without forethought and have a high potential for self-harm (e.g., darting in front of traffic) and a desire for immediate gratification (DSM 5). See Table 8.2 for full DSM 5 criteria for ADHD.

Referrals for neuropsychological testing are frequently recommended for ADHD diagnosis. However, testing is only likely to be helpful in cases of diagnostic uncertainty. If screening tests are desired to assist in symptom gathering, they may be obtained for free on the website for the Canadian ADHD Resource Alliance at www.caddra.ca as noted above. Per CADDRA guidelines, in order to ensure an accurate diagnosis in the primary care setting, the physician must:

1. Ensure that patients meet symptom criteria in Table 8.2.
2. Document age of onset of symptoms prior to the age of 12.

Table 8.2 DSM 5 criteria for ADHD in adults

A. A persistent pattern of inattention and/or hyperactivity-impulsivity that interferes with functioning or development, as characterized by (1) and/or (2).	
1. *Inattention*: Five or more symptoms have persisted for at least 6 months to a degree that negatively impacts social and academic or occupational activities.	2. *Hyperactivity and impulsivity*: Five or more symptoms have persisted for at least 6 months to a degree that negatively impacts social and academic or occupational activities.
Often fails to give close attention to details or makes careless mistakes in schoolwork	Often fidgets with hands or feet or squirms in seat
Often has difficulty sustaining attention in tasks or play activities	Often leaves seat in classroom when remaining seated is expected
Often does not seem to listen when spoken directly to	Often runs about or climbs excessively in situations where it is inappropriate
Often does not follow through on instructions and fails to finish schoolwork	Often has difficulty playing or engaging in leisure activities quietly
Often has difficulty organizing tasks and activities	Often is "on the go" or often acts as if "driven by a motor"
Often avoids, dislikes, or reluctantly engages in tasks requiring sustained mental effort	Often talks excessively
Often loses things necessary for activities (e.g., school assignments, pencils, or books)	Often blurts out answers to questions before the questions have been completed
Often is distracted by extraneous stimuli	Often has difficulty awaiting turn
Often is forgetful in daily activities	Often interrupts or intrudes on others (e.g., butts into conversations or games)
B. Several inattentive or hyperactive-impulsive symptoms were present prior to the age of 12.	
C. Several inattentive or hyperactive-impulsive symptoms are present in two or more settings (e.g., home, school, or work).	
D. There is clear evidence that the symptoms interfere with, or reduce the quality of, social, academic, or occupational functioning.	
E. The symptoms do not occur exclusively during the course of schizophrenia or another psychotic disorder and are not better explained by another mental disorder (e.g., mood disorder, anxiety disorder, dissociative disorder, personality disorder, substance intoxication or withdrawal).	

3. Document impairment in two roles of functioning: social, occupational, and/or academic.
4. Document that no better, alternative explanation for the symptoms, either medical, psychiatric, or social/circumstantial, exists.

8.3.1 Treatment

The treatment protocols for ADHD differ from those used for children (not covered in this book). Prior to treatment for ADHD, particularly pharmacological treatment, any psychiatric comorbidities must be addressed. This is especially important in the cases of comorbid bipolar disorder due to an overlapping clinical presentation [9, 15] and for substance use disorders, as the risk in using of stimulants can be high in that population [12]. Stimulants can also be problematic in patients with psychotic disorders as well as certain patients with anxiety or obsessive-compulsive disorders.

Both pharmacologic and psychotherapeutic approaches can be used in the treatment of ADHD in adults. As of this writing, there is no accepted consensus on when to offer therapy, medications, or both. However, due to the relative safety and low risk of psychotherapy, it is reasonable to offer that to any patient with ADHD. In addition to treatment of the primary symptoms, psychotherapy can help the patient deal with fallout from the psychosocial dysfunction of the illness. Many patients will prefer to try psychotherapy alone at first; since developing inherent coping skills can be empowering, those who wish to try alone initially can be encouraged to do so. If psychotherapy fails to give the patient the desired improvement, the addition of medications should be encouraged. The treatment recommended for ADHD is cognitive behavioral therapy (CBT) and should target executive functioning. Symptoms such as time management and organizational skills are the symptoms that are targeted [3]. Other therapies can be helpful for ADHD, such as occupational therapy [1]. See Fig. 8.1 for an algorithmic approach to seeing patients in the primary care setting who complain of ADHD symptoms.

8.4 Treatment

8.4.1 Pharmacology

Generally speaking, there are three categories of medications that are used to treat ADHD:

1. Stimulants.
   (a) Amphetamines.
   (b) Methylphenidate.
2. Antidepressants and other non-stimulants.
3. Alpha-agonist medications (e.g., guanfacine, clonidine).

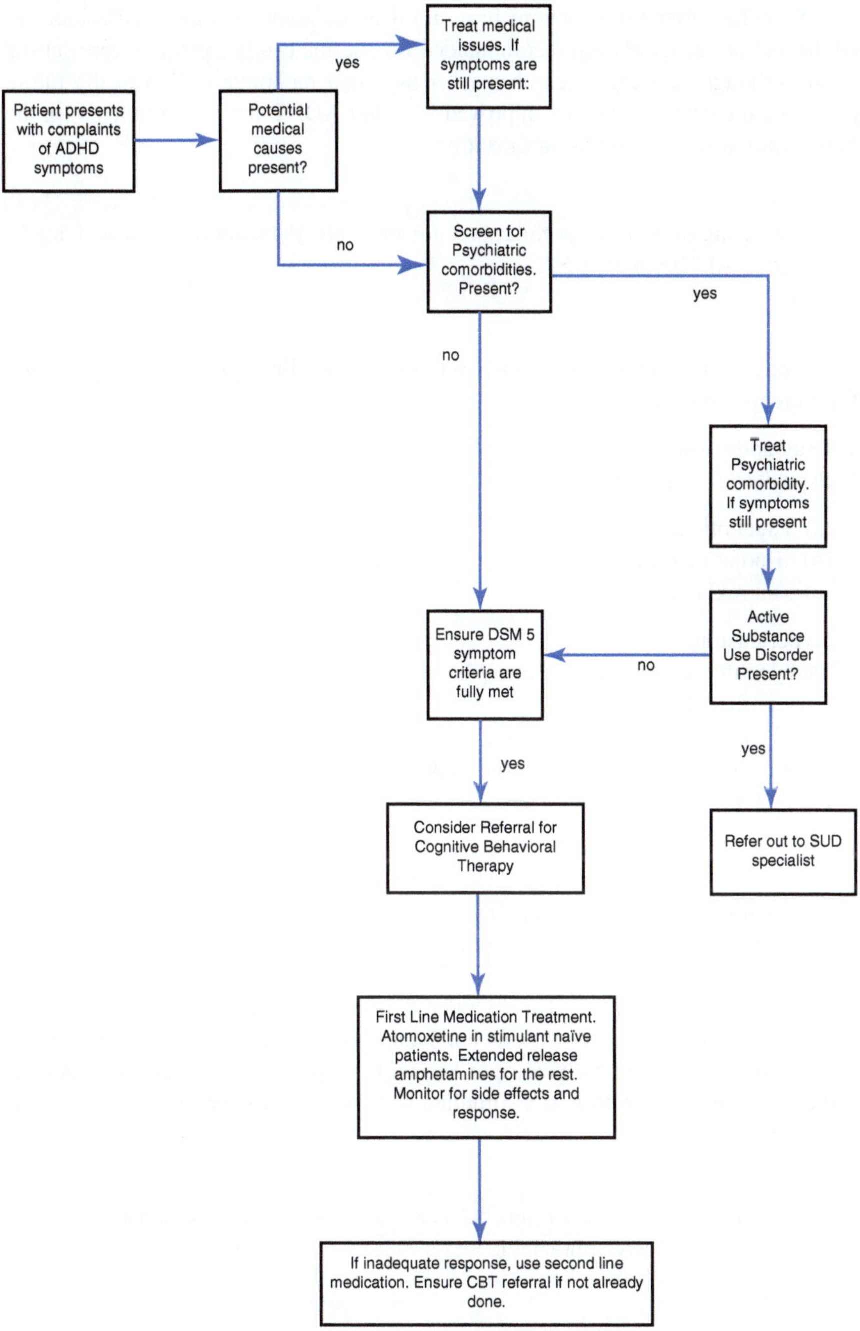

Fig. 8.1 Algorithmic approach to ADHD in the primary care setting

The alpha-agonist medications have not been demonstrated to be efficacious in adults and are generally not recommended for routine use in a primary care setting [3, 8] although ongoing research may change that recommendation in the future [10]. The medications that are approved for adult ADHD are the stimulants (in the long-acting form) as well as atomoxetine.

Long-acting stimulant formulations are the only FDA-approved stimulants for adult ADHD in the USA.

Using a non-stimulant (e.g., atomoxetine) as a first-line option may be preferred for patients with a history of:

1. Drug addiction.
2. Psychiatric comorbidity.
   (a) Psychotic disorder.
   (b) Bipolar disorder.
   (c) Anorexia nervosa.
3. Hypertension.
4. Tachycardia or other cardiac arrhythmia.
5. Seizure disorder.
6. Tic disorder or Tourette syndrome.
7. Prior history of nonresponse to stimulants.
8. Patients who are stimulant naive.

Both stimulants and atomoxetine are effective for adult ADHD. Stimulants may have a higher response rate than atomoxetine [7]. An important difference between them is that stimulants work immediately, while atomoxetine can take several weeks before improvement is noted. Atomoxetine works by blocking the reuptake of norepinephrine. See Table 8.3 for the use of atomoxetine in adults.

The efficacy of stimulants (methylphenidate) and amphetamines are likely similar, although some data suggests that amphetamines might have a higher effect size. More importantly, patients have been known to respond to one class of stimulant and not the other. Therefore, if a stimulant is chosen and then patient fails one, the other should be tried [5].

Careful diagnosis is important, because these medications would not have helped Ms. G. in any appreciable way.

Table 8.3 Atomoxetine in adult ADHD

Initial dose (maintain for a minimum of 3 days)	Target dose	Maximum dose (consider if inadequate response after 2–4 weeks)
40 mg/day	80 mg/day	100 mg/day

Amphetamines work for ADHD by increasing dopamine and norepinephrine release as well as blocking their reuptake. See Table 8.4 for a list of amphetamines that are considered first line for adult ADHD and Table 8.5 for a list of other stimulants that are also considered first line for adult ADHD. Table 8.6 contains amphetamines that are considered second line for ADHD and Table 8.7 stimulants that are second line. The need for twice-daily dosing of these medications precludes them from being recommended as first-line agents. Note that brand names are included to minimize confusion concerning the different formulations available.

As with any psychiatric medication, it is important to periodically assess whether the medication is working and whether a titration up or down, or even taking a medication holiday, is warranted. Much of these decisions will be made in concert with the patient and their report on how well the medication is working, as well as side effects they are experiencing. Patients who want a break off the medication should be encouraged to try it during weekends and vacation where it won't affect their functioning at work. Some patients will be able to simply stop the medications during a drug holiday and then restart. However, other patients may experience withdrawal effects and a taper may be recommended in those people.

Patients who experience delayed sleep onset may need to have the dose reduced and/or given earlier in the morning. Patients who experience other side effects, such as decreased appetite, headache, jitteriness, irritability, or anxiety, may need to have their dosages adjusted downward or switched to atomoxetine.

Because atomoxetine is related to antidepressant medication, patients should generally remain on it even on weekends, breaks and holidays, etc.

Table 8.4 First-line amphetamines for adult ADHD

Brand name	Generic name/ingredients	Duration of effect	Starting dose	Titration dose	Maximum dose	Notes
Adderall XR[a]	Amphetamine-dextroamphetamine (amphetamine mixed salts)	12 hours	5–10 mg/day	5 mg/week	40 mg/day	Food (especially fat) lowers blood levels. Available in 5, 10, 15, 20, 25, 30 mg caps
Mydayis	Amphetamine-dextroamphetamine (amphetamine mixed salts)	16 hours	12.5 mg/day	12.5 mg/week	50 mg/day	Once-daily med. Give first thing in AM. Available in 12.5, 25, 37.5, and 50 mg caps
Vyvanse	Lisdexamfetamine	12 hours	20–30 mg/day	10–20 mg/week	70 mg/day	Becomes d-amphetamine after cleavage. Available in 10, 20, 30, 40, 50, 60,70 mg caps

[a] Note: Multiply Concerta dose by 0.55 to get equivalent Adderall dose

Table 8.5 First-line stimulants for ADHD

Brand name	Generic name/ingredients	Duration of effect	Starting dose	Titration dose	Maximum dose	Notes
Concerta[a]	Methylphenidate ER	12 hours	18 mg/day	18 mg/week	72 mg/day	Not approved for adults >65 years. Available in 18, 36, 54, 72 mg caps
Ritalin LA	Methylphenidate	8 hours	20 mg/day	10 mg/week	60 mg daily	Given once daily. Biphasic release. The capsule may be opened, but the beads inside must not be chewed or crushed. Available in 10, 20, 30, 40, 60 mg caps
Metadate CD	Methylphenidate (30%) + methylphenidate ER (70%)	8 hours	20 mg/day	10–20 mg/week	60 mg daily	Given once daily. Biphasic release of immediate and extended release. Available in 10, 20, 30, 40, 50, and 60 mg caps
Focalin XR	Dexmethylphenidate	12 hours	Patients naïve to methylphenidate: 10 mg daily	10 mg/week	40 mg/day	Dexmethylphenidate is the more active enantiomer and is > = 2x as potent as methylphenidate
			Patients currently taking methylphenidate: One-half daily dose of methylphenidate	10 mg/week	40 mg/day	

[a] Note: Multiply Adderall XR dose by 1.82 to get equivalent Concerta dose

Table 8.6 Second-line amphetamines for adult ADHD

Brand name	Generic name/ ingredients	Duration of effect	Starting dose	Titration dose	Maximum dose	Notes
Dexedrine	Dextroamphetamine	6 hours	5 mg once or twice daily	5 mg/ week	40 mg/day	Available in 5, 10, 15 mg caps
Dexedrine Spansule	Dextroamphetamine	8 hours	5 mg once or twice daily	5 mg/ week	40 mg/day	Available in 5, 10, 15 mg caps

Table 8.7 Second-line stimulants for adult ADHD

Brand name	Generic name/ ingredients	Duration of effect	Starting dose	Titration dose	Maximum dose	Notes
Ritalin	Methylphenidate	4 hours	5 mg bid to tid	5 mg/week	60 mg	Is given bid or tid. Available in 5, 10, 20 mg tabs
Ritalin SR	Methylphenidate	6 hours	20 mg	20 mg (add 2 pm dose)	60 mg	May need to be bid. Available in 20 mg tab
Metadate ER	Methylphenidate ER	6 hours	20 mg/ day	20 mg/ week	60 mg daily	May need to be given bid. Available as 20 mg cap

8.5 When to Refer

Many patients with ADHD are successfully able to be managed in the primary care setting, and there is no compelling evidence regarding when referral to a psychiatrist should take place [13]. Referrals to a specialist should be made when comorbidities present are of the type that usually necessitates referral. This would include an active substance use disorder, uncontrolled mood, anxiety, or obsessive-compulsive and related disorders that are unable to be managed. In cases where there is diagnostic uncertainty or evidence that the ADHD symptoms are secondary to other psychiatric disorders, as in the case of Ms. G., specialty referral should be initiated. If a patient fails all three first-line options, atomoxetine, first-line stimulants, and first-line amphetamines, that should trigger referral as well. Concerns about diversion of stimulant medication will typically trigger a referral, especially when routine drug screening and monitoring is prohibitive. As always, the clinician's level of comfort is always a factor in deciding when to refer out.

As cognitive behavioral therapy can be useful in ADHD treatment, referrals can be suggested for therapy for any patient will to participate.

References

1. Adamou M, Asherson P, Arif M, Buckenham L, Cubbin S, et al. Recommendations for occupational therapy interventions for adults with ADHD: a consensus statement from the UK adult ADHD network. BMC Psychiatry. 2021;21(1):72. https://doi.org/10.1186/s12888-021-03070-z. PMID: 33541313; PMCID: PMC7863422.
2. Anbarasan D, Kitchin M, Adler LA. Screening for adult ADHD. Curr Psychiatry Rep. 2020;22(12):72. https://doi.org/10.1007/s11920-020-01194-9.
3. CADDRA – Canadian ADHD Resource Alliance: Canadian ADHD Practice Guidelines, 4.1 Edition, Toronto ON; CADDRA, 2020.
4. Chang Z, Lichtenstein P, D'Onofrio BM, Sjölander A, Larsson H. Serious transport accidents in adults with attention-deficit/hyperactivity disorder and the effect of medication: a population-based study. JAMA Psychiatry. 2014;71(3):319–25. https://doi.org/10.1001/jamapsychiatry.2013.4174. PMID: 24477798; PMCID: PMC3949159.
5. Cortese S. Pharmacologic treatment of attention deficit-hyperactivity disorder. N Engl J Med. 2020;383(11):1050–6. https://doi.org/10.1056/NEJMra1917069.
6. Cox DJ, Madaan V, Cox BS. Adult attention-deficit/hyperactivity disorder and driving: why and how to manage it. Curr Psychiatry Rep. 2011;13(5):345–50. https://doi.org/10.1007/s11920-011-0216-0.
7. Faraone SV. Using Meta-analysis to Compare the Efficacy of Medications for Attention-Deficit/Hyperactivity Disorder in Youths. P T. 2009;34(12):678–94. PMID: 20140141; PMCID: PMC2810184.
8. Faraone SV, Banaschewski T, Coghill D, Zheng Y, Biederman J, et al. The World Federation of ADHD International Consensus Statement: 208 Evidence-based conclusions about the disorder. Neurosci Biobehav Rev. 2021;128:789–818. https://doi.org/10.1016/j.neubiorev.2021.01.022. Epub 2021 Feb 4. PMID: 33549739; PMCID: PMC8328933.
9. Goodman DW, Thase ME. Recognizing ADHD in adults with comorbid mood disorders: implications for identification and management. Postgrad Med. 2009;121(5):20–30. https://doi.org/10.3810/pgm.2009.09.2049.
10. Naya N, Sakai C, Okutsu D, Kiguchi R, Fujiwara M, Tsuji T, Iwanami A. Efficacy and safety of guanfacine extended-release in Japanese adults with attention-deficit/hyperactivity disorder: Exploratory post hoc subgroup analyses of a randomized, double-blind, placebo-controlled study. Neuropsychopharmacol Rep. 2021;41(1):26–39. https://doi.org/10.1002/npr2.12152. Epub 2020 Dec 10. PMID: 33305542; PMCID: PMC8182954
11. Oliva F, Mangiapane C, Nibbio G, Berchialla P, Colombi N, Vigna-Taglianti FD. Prevalence of cocaine use and cocaine use disorder among adult patients with attention-deficit/hyperactivity disorder: A systematic review and meta-analysis. J Psychiatr Res. 2020:S0022–3956(20)31080–3. https://doi.org/10.1016/j.jpsychires.2020.11.021. Epub ahead of print
12. Perugi G, Pallucchini A, Rizzato S, De Rossi P, Sani G, Maremmani AG, Pinzone V, Maremmani I. Pharmacotherapeutic strategies for the treatment of attention-deficit hyperactivity (ADHD) disorder with comorbid substance-use disorder (SUD). Expert Opin Pharmacother. 2019;20(3):343–55. https://doi.org/10.1080/14656566.2018.1551878. Epub 2018 Dec 4
13. Post RE, Kurlansik SL. Diagnosis and management of adult attention-deficit/hyperactivity disorder. Am Fam Physician. 2012;85(9):890–6.
14. Prakash J, Chatterjee K, Guha S, Srivastava K, Chauhan VS. Adult attention-deficit Hyperactivity disorder: From clinical reality toward conceptual clarity. Ind Psychiatry J. 2021;30(1):23–8. https://doi.org/10.4103/ipj.ipj_7_21. Epub 2021 Jun 10. PMID: 34483520; PMCID: PMC8395556.
15. Salvi V, Ribuoli E, Servasi M, Orsolini L, Volpe U. ADHD and Bipolar Disorder in Adulthood: Clinical and Treatment Implications. Medicina (Kaunas). 2021;57(5):466. https://doi.org/10.3390/medicina57050466. PMID: 34068605; PMCID: PMC8151516.

16. Sandstrom A, Perroud N, Alda M, Uher R, Pavlova B. Prevalence of attention-deficit/hyperactivity disorder in people with mood disorders: a systematic review and meta-analysis. Acta Psychiatr Scand. 2021;143(5):380–91. https://doi.org/10.1111/acps.13283. Epub 2021 Feb 15
17. Sibley MH, Arnold LE, Swanson JM, Hechtman LT, Kennedy TM, Owens E, Molina BSG, Jensen PS, Hinshaw SP, Roy A, Chronis-Tuscano A, Newcorn JH, Rohde LA, MTA Cooperative Group. Variable Patterns of Remission From ADHD in the Multimodal Treatment Study of ADHD. Am J Psychiatry. 2021:appiajp202121010032. https://doi.org/10.1176/appi.ajp.2021.21010032. Epub ahead of print.

Chapter 9
Eating Disorders in the Medical Setting

9.1 Introduction and Epidemiology

Case Example 9.1
Ms. J. is a 21-year-old college student, home during her summer break, and presents to her family physician with complaints of intermittent dizziness and fatigue. Her mother also states that she is concerned about the patient's weight, as while she has always been tall and thin, she has looked particularly thin after this last semester. When asked about her appetite, she seems guarded, stating that her appetite is low but that she eats just fine. She says that her last menstrual period was 4 months ago, but there is no chance she is pregnant. The physical exam is remarkable for a thin appearance, pedal edema, sinus bradycardia, and the appearance of lanugo. Her BMI is 16. She is noted to have a constricted affect on mental status exam. Laboratory results are remarkable for mild hypokalemia and low prealbumin. She does not like to discuss her weight but, when asked directly, does state that she could stand to lose 5 pounds. She is diagnosed with a probable anorexia nervosa and referred for intake to a local eating disorders program that will see her that day in the psychiatric emergency room.

The focus of this chapter is somewhat uniquely positioned in this book. The purpose of most of the information presented has been to introduce psychiatric disorders to the clinicians in primary medical settings, enabling them to initiate treatment and understand when it is time to refer to psychiatric specialists. However, eating disorders (ED), especially anorexia nervosa (AN), are severe and deadly disorders with significant mortality rates. Bulimia nervosa (BN) may not have as high a mortality rate as AN, but their significant overlap in symptomology will often necessitate a

R. Hudak, J. M. Gannon, *Handbook of Psychiatric Disorders in Adults in the Primary Care Setting*, Current Clinical Practice,
https://doi.org/10.1007/978-3-030-98709-1_9

similar, urgent response. As a result, patients with these disorders must be referred to psychiatric specialists upon identification and diagnosis. There is going to be little role in management and treatment of these disorders in primary care settings. Even many psychiatric settings are not properly equipped to deal with these disorders when they present acutely, meaning that specialty eating disorders programs are typically where patients are ultimately treated. As a result, the goal of this chapter is to provide basic information on these disorders, helping primary care physicians and clinicians improve their recognition of these disorders, stress the importance of proper referrals, and provide basic information on the treatments that they can expect their patients to receive when in eating disorder treatment. A third eating disorder, binge-eating disorder (BED), also presents commonly in the primary care setting, and appropriate medical treatment can often be initiated and delivered there. However, even those patients require mental health referrals as registered dieticians and therapists with expertise in ED are critical to recovery.

Eating disorders are common, with one in eight people meeting criteria for an eating disorder by the age of 20, with five million Americans effected by ED every year [1]. Anorexia nervosa is approximately 10 to 20 times more common in females than males, with an onset of late adolescence being most typical. It occurs in about 0.5% to 1% of adolescents, although some studies show rates of 2% to 4% [5]. Younger patients who receive prompt and appropriate intervention have the best chance of a full recovery [12] with >70% of adolescents having a full and lasting recovery 5 years later [10]. However, 5% of patients die, and a quarter of patients have poor outcomes, with many patients having ongoing issues including developing bulimic symptoms [12]. These statistics further emphasize the need for specialized referral for all AN patients. Patients with AN will occasionally engage in rumination behaviors—the purposeful regurgitation of swallowed food, chewing it, and then re-swallowed or spit out. If rumination occurs outside the context of AN or BN, it is given as a separate diagnosis—rumination disorder. Not all patients with AN are underweight: an even more common category is atypical anorexia nervosa in which patients have all of the symptoms of AN but their weight is within or above the normal range. These patients are formally diagnosed by DSM 5 with "Other Specified Feeding or Eating Disorder."

Significantly low weight in anorexia nervosa is defined as less than minimally normal or, for children and adolescents, less than minimally expected.

Bulimia nervosa (BN), another potentially life-threatening eating disorder, is more common than AN in the general population affecting approximately 1.5% of females [8] although one in five college women reports some bulimic-type behavior. BN can present in normal-weight or obese patients. The usual age of onset is adolescence or early adulthood, and long-term follow-up indicates that the number of women who meet criteria for the disorder decreases over time, but 30% continue to engage in binge-eating and purging behaviors [12]. Onset of illness in adolescence may portend a better prognosis than onset later in life [2], but this is an illness with considerable variability in its natural course [12]. Some patients present only with purging behavior without binging behavior. This is termed purging disorder and is given a formal DSM 5 diagnosis of “Other Specified Feeding or Eating Disorder.”

Binge-eating disorder (BED) is a new disorder that was just added to the DSM 5 and may be the most common of the eating disorders [4]. It usually begins in adolescence and is more common in men than the other eating disorders, with about a third of BED patients being men [1]. The medical complications of this disorder are similar to that of obesity, but BED should not be confused with overeating and obesity. The behaviors of binge eating are identical to what is seen in BN but without the compensatory purging behavior [1]. The symptoms tend to remit and reoccur over time. Proper recognition and diagnosis are critical, because treatments aimed at weight loss strategies will actually increase BED symptomatology. If the binge eating only occurs at night after awakening from sleep, this is termed night eating syndrome and is again given a formal DSM 5 diagnosis of “Other Specified Feeding or Eating Disorder.”

9.2 Eating Disorders in the Medical Setting

The role of the physician in the primary care setting regarding eating disorders is generally going to be one of recognition, ensuring proper referral, and coordinating with ED specialists on dealing with the medical sequelae. For the proper recognition of AN, clinicians must be suspicious when a patient presents with unexplained weight loss that is not accounted for by a medical condition. AN patients have an intense fear of becoming fat, although they will often not admit that fact initially, meaning that clinical suspicion is necessary when appropriate. Therefore, it can take some diligence to uncover an AN diagnosis. Regardless of how thin patients are, they will see themselves as overweight and needing to lose more weight. As the disorder progresses, they will have significant secondary medical problems, including sudden cardiac death, endocrine issues (especially amenorrhea and other reproductive hormone dysfunctions), decreased bone mineral density, hypothermia, bradycardia, orthostasis, significant GI complaints (nausea, pain, constipation or diarrhea, and dysphagia), and neutropenia among others [7]. Laboratory values are also abnormal: More than half of patients have low prealbumin, 30% have vitamin D deficiency, 42.5% are hypokalemic, and 33.3% have metabolic alkalosis. AN patients who also binge and purge may have longer QTc intervals although patients who restrict only tend to have normal QTc [3]. When there is suspicion for AN in the primary care setting, a careful medical exam and appropriate laboratory studies is essential alongside a referral to a psychiatric specialist. Comorbid AN and alcohol use disorder is a particularly serious concern, as these patients are unable to develop the compensatory fatty liver and can quickly progress to cirrhosis.

Despite their desire for thinness, many patients with bulimia nervosa are of normal body weight and may be either overweight or underweight as well.

Ms. J. should be carefully screened for abuse of diuretics, laxatives, and self-induced vomiting, including the abuse or emetics. If she is diabetic, potential purging via underdosing of insulin must be examined.

Patients with BN have a significantly increased morbidity and mortality attributable to purging behaviors, which typically consist of vomiting, laxative abuse, and diuretic abuse. Patients are at elevated risk of cardiac disease of any etiology [11]. Electrolyte disturbances are common and require frequent, sometimes daily screening [6]. Hypokalemia, hyponatremia, hypochloremia, and metabolic alkalosis are commonly present [3]. Russell's sign is a classic marker of BN. It is a callus on the knuckle of the dominant hand induced by sticking their finger down their throat and is usually not seen as patients are often able to self-induce vomiting. Numerous dental complications can also be seen in BN, including erosive tooth wear, gingivitis, and gingival recession [9]. Other sequelae of chronic purging by vomiting include pharyngitis, parotid hypertrophy, pneumomediastinum and aspiration, esophageal abnormalities such as Mallory-Weiss tears and Barret esophagus, irregular menses (rather than the amenorrhea of AN), and a pseudo-Bartter syndrome from chronic dehydration [6]. As with AN, a careful medical exam and laboratory studies are essential in bulimia due to these potentially fatal medical complications followed by a referral to psychiatric specialists.

Binge-eating disorder is the most common of the eating disorders, and its major medical complications include obesity with the typical complications of metabolic syndromes including type II diabetes and increases in diastolic blood pressure, heart disease, and stroke [4]. BED also poses a higher risk of amenorrhea or oligomenorrhea, potentially indicating endocrine dysfunction [4]. Physicians in the primary care setting are well-equipped to manage the medical complications from the chronic obesity that is a result of BED. In addition, there is an FDA-approved pharmacological treatment (lisdexamfetamine—see below) that many clinicians in the primary care setting would be comfortable prescribing. However, referral to a qualified therapist or eating disorder specialist is still recommended as the therapy for BED is specific to the disorder; typical strategies for obesity can backfire and make BED symptoms worse.

9.3 Diagnosis and Presentation of Eating Disorders

9.3.1 *Anorexia Nervosa*

The weight loss in AN is achieved either solely via restriction of calories or the patient may incorporate binging and purging behaviors. There are slightly different medical complications of both subtypes.

The diagnosis of AN occurs when the individual voluntarily and intentionally loses weight to an unhealthy level while experiencing a great deal of fear about becoming fat. The patient perceives themselves as overweight. If they do think they are thin, they feel that parts of their body are fat. Medical complications of this severe weight loss are typical in these patients. The patients may engage in checking rituals regarding food: calorie counting, cutting food into tiny portions, or hiding food. They will often engage in frequent weighing (which can occur multiple times throughout the day), measuring body parts, and checking their appearance in mirrors. Many of these behaviors can mimic checking rituals seen in body dysmorphic disorder, but eating disorders are considered to be separate disorders. Most of the dysfunctional behavior occurs in private; patients will do their best to hide what is going on. Some binging and purging behavior may be noted. In some patients, purging behavior can take the form of excessive exercise. Patients will often present initially with medical complications from weight loss, including amenorrhea, hypothermia, bradycardia, edema, or the presence of lanugo. Patients with AN are often described as rigid, perfectionistic, depressive, anxious, and displaying a lack of interest in sex [12]. See Table 9.1 for diagnostic criteria for anorexia nervosa.

Table 9.1 DSM 5 diagnostic criteria for anorexia nervosa

A. Restriction of energy intake relative to requirements, leading to a significantly low body weight in the context of age, sex, developmental trajectory, and physical health. Significantly low body weight is defined as less than minimally normal or, for children and adolescents, less than minimally expected
B. Intense fear of gaining weight or of becoming fat, or persistent behavior that interferes with weight gain, even though at a significantly low weight
C. Disturbance in the way in which one's body weight or shape is experienced, undue influence of body weight or shape on self-evaluation, or persistent lack of recognition of the seriousness of the current low body weight

Note: Patients may be **restricting type** in which weight loss is solely achieved through restricting behaviors and **binge-eating/purging type** in which they engage in binge eating and/or purging (e.g., self-induced vomiting or the misuse of diuretics, laxatives, or enemas)

While it can sometimes appear difficult to distinguish overexercising due to anorexic behavior from exercising due to extreme sports (such as ultra-marathon running or triathlon training), endurance athletes tend to be more focused on health rather than weight loss. They will usually engage in behavior to increase calorie intake to facilitate their activity (e.g., carbohydrate replacement immediately after exercise).

9.4 Bulimia Nervosa

The diagnosis of bulimia nervosa depends on binge-eating behaviors that occur at least on a weekly basis and consists of an excessive intake of food during a discrete (i.e., less than 2-hour) period of time. The behaviors occur over a period of 3 months or more. The binging occurs with the person feeling a distinct lack of control over their behavior. A compensatory behavior of some sort will occur in response to the binging; this can include self-induced vomiting, laxative abuse, diuretic abuse, use of enemas, or dieting and exercising when not engaging in the binge/purge behaviors. Other methods may be employed as well, such as the use of thyroid medication or (in diabetic patients) underdosing insulin. The type of food the person binges can vary. Most patients with BN are either normal weight, but they may be slightly over- or underweight as well. Because patients with BN can have significant laboratory and/or EKG changes, appropriate medical work-ups are vital when this disorder is recognized. See Table 9.2 for diagnostic criteria for bulimia nervosa.

Table 9.2 DSM 5 diagnostic criteria for bulimia nervosa

A. Recurrent episodes of binge eating. An episode of binge eating is characterized by both of thefollowing: 1. Eating, in a discrete period of time (e.g., within a 2-hour period), an amount of food that is definitely larger than what most individuals would consume in a similar period of time under similar circumstances 2. A sense of lack of control over eating during the episode (e.g., a feeling that one cannot stop eating or control how much one is eating)
B. Recurrent inappropriate compensatory behaviors in order to prevent weight gain, such as self-induced vomiting; misuse of laxatives, diuretics, or other medications; fasting; or excessive exercise
C. The binge-eating and inappropriate compensatory behaviors both occur, on average, at least once a week for 3 months
D. Self-evaluation is unduly influenced by body shape and weight
E. The disturbance does not exclusively occur during anorexia nervosa

The symptoms of binging and purging in BN are similar to the symptoms of binging and purging subtype of anorexia nervosa. The difference is that patients with BN are near normal weight rather than being underweight.

9.5 Binge-Eating Disorder

Binge-eating disorder (BED) is the most common of the eating disorders and is characterized by eating large amounts of food in discrete periods of time without the compensatory purging behaviors that are seen in BN. Like BN, the behaviors must occur over a period of 3 months or more. The binging behaviors are essentially the same as seen in BN—the person eats more rapidly and consuming more food than usual to the point of discomfort. As with all of the eating disorders, there is significant shame associated with the symptoms. Patients with BED have a risk of secondary obesity with typical complications such as heart disease, diabetes, and stroke. However, the treatment for BED is markedly different than that for obesity, so careful diagnosis is critical. The focus for treatment is to reduce binge behavior rather than focusing on weight reduction which can actually worsen BED. There is an FDA-approved medication for BED (lisdexamfetamine) that is fairly straightforward to prescribe, and since practitioners in the primary care setting are well-equipped to treat medical complications of obesity, BED may be able to be treated medically in the primary care setting. However, because the therapy for binging is specialized, referral for specialized therapy is still strongly encouraged. Please see Table 9.3 for DSM criteria for BED.

9.6 Treatment

The treatment for eating disorders generally involves:

1. Nutritional rehabilitation—This typically involves weight restoration which can occur in an inpatient or ambulatory setting. Brief hospitalizations have not been

Table 9.3 DSM criteria for binge-eating disorder

A. Recurrent episodes of binge eating. An episode of binge eating is characterized by both of the following: 1. Eating, in a discrete period of time (e.g., within any 2-hour period), an amount of food that is defiantly larger than what most people would eat in a similar period of time under similar circumstances 2. A sense of lack of control over eating during the episode (e.g., a feeling that one cannot stop eating or control what or how much one is eating)
B. The binge-eating episodes are associated with three or more of the following: 1. Eating much more rapidly than usual 2. Eating until feeling uncomfortably full 3. Eating large amounts of food when not feeling physically hungry 4. Eating alone because of feeling embarrassed by how much one is eating 5. Feeling disgusted with oneself, depressed, or very guilty afterward
C. Marked distress regarding binge eating is present
D. The binge eating occurs, on average, at least once a week for 3 months
E. The binge eating is not associated with the recurrent use of inappropriate compensatory behavior as in bulimia nervosa and does not occur exclusively during the course of bulimia nervosa or anorexia nervosa

demonstrated to produce good outcomes, and discharging patients when they are closer to healthy weights improves the prognosis [12]. Patients need to be carefully monitored for refeeding syndrome following prolonged starvation.
2. Psychotherapy—Numerous types of psychotherapy are used including cognitive behavioral therapy, family-based therapy, and group-based therapies.
3. Treatment can be given in inpatient, partial, intensive outpatient, or outpatient settings depending on the patient's medical state and current needs.
4. Pharmacotherapy is generally not used for AN, and antidepressants have little benefit in low-weight AN patients (however, SSRIs can be useful for comorbid disorders such as OCD). Medications to increase appetite in AN patients are *not* recommended. **Fluoxetine** is FDA approved for BN and may be useful at doses similar to that of OCD—60–80 mg/day [12]. Dosing for fluoxetine would typically start at 10–20 mg per day and titrated by 20 mg weekly until the 60–80 mg daily dose is reached. **Lisdexamfetamine** is approved for the treatment of BED. It is typically started at a 30 mg dose, increasing by 20 mg per week until a dose of 50–70 mg per day is achieved.
5. Aftercare is a vital part of eating disorder treatment. Symptoms of anxiety or depression can emerge as the patient recovers, as well as the fact that relapse is common if the patients do not remain engaged in psychotherapy [1].

9.7 When to Refer

As has been stated about, virtually all eating disorder patients should be referred to psychiatric specialists. Psychotherapy is a cornerstone of treatment for all eating disorders and needs to be performed by those with expertise. The role in the primary care setting will typically be to ensure that the patient's referral is made with the proper urgency. In other words, people with metabolic abnormalities or other potential life-threatening issues demand emergency treatment and referral. These patients are often admitted to med/surg hospitals with psychiatric consults and then transferred to specialty eating disorders programs. Patients who are not severely underweight and do not have metabolic abnormalities requiring urgent treatment can be referred to outpatient treatment providers.

For patients with BN who are eligible for outpatient therapy (i.e., without significant medical or metabolic issues), physicians in the primary care setting may want to prescribe fluoxetine as outlined above. This would typically include coordination of medical and psychotherapeutic care and treatment plan with eating disorder therapists.

As stated above, BED is the eating disorder that may be well served by treatment in the primary care setting as PCPs are well versed in treating the medical comorbidities of the disorder. If the PCP is comfortable prescribing lisdexamfetamine (see above for dosing) and following their state's protocols for Schedule II medications, pharmacotherapy may occur in the primary care setting. However, as the psychotherapy and approach to BED is very different than that of obesity, patients will still require referrals to qualified therapists, and the prescribing physician would still need to coordinate the medications with the eating disorder treatment team according to the patient's treatment plan and progress.

9.8 Conclusion

Eating disorders are serious psychiatric disorders with significant morbidity and mortality. While there are two medications approved (for bulimia nervosa and binge-eating disorder), the mainstay of treatment for eating disorders remains a comprehensive psychotherapeutic approach, treating psychological, family, and nutritional issues. Prompt and appropriate referrals to psychiatric specialists are standard treatment approaches for patients seen in the primary care setting.

References

1. Balasundaram P, Santhanam P. Eating Disorders. In: StatPearls [Internet]. Treasure Island (FL): StatPearls Publishing; 2021.
2. Fisher M. The course and outcome of eating disorders in adults and in adolescents: a review. Adolesc Med. 2003;14(1):149–58.
3. Mehler PS, Blalock DV, Walden K, Kaur S, McBride J, Walsh K, Watts J. Medical findings in 1,026 consecutive adult inpatient-residential eating disordered patients. Int J Eat Disord. 2018;51(4):305–13. https://doi.org/10.1002/eat.22830. Epub 2018 Feb 8.
4. Mitchell JE. Medical comorbidity and medical complications associated with binge-eating disorder. Int J Eat Disord. 2016;49(3):319–23. https://doi.org/10.1002/eat.22452. Epub 2015 Aug 27.
5. Moore CA, Bokor BR. Anorexia Nervosa. In: StatPearls [Internet]. Treasure Island (FL): StatPearls Publishing; 2021.
6. Nitsch A, Dlugosz H, Gibson D, Mehler PS. Medical complications of bulimia nervosa. Cleve Clin J Med. 2021;88(6):333–43. https://doi.org/10.3949/ccjm.88a.20168.
7. Puckett L, Grayeb D, Khatri V, Cass K, Mehler P. A comprehensive review of complications and new findings associated with anorexia Nervosa. J Clin Med. 2021;10(12):2555. https://doi.org/10.3390/jcm10122555. PMID: 34207744; PMCID: PMC8226688.
8. Ranalli DN, Studen-Pavlovich D. Eating Disorders in the adolescent patient. Dent Clin N Am. 2021;65(4):689–703. https://doi.org/10.1016/j.cden.2021.06.009. Epub 2021 Aug 2.
9. Rangé H, Colon P, Godart N, Kapila Y, Bouchard P. Eating disorders through the periodontal lens. Periodontol 2000. 2021;87(1):17–31. https://doi.org/10.1111/prd.12391.
10. Strober M, Freeman R, Morrell W. The long-term course of severe anorexia nervosa in adolescents: survival analysis of recovery, relapse, and outcome predictors over 10-15 years in a prospective study. Int J Eat Disord. 1997;22(4):339–60. https://doi.org/10.1002/(sici)1098-108x(199712)22:4<339::aid-eat1>3.0.co;2-n.
11. Tith RM, Paradis G, Potter BJ, Low N, Healy-Profitós J, He S, Auger N. Association of Bulimia Nervosa with Long-term Risk of cardiovascular disease and mortality among women. JAMA Psychiat. 2020;77(1):44–51. https://doi.org/10.1001/jamapsychiatry.2019.2914. PMID: 31617882; PMCID: PMC6802370.
12. Yager J, Devlin MJ, Halmi KA, et al. Treatment of patients with eating Disorders. 3rd ed. American Psychiatric Association Steering Committee on Practice Guidelines; 2010.

Chapter 10
Autism in the Primary Care Setting

10.1 Introduction and Epidemiology

Case Example 10.1
Mr. K. is a 27-year-old male in an outpatient family practice clinic. He is well known for creating multiple difficulties in the practice setting. He is generally well liked by the office staff despite the amount of time he costs them, and his behavior is never inappropriate. However, he typically has numerous, disparate physical complaints that are hard to resolve in any one visit. Constipation is one main, ongoing complaint and is a real, documented problem. During physical exams, he constantly expresses fear about possible pain from routine exam maneuvers, and he generally refuses blood draws. He calls the office staff multiple times a day, to complain of new problems. Many of these are not physical in nature but are related to social circumstances. He also calls numerous times after an appointment to ask for his directions to be repeated.

While autism spectrum disorder (ASD) is commonly seen in the medical setting, the focus of this chapter is somewhat different than other chapters in this book. The first aim of this chapter is to help familiarize medical providers with the symptoms and presentation of ASD, including when to refer patients for expert evaluation and diagnosis. Typically, most physicians would not be expected to diagnose ASD in patients in the medical setting. Being that it is a neurodevelopmental disorder, ASD is present and potentially diagnosable in very young patients. However, not all adults with ASD will come with a previously made diagnosis from childhood. It is not at all unusual for the diagnosis to be missed in childhood initially, only to be made in adulthood when the patient is suffering from problems that are not easily

R. Hudak, J. M. Gannon, *Handbook of Psychiatric Disorders in Adults in the Primary Care Setting*, Current Clinical Practice,
https://doi.org/10.1007/978-3-030-98709-1_10

explained by other psychiatric disorders. It is not typically the role of the primary care physician to be responsible for making this diagnosis in such patients. Rather, patients are typically referred out to mental health professionals who can fully evaluate and diagnose potential ASD in patients. The second aim of this chapter is one of accommodation: people who are on the spectrum often have different needs than patients who are neurotypical. The authors are frequently asked by physicians how to accommodate such individuals in their practice settings. An understanding of the presentation of ASD can make a marked difference in the ability to manage these patients. Suggestions on modifications specific to ASD patients will be given.

There are no pharmacologic treatments for the core features of ASD—psychiatric medications are typically given to treat manifestations that result from the presence of the disorder (e.g., people with ASD often suffer from increased anxiety) as well as comorbid conditions. Psychotherapy with therapists familiar with ASD can help with numerous consequences of the disorder, including everything from improving social skills to helping individuals learn independent living skills. It is relevant to note that much of the literature on ASD is focused on it as a childhood illness. These children obviously grow up to become adults, but with the advocacy and medical establishment being successful at increasing awareness on ASD in children, there is much less focus on adults. Therefore, much of the literature is not directly relevant to adults with ASD.

Autism spectrum disorder is a neurodevelopmental disorder that is present early in childhood. The presentation of the disorder varies greatly in different individuals, and the core features of the disorder may be dominant in certain circumstances while being masked in others, complicating diagnosis. This can show up in numerous ways. For example, one individual with ASD may show limited or no eye contact in social settings, while another displays increased and inappropriate eye contact. In both cases, the patient demonstrates a deficit in social functioning, but it manifests in exactly the opposite way. In addition, yet another patient may have more socially acceptable amounts and types of eye contact but show deficits in other arenas.

Rates of ASD have been increasing over the last two decades, and the reasons for this have been the subject of some controversy. Increased recognition, better screening, and better neuropsychological rating scales likely are strong contributors to this trend. It is now estimated that 1 in 68 children have a diagnosis of ASD [3], but the rates in adults are less clear. Certainly, the rate in adults is likely to be higher as many individuals are not diagnosed until adulthood. This is especially common in females where the diagnosis is more likely to be overlooked.

Prior to DSM 5, autism, Asperger's, and pervasive developmental disorder were three different disorders with three different sets of diagnostic criteria. DSM currently only recognizes autism spectrum disorder as a single diagnosis to better reflect the fact that ASD is a single diagnostic entity with core features of deficits in social communication and interaction as well-restricted repetitive patterns of interest, behavior, or activities that can all appear in varying degrees across the spectrum in different individuals.

10.2 Autism Spectrum Disorder in the Medical Setting

"What am I to do? To have anything like a reasonable quality of life, my life is abominably high maintenance. I can't find a medical doctor who is willing to work with me without the drugs that I get all the side effects for, unpredictable intended side effects, and wild card effects that don't show up in the literature at all. I don't know how to live in this world, never mind participate in it" [9].

The above is a quote from a patient that illustrates some of the frustration and medical issues that people with ASD feel. These complaints could easily be voiced by Mr. K. from Case Example 10.1 as well. It can be difficult for physicians to tailor their practice habits to patients on the spectrum, and this section is meant to aid physicians with additional tools to improve patient outcomes as well as practice efficiency. This is vital, because patients with ASD are not only higher utilizers of outpatient primary care visits, but their healthcare needs are less likely to be met, including the fact that women with ASD are less likely to receive screening for cervical cancer [10]. People with ASD are also more likely to suffer from immune conditions, gastrointestinal and sleep disorders, seizure disorders, obesity, dyslipidemia, hypertension, and diabetes [4]. See Table 10.1. They are more likely to state that their healthcare needs are not being met and that they receive less communication from their healthcare providers [9].

The core features of ASD can also lead to other difficulties in obtaining proper medical care, which is a likely contributor to increased health risks. These can include [6]:

- *Sensory processing concerns*. Patients with ASD can have markedly high levels of pain tolerance, or conversely, they may have a decreased pain tolerance (i.e., unable to tolerate routine blood draws). Patients may take longer to report physical symptoms as a result of high pain tolerance.

Table 10.1 Rate of medical disorders in patients with ASD compared to the general population [5]

Disorder	Rate in ASD	Rate in general population
Seizure disorder	19.4%	2.19%
CNS disorders (non-seizure)	12.4%	1.19%
Bowel disorders (excl. IBD)	11.7%	4.55
Inflammatory bowel disease	0.83%	0.54%
Diabetes type 1	0.79%	0.34%
Sleep disorders	1.1%	0.14%

- *Other sensory processing concerns*: Patients with ASD commonly report problems with hyperacusis (decreased tolerance to loud sounds) or misophonia (decreased tolerance to specific sounds) that can lead to difficulties tolerating healthcare settings.
- *Executive dysfunction.* This can occur even in patients with high IQs or high-functioning ASD patients, leading to difficulties keeping, remembering, or being on time for appointments or organizing their physical complaints or history in a coherent manner.
- *Increased anxiety.* This can make it harder for patients to tolerate sitting in waiting rooms.
- *Increased rates of comorbid psychiatric disorders.* Higher rates of coexisting psychiatric disorders, including ADHD, bipolar disorder, major depressive disorder, and schizophrenia [8], can add to the complexity in treating these individuals.

Mr. K.'s aversion to needles could be due to anxiety (i.e., a needle phobia), a sensory processing concern, or both.

There are numerous modifications that can be done in the primary care setting that will not only improve patient outcomes but improve physician efficiency when seeing patients on the spectrum as well. Applying these strategies would greatly improve office efficiency in patients like Mr. K. These may include [1, 2, 6]:

- Scheduling when the office is less busy can reduce problems with sensory stimulation. Consider a separate waiting room for these individuals or other ways to decrease sound and noise.
- As patients may be slow in engaging with new providers, consider scheduling multiple visits upon initiation of services and/or scheduling more time for visits.
- Support persons should be allowed and encouraged to accompany the patient. However, if the patient asks for privacy, this should be respected even over caregiver request. Even if the adult patient has a legal guardian of person, physicians can perform histories and physicals, as well as discuss treatment plans in most places. Depending on specific rules in your locale, initiation or changes in treatment plan may need to be discussed with a guardian first, however.
- Patients with ASD may have varied needs regarding communication. Consider preparing various types of communication that may be beneficial to your patient. For example, visual aids and diagrams may be of benefit in many patients.
- Be prepared to explain exam procedures and instructions fully and ensure that the patient understands. Even high IQ and high-functioning individuals can have executive deficits that make the ability to comply and follow problematic. Simpler language can help here. Patients may be less educated than their peers as they may be less likely to discuss personal or medical issues with friends or family.
- Patients with ASD are more likely than the general population to have gender identity concerns. Ensure that these issues are discussed and addressed appropriately and that proper pronouns are used and charted.

- Be prepared to discuss issues that are not often addressed in other populations. For example, patients may need to be educated on appropriate and inappropriate settings for masturbation.
- Screen carefully for sexual abuse, as these patients are much more prone to sexual assault and resultant sequelae, including sexually transmitted infections, trauma and PTSD concerns, etc.
- Have prepared a list of resources, mental health referrals, and community supports for these individuals.
- Use concrete language and avoid idioms, irony, and jokes with your patients as they may be less likely to understand them.
- Teach your patient to be a better patient. A guide that has been published that helps patients prepare for medical appointments can be found here: https://autisticadvocacy.org/wp-content/uploads/2014/07/ASAN-healthcare-toolkit-final.pdf

> When seeing patients with ASD, use concrete language and avoid irony, jokes, etc.

10.3 Diagnosis and Presentation of Autism Spectrum Disorder

The behavioral features of ASD are present early in life—usually during the first or second year of life—although they may not be recognized or formally diagnosed until much later in life. It is not a degenerative disorder, and compensation for deficits can continue throughout the lifespan. Because the individual may have significant deficits in one area and little to no deficits in others, ASD can look very different in different individuals. The deficits that they have in emotional awareness and communication skills can make history gathering difficult. ASD is often not diagnosed until adulthood or missed completely for this reason, especially in female patients. Many ASD traits are also found in the general population which can contribute to this under recognition [7].

To make a diagnosis of ASD, the patient must demonstrate impairment in social communication and social interaction, as well as have restricted, repetitive patterns of behavior. See Table 10.2 for the DSM 5 diagnostic criteria.

As noted above, anxiety and depression are more common in ASD than in the general population. As a result, ASD traits, such as extreme distress at small changes or difficulty with transitions, can lead to a significant increase in anxiety. This can manifest as behavioral outbursts or explosive behavior in some individuals. The highly restricted repetitive patterns of behavior can look like obsessive-compulsive symptoms; however, this is not considered OCD and is approached quite differently as a result (there is a high comorbidity with ASD and OCD, however).

It would be extremely unusual for a diagnosis of ASD to be made in the primary care setting in adult patients. We recommend that if a patient is noted to have

Table 10.2 DSM 5 diagnostic criteria for autism spectrum disorder

Persistent deficits in social communication and social interaction across multiple contexts as manifested by: 1. Deficits in social-emotional reciprocity (e.g., abnormal social approach, failure of normal back and forth conversation, reduced sharing of emotions or interests, failure to initiate or respond to social interaction) 2. Deficits in nonverbal communications behaviors used for social interaction (e.g., poorly integrated verbal and nonverbal communication, abnormalities in eye contact, body language, and deficits in understanding body language and gestures, to a total lack of facial expressions and nonverbal communication) 3. Deficits in developing, maintaining, and understanding relationships (e.g., adjusting behavior to social context, difficulty in making friends, absence of interest in peers)
Restricted, repetitive patterns of behavior, interests, or activities as manifested by at least two of the following: 1. Stereotyped or repetitive motor movements, use of objects, or speech (e.g., simple motor stereotypies, lining up toys or flipping objects, echolalia, idiosyncratic phrases) 2. Insistence on sameness, inflexible adherence to routine, or ritualized patterns of verbal or nonverbal behavior (e.g., extreme distress at small changes, difficulty with transitions, rigid thinking patterns, needing to eat the same foods to take the same routes every day) 3. Highly restricted, fixated interests that are abnormal in intensity or focus (e.g., strong attachment to or preoccupation with unusual objects, excessively circumscribed or perseverative interests) 4. Hyper- or hyporeactivity to sensory input or unusual interest in sensory aspects of the environment (e.g., apparent indifference to pain or temperature, adverse response to specific sounds or textures, excessive smelling or touching of objects, visual fascination with lights and movement)
Symptoms must be present in the early developmental period (but may not manifest until social demands exceed limited capacity or may be masked by learned strategies later in life)
Symptoms cause clinically significant impairment in social, occupational, or other important areas of functioning
Symptoms are not better explained by intellectual disability or global developmental delay. Intellectual disability and ASD often occur together and in these individuals' social communication should be below expected developmental level

difficulties in social communication and interaction or restricted and repetitive patterns of behavior, a referral to a mental health specialist be given so that a full evaluation can be made.

10.4 Treatment

Treatment of ASD patients for psychiatric issues will be briefly discussed here, as these patients should be referred to psychiatry, with a few exceptions (For example, a well-known patient with a clear, acute onset of major depressive disorder may have medical treatment initiated in the primary care setting). The diagnosis of other psychiatric disorders in ASD patients can be challenging, which is another reason that psychiatric evaluation is recommended in any patient where the diagnosis isn't perfectly clear.

There is currently no available treatment for the core symptoms of autism. In fact, many individuals on the spectrum do not consider themselves to have a disorder and simply view themselves as atypical, having a brain that interacts with the world in a way that is different than "neurotypicals". This should not minimize the severe impairment that is possible in this disorder, however.

The treatment for ASD is typically focused on improving learning and coping skills around the core symptoms of ASD and involves interventions such as psychoeducation, social coaching to enhance social skills, instruction on self-care skills, and recognition and understanding of both their own and others' thoughts and feelings [8]. The treatment of anxiety symptoms is especially important, and therapists specializing in the care of ASD have modified techniques they use to make cognitive behavioral therapy more translatable to the individual. Social behavioral therapy targets emotional regulation, social skills, and communication, while applied behavioral analysis (ABA) employs structured techniques to improve language, cognitive skills, sensorimotor skills, social interactions, and living skills and targets problematic behaviors [8].

There are only two medications approved for use in the treatment of ASD in the USA: aripiprazole is approved for the treatment of irritability associated with ASD, while risperidone is approved for the treatment of irritability associated with autism in children and adolescents aged 5–16 years. However, the irritability associated with ASD is often secondary to increased anxiety, typically in response to an environmental stimulus. As a result, the use of antipsychotics for explosive outbursts in ASD may not be the best first-line option in many patients due to their side effect burden. Often, selective serotonin reuptake inhibitors (SSRIs) are used first line to reduce the excessive anxiety associated with ASD, thereby reducing the outbursts. Children with ASD may be more sensitive to SSRI side effects than adults are. Even adults who have had side effects to SSRIs as children can typically be rechallenged with SSRIs in adulthood safely. Therefore, the old saw that people with ASD cannot tolerate SSRIs may not be true in adults.

As Mr. K. does not have irritability or aggressive outbursts, the use of aripiprazole or risperidone would not be indicated at all; an SSRI may help with his heightened anxiety.

10.5 When to Refer

Patients are not typically diagnosed with ASD in the primary care setting. If the suspicion of ASD is raised, a referral to mental health specialist is warranted. Due to the high rate of comorbidity with other psychiatric disorders and the difficulty in proper diagnosis and treatment of those disorders in the ASD population, the threshold for referral to a mental health specialist is going to be far lower than it is for other patients. Patients in need of ASD-specific therapies are referred to appropriate specialists. Patients with explosive outbursts or excessive anxiety may have pharmacological treatment initiated in the primary care setting. Typically, this will involve the use of SSRIs for excessive anxiety or behavioral outbursts, or occasionally the use of antipsychotics, especially risperidone or aripiprazole (see Chap. 2 on Excessive Anxiety for a detailed guide on prescribing medications for anxiety). However, the difficulty in diagnosis, managing side effects, and treatment response in this cohort may necessitate referral in all but the most straightforward and treatment-responsive patients.

References

1. Abells D, Kirkham YA, Ornstein MP. Review of gynecologic and reproductive care for women with developmental disabilities. Curr Opin Obstet Gynecol. 2016;28(5):350–8. https://doi.org/10.1097/GCO.0000000000000299.
2. Brigham KS, Plante AA. Gynecology. In: The Massachusetts General Hospital guide to medical Care in Patients with autism Spectrum disorder. Cham: Humana Press; 2018. p. 193–206.
3. Christensen DL, Baio J, Van Naarden Braun K, Bilder D, Charles J, Constantino JN, Daniels J, Durkin MS, Fitzgerald RT, Kurzius-Spencer M, Lee LC, Pettygrove S, Robinson C, Schulz E, Wells C, Wingate MS, Zahorodny W, Yeargin-Allsopp M, Centers for Disease Control and Prevention (CDC). Prevalence and characteristics of autism spectrum disorder among children aged 8 years--Autism and developmental disabilities monitoring network, 11 Sites, United States, 2012. MMWR Surveill Summ. 2016;65(3):1–23. https://doi.org/10.15585/mmwr.ss6503a1. Erratum in: MMWR Morb Mortal Wkly Rep. 2016;65(15):404. Erratum in: MMWR Morb Mortal Wkly Rep. 2018 Nov 16;67(45):1279. PMID: 27031587; PMCID: PMC7909709.
4. Croen LA, Zerbo O, Qian Y, Massolo ML, Rich S, Sidney S, Kripke C. The health status of adults on the autism spectrum. Autism. 2015;19(7):814–23. https://doi.org/10.1177/1362361315577517. Epub 2015 Apr 24
5. Kohane IS, McMurry A, Weber G, MacFadden D, Rappaport L, Kunkel L, Bickel J, Wattanasin N, Spence S, Murphy S, Churchill S. The co-morbidity burden of children and young adults with autism spectrum disorders. PLoS One. 2012;7(4):e33224. https://doi.org/10.1371/journal.pone.0033224. Epub 2012 Apr 12. PMID: 22511918; PMCID: PMC3325235.
6. Kucherer S. Personal communication 2020.
7. Ruzich E, Allison C, Smith P, et al. Measuring autistic traits in the general population: a systematic review of the Autism-Spectrum Quotient (AQ) in a nonclinical population sample of 6,900 typical adult males and females. Mol Autism. 2015;6(2) https://doi.org/10.1186/2040-2392-6-2.
8. Sharma SR, Gonda X, Tarazi FI. Autism Spectrum disorder: classification, diagnosis and therapy. Pharmacol Ther. 2018;190:91–104. https://doi.org/10.1016/j.pharmthera.2018.05.007. Epub 2018 May 12.
9. Volkmar FR, Reichow B, McPartland JC. Adolescents and adults with autism spectrum disorders. New York: Springer; 2014.
10. Zerbo O, Qian Y, Ray T, Sidney S, Rich S, Massolo M, Croen LA. Health care service utilization and cost among adults with autism spectrum disorders in a US integrated health care system. Autism Adulthood. 2019;1(1):27–36.

Index

R. Hudak, J. M. Gannon, *Handbook of Psychiatric Disorders in Adults in the Primary Care Setting*, Current Clinical Practice,
https://doi.org/10.1007/978-3-030-98709-1

MIX
Papier aus verantwortungsvollen Quellen
Paper from responsible sources
FSC® C105338

If you have any concerns about our products,
you can contact us on
ProductSafety@springernature.com

In case Publisher is established outside the EU,
the EU authorized representative is:
Springer Nature Customer Service Center GmbH
Europaplatz 3, 69115 Heidelberg, Germany

Printed by Libri Plureos GmbH
in Hamburg, Germany